Medical Statistics from Scratch

An Introduction for Health Professionals

Third Edition

David Bowers

*Honorary Lecturer, Leeds Institute of Health Sciences,
School of Medicine, University of Leeds, UK*

WILEY Blackwell

Registered office: John Wiley & Sons, Ltd, The Atrium, Southern Gate, Chichester, West Sussex, PO19 8SQ, UK

Editorial offices: 9600 Garsington Road, Oxford, OX4 2DQ, UK
        The Atrium, Southern Gate, Chichester, West Sussex, PO19 8SQ, UK
        111 River Street, Hoboken, NJ 07030-5774, USA

For details of our global editorial offices, for customer services and for information about how to apply for permission to reuse the copyright material in this book please see our website at www.wiley.com/wiley-blackwell

Library of Congress Cataloging-in-Publication Data

Bowers, David, 1938- author.
  Medical statistics from scratch : an introduction for health professionals / David Bowers. – Third edition.
      p. ; cm.
  Includes bibliographical references and index.
  ISBN 978-1-118-51938-7 (pbk.)
  I. Title.
  [DNLM: 1. Biometry. 2. Statistics as Topic–methods. WA 950]
  RA409
  610.72'7 – dc23
                                2014020550

A catalogue record for this book is available from the British Library.

Wiley also publishes its books in a variety of electronic formats. Some content that appears in print may not be available in electronic books.

Cover image courtesy of the author.

Typeset in 10/12pt Minion by Laserwords Private Limited, Chennai, India
Printed and bound in Malaysia by Vivar Printing Sdn Bhd

2   2015

Brief Contents

Contents

Preface to the 3rd Edition

The 1st edition of this book was published in 2002 and the 2nd edition in 2008. I was surprised when I discovered it was quite such a long time ago. Where did the time go! Anyway, over the course of the last five years, I have received many favourable comments from readers of my book, which of course is immensely gratifying. I must be doing something right then.

This edition contains a completely new chapter (on diagnostic tests), there is a quite a lot of new material and most of the chapters have received an extensive re-write. I have also updated virtually all of the examples drawn from the journals and added many new exercises. I hope that this gives the book a fresh feel – as well as a new lease of life.

The book should appeal, as before, to everybody in health care (students and professionals alike) including nurses, doctors, health visitors, physiotherapists, midwives, radiographers, dieticians, speech therapists, health educators and promoters, chiropodists and all those other allied and auxiliary professionals. It might possibly also be of interest to veterinary surgeons, one of whom reviewed my proposal fairly enthusiastically.

My thanks to Jon Peacock and all the others at Wiley who have shepherded me along in the past and no doubt will do so in the future. I must also thank Barbara Noble, who patiently acted as my first-line copyeditor. She read through my manuscript, discovered quite a few errors of various sorts and made many valuable suggestions to improve readability. Any remaining mistakes are of course mine.

I also want to acknowledge my great debt to Susanne, who always encourages me, enthusiastically, in everything I attempt.

Finally, I would like to mention another book which might be of interest to any readers who are thinking of embarking on research for the first time – *Getting Started in Health Research*, Bowers *et al.*, Wiley, 2012. This book covers both quantitative and qualitative research. It will guide you through the research process, from the very first idea to the interpretation of your results and your conclusions.

David Bowers, 2013

Preface to the 2nd Edition

This book is a 'not-too-mathematical' introduction to medical statistics. It should appeal to anyone training or working in the health care arena – whatever his or her particular discipline is – who wants either a simple introduction to the subject or a gentle reminder of stuff that they might have forgotten. I have aimed the book at:

- students doing either a first degree or a diploma in clinical and health care courses

- students doing post-graduate clinical and health care studies

- health care professionals doing professional and membership examinations

- health care professionals who want to brush up on some medical statistics generally or who want a simple reminder of a particular topic

- anybody else who wants to know a bit of what medical statistics is about.

The most significant change in this edition is the addition of two new chapters, one on measuring survival and the other on systematic review and meta-analysis. The ability to understand the principles of survival analysis is important, not least because of its popularity in clinical research and consequently in the clinical literature. Similarly, the increasing importance of evidence-based clinical practice means that systematic review and meta-analysis also demand a place. In addition, I have taken the opportunity to correct and freshen the text in a few places, as well as adding a small number of new examples. My thanks to Lucy Sayer, my editor at John Wiley & Sons, for her enthusiastic support, to Liz Renwick and Robert Hambrook and all the other people in Wiley for their invaluable help and my special thanks to my copyeditor Barbara Noble for her truly excellent work and enthusiasm (of course, any remaining errors are mine).

I am happy to get any comments from you. You can e-mail me at: d.bowers@leeds.ac.uk.

Preface to the 1st Edition

This book is intended to be an introduction to medical statistics but one which is not too mathematical – in fact, it has the absolute minimum of maths. The exceptions however are Chapters 17 and 18, which have maths on linear and logistic regressions. It is really impossible to provide material on these procedures without some maths, and I hesitated about including them at all. However, they are such useful and widely used techniques, particularly logistic regression and its production of odds ratios, which I felt they must go in. Of course, you do not *have* to read them. It should appeal to anyone training or working in the health care arena – whatever his or her particular discipline is – who wants a simple, not-too-technical introduction to the subject. I have aimed the book at:

- students doing either a first degree or a diploma in health care-related courses

- students doing post-graduate health care studies

- health care professionals doing professional and membership examinations

- health care professionals who want to brush up on some medical statistics generally or who want a simple reminder of a particular topic

- anybody else who wants to know a bit of what medical statistics is about.

I intended originally to make this book as an amalgam of two previous books of mine, *Statistics from Scratch for Health Care Professionals* and *Statistics Further from Scratch*. However, although it covers a lot of the same material as in those two books, this is in reality a completely new book, with a lot of extra stuff, particularly on linear and logistic regressions. I am happy to get any comments and criticisms from you. You can e-mail me at: slothist@hotmail.com.

Introduction

My purpose in writing this book is to offer a guide to all those health care students and professionals out there, who either want to get started in medical statistics or who would like (or need) to refresh their understanding of one or more medical statistics topics. I have tried to keep the mathematics to a minimum, although this is a bit more difficult with the somewhat challenging material on modelling in later chapters.

I have used lots of appropriate examples drawn from clinical journals to illustrate the ideas and lots of exercises which the readers may wish to work through to consolidate their understanding of the material covered (the solutions are at the end of this book).

I have included some outputs from SPSS and Minitab which I hope will help the readers interpret the results from these statistical programmes.

Finally, for any tutors who are using this book to introduce their students to medical statistics, I am always very pleased to receive any comments or criticisms they may have which will help me improve the book in the future editions. My e-mail address is d.bowers@leeds.ac.uk.

I

Some Fundamental Stuff

1

First things first – the nature of data

Learning objectives

When you have finished this chapter, you should be able to:

- Explain the difference between nominal, ordinal and metric data.

- Identify the type of any given variable.

- Explain the non-numeric nature of ordinal data.

Variables and data

Let's start with some numbers. Have a look at Figure 1.1.

These numbers are actually the birthweights of a sample of 100 babies (measured in grams). We call these numbers *sample data*. These data arise from the variable *birthweight*. To state the blindingly obvious, a variable is something whose value can vary. Other variables could be blood type, age, parity and so on; the values of these variables can change from one individual

---

Medical Statistics from Scratch: An Introduction for Health Professionals, Third Edition. David Bowers.
© 2014 John Wiley & Sons, Ltd. Published 2014 by John Wiley & Sons, Ltd.

2240	4110	3590	2880	2850	2660	4040	3580	1960	3550
3050	3130	2660	3150	3220	3990	4020	3040	3460	4230
4110	2780	2840	3660	3580	2780	3560	2350	2720	2460
3200	2650	3000	3170	3500	2400	3300	3740	2760	3840
3740	2380	3300	3480	3740	3770	2520	3570	3400	3780
3040	3170	3300	3560	3180	2920	4000	2700	3680	2500
2920	2980	3780	2650	2880	4550	3570	1620	3000	3700
4080	3280	3800	2800	2560	2740	3180	3200	3120	4880
2800	3640	4020	3080	2590	3360	3630	3740	2960	3300
3090	3600	3720	2840	3320	2940	3640	2720	3220	4140

Figure 1.1   Some numbers. Actually, the birthweight (g) of a sample of 100 babies. Data from the Born in Bradford Cohort Study. Born in Bradford, Bradford Institute for Health Research, Bradford Teaching Hospitals NHS Foundation Trust

to the other. When we measure a variable, we get data – in this case, the variable birthweight produces birthweight *data*.

Figure 1.2 contains more sample data, in this case, for the *gender* of the same 100 babies.

M	M	F	F	M	M	F	F	M	M
M	M	M	F	M	M	F	F	M	M
F	F	M	M	F	F	M	F	F	F
M	M	F	F	M	M	M	M	F	F
M	M	F	F	M	F	F	F	F	F
F	M	F	M	M	M	F	F	M	F
F	F	M	M	M	F	M	M	M	F
M	F	M	M	M	M	M	M	M	M
M	F	M	M	M	F	F	M	M	F
M	F	M	F	M	M	F	F	M	F

Figure 1.2   The gender of the sample of babies in Figure 1.1

Moreover, Figure 1.3 contains sample data for the variable *smoked while pregnant*.

The data in Figures 1.1, 1.2 and 1.3 are known as *raw* data because they have not been organised or arranged in any way. This makes it difficult to see what interesting characteristics or features the data might contain. The data cannot tell its story, if you like. For example, it is not easy to observe how many babies had a low birthweight (less than 2500 g) from Figure 1.1, or what proportion of the babies were female from Figure 1.2. Moreover, this is for only 100 values. Imagine how much more difficult it would be for 500 or 5000 values. In the next four chapters, we will discuss a number of different ways that we can organise data so that it can tell its story. Then, we can see more easily what is going on.

No	No	No	No	No	No	No	No	Yes	No
No	No	No	No	No	No	No	No	Yes	No
No	No	No	No	No	Yes	No	No	No	No
Yes	No	Yes	No	No	No	No	No	No	No
No	No	No	No	No	No	No	No	No	No
No	No	No	Yes	Yes	No	No	No	No	No
No	No	Yes	No	No	Yes	No	No	No	No
Yes	No	No	No	Yes	Yes	No	No	Yes	No
No	No	No	No	No	No	No	No	No	No
No	Yes	No	No	No	Yes	No	No	Yes	No

Figure 1.3 The variable 'smoked while pregnant?' for the mothers of the babies in Figure 1.1

Exercise 1.1. Why do you think that the data in Figures 1.1, 1.2 and 1.3 are referred to as 'sample data'?

Exercise 1.2. What percentage of mothers smoked during their pregnancy? How does your value contrast with the evidence which suggests that about 20 per cent of mothers in the United Kingdom smoked when pregnant?

Of course, we gather data not because it is nice to look at or we've got nothing better to do but because we want to answer a question. A question such as 'Do the babies of mothers who smoked while pregnant have a different (we're probably guessing lower) birthweight than the babies of mothers who did not smoke?' or 'On average, do male babies have the same birthweight as female babies?' Later in the book, we will deal with methods which you can use to answer such questions (and ones more complex); however, for now, we need to stick with variables and data.

Where are we going ... ?

- This book is an introduction to medical statistics.

- Medical statistics is about doing things with data.

- We get data when we determine the value of a variable.

- We need data in order to answer a question.

- What we can do with data depends on what type of data it is.

The good, the bad, and the ugly – types of variables

There are two major types of variable – *categorical* variables and *metric* variables; each of them can be further divided into two subtypes, as shown in Figure 1.4.

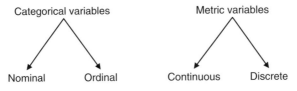

Figure 1.4 Types of variables

Each of these variable types produces a different type of data. The differences in these data types are of great importance – some statistical methods are appropriate for some types of data but not for others, and applying an inappropriate procedure can result in a misleading outcome. It is therefore critical that you identify the sort of variable (and data) you are dealing with *before* you begin any analysis, and we need therefore to examine the differences in data types in a bit more detail. From now on, I will be using the word 'data' rather than 'variable' because it is the data we will be working with – but remember that data come from variables. We'll start with categorical data.

Categorical data

Nominal categorical data

Consider the gender data shown in Figure 1.2. These data are *nominal categorical* data (or just nominal data for short).

The data are 'nominal' because it usually relates to *named* things, such as occupation, blood type, or ethnicity. It is particularly *not* numeric. It is 'categorical' because we allocate each value to a specific category. Therefore, for example, we allocate each M value in Figure 1.2 to the category Male and each F value to the category Female. If we do this for all 100 values, we get:

Male   56
Female   44

Notice two things about this data, which is typical of all nominal data:

- The data do not have any units of measurement.[1]

- The ordering of the categories is *arbitrary*. In other words, the categories cannot be ordered in any meaningful way.[2] We could just as easily have written the number of males and females in the order:

---

[1] For example, cm, seconds, ccs, or kg, etc.
[2] We are excluding trivial arrangements such as alphabetic.

Female   44
Male   56

By the way, allocating values to categories by hand is pretty tedious as well as error-prone, more so if there are a lot of values. In practice, you would use a computer to do this.

> **Exercise 1.3.**   Suggest a few nominal variables.

Ordinal categorical data

Let's now consider data from the Glasgow Coma Scale (GCS) (which some of you may be familiar with). As the name suggests, this scale is used to assess the level of consciousness after head injury. A patient's GCS score is judged by the sum of responses in three areas: eye opening response, verbal response, and motor response. Notice particularly that these responses are *assessed* rather than measured (as weight, height or temperature would be). The GCS score can vary from 3 (deeply unconscious) to 15 (fully conscious). In other words, there are 13 possible categories of consciousness.[3]

Suppose that we have two motor-cyclists, let us call them Wayne and Kylie, who have been admitted to the Emergency Department with head injuries following a road traffic accident. Wayne has a GCS of 5 and Kylie a GCS of 10. We *can* say that Wayne's level of consciousness is *less* than that of Kylie (so we can order the values) but *we can't say exactly by how much*. We certainly cannot say that Wayne is exactly half as conscious as Kylie. Moreover, the levels of consciousness between adjacent scores are not necessarily the same; for example, the difference in the levels of consciousness between two patients with GCS scores of 10 and 11 may not be the same as that between patients with scores of 11 and 12. It's therefore important to recognise that we cannot quantify these differences.

GCS data is *ordinal categorical* (or just *ordinal*) data. It is ordinal because the values can be meaningfully ordered, and it is categorical because each value is assigned to a specific category. Notice two things about this variable, which is typical of all ordinal variables:

- The data do not have any units of measurement (so the same as that for nominal variables).

- The ordering of the categories is *not* arbitrary, as it is with nominal variables.

The *seemingly* numeric values of ordinal data, such as GCS scores, are not in fact real numbers but only *numeric labels* which we attach to category values (usually for convenience or for data entry to a computer). The reason is of course (to re-emphasise this important point) that GCS data, and the data generated by most other scales, are *not properly measured* but *assessed* in

---

[3]The scale is now used by first responders, paramedics and doctors, as being applicable to all acute medical and trauma patients.

some way by a clinician or a researcher, working with the individual concerned.[4] This is a characteristic of all ordinal data.

Because ordinal data are not real numbers, it is not appropriate to apply any of the rules of basic arithmetic to this sort of data. You should not add, subtract, multiply or divide ordinal values. This limitation has marked implications for the sorts of analyses that we can do with such data – as you will see later in this book. Finally, we should note that ordinal data are almost always integer, that is, they have whole number values.

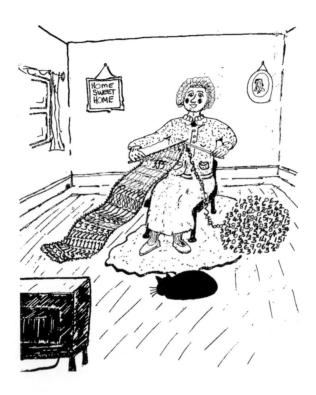

Exercise 1.4. Suggest a few more scales with which you may be familiar from your clinical work.

Exercise 1.5. Explain why it would not really make sense to calculate an average GCS for a group of head injury patients.

---

[4]There are some scales which may involve *some* degree of proper measurement, but these still produce ordinal values if even one part of the score is determined by a non-measured element.

Metric data

Discrete metric data

Consider the data in Figure 1.5. This shows the parity[5] of the mothers of the babies whose birthweights are shown in Figure 1.1.

0	0	2	0	0	3	3	1	0	3
0	0	0	0	1	0	3	2	3	1
2	2	3	1	10	0	1	0	1	5
1	0	1	0	0	0	0	0	0	0
2	0	0	0	2	1	0	2	2	0
1	0	0	0	0	0	1	0	0	0
0	0	2	2	3	2	2	0	3	1
0	4	0	0	2	1	0	0	0	1
3	3	0	3	0	0	6	0	1	0
2	2	1	2	4	1	0	2	1	0

Figure 1.5 Parity data (number of viable pregnancies) for the mothers whose babies' birthweights are shown in Figure 1.1

Discrete metric data, such as that shown in Figure 1.5, comes from *counting*. Counting is a form of measurement – hence the name 'metric'. The data is 'discrete' because the values are in discrete steps; for example, 0, 1, 2, 3 and so on. Parity data comes from counting – probably by asking the mother or by looking at records. Other examples of discrete metric data would include number of deaths, number of pressure sores, number of angina attacks, number of hospital visits and so on. The data produced are real numbers, and in contrast to ordinal data, this means that the difference between parities of 1 and 2 is exactly the same as the difference between parities of 2 and 3, and a parity of 4 is exactly twice a parity of 2.

In short:

- Metric discrete variables can be *counted* and can have units of measurement – 'numbers of things'.

- They produce data which are real numbers and are invariably integers (i.e. whole numbers).

---

[5] Number of pregnancies carried to a viable gestational age – 24 weeks in the United Kingdom, 20 weeks in the United States.

Continuous metric data

Look back at Figure 1.1 – the birthweight data.

Birthweight is a *metric continuous* variable because it can be measured. For example, if we want to know someone's weight, we can use a weighing machine; we don't have to look at the individual and make a guess (which would be approximate) or ask them how heavy they are (very unreliable). Similarly, if we want to know their diastolic blood pressure, we can use a sphygmomanometer.[6] Guessing or asking is not necessary. But, what do we mean by 'continuous'? Compare a digital clock with a more old-fashioned analogue clock. With a digital clock, the seconds are indicated in discrete steps: 1, 2, 3 and so on. With the analogue clock, the hand sweeps around the dial in a smooth, continuous movement. In the same way, weight is a continuous variable because the values form a continuum; weight does not increase in steps of 1 g.

Because they can be properly measured, these data *are* real numbers. In contrast to ordinal values, the difference between any pair of adjacent values, say 4000 g and 4001 g is exactly the same as the difference between 4001 g and 4002 g, and a baby who weighs 4000 g is exactly twice as heavy as a baby of 2000 g. Some other examples of metric continuous data include blood pressure (mmHg), blood cholesterol (μg/ml), waiting time (minutes), body mass index (kg/m^2), peak expiry flow (l per min) and so on. Notice that all of these variables have units of measurement attached to them. This is a characteristic of all metric continuous data.

Because metric data values are real numbers, you can apply all of the usual mathematical operations to them. This opens up a much wider range of analytic possibilities than is possible with either nominal or ordinal data – as you will see later.

To sum up:

- Metric continuous data result from *measurement* and they have units of measurement.

- The data are real numbers.

These properties of both types of metric data are markedly different from the characteristics of nominal and ordinal data.

Exercise 1.6.   Suggest a few continuous metric variables which you are familiar with. What is the difference between assessing the value of something and measuring it?

Exercise 1.7.   Suggest a few discrete metric variables which you are familiar with.

Exercise 1.8.   What is the difference between continuous and discrete metric data? Somebody shows you a six-pack egg carton. List (a) the possible number of eggs that the carton could contain; and (b) the number of possible values for the weight of the empty carton. What do you conclude?

---

[6] We call the device that we use to obtain the measured value, for example, a weighing scale, a sphygmomanometer, or a tape measure, etc. a *measuring instrument*.

How can I tell what type of variable I am dealing with?

The easiest way to tell whether data is metric is to check whether it has *units* attached to it, such as g, mm, °C, µg/cm³, *number of* pressure sores and *number of* deaths. If not, it may be ordinal or nominal – the former if the values can be put in any meaningful order. Figure 1.6 is an aid to variable-type recognition.

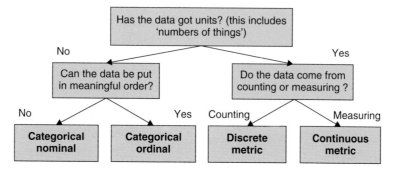

Figure 1.6 An algorithm to help identify data type

Exercise 1.9. Four migraine patients are asked to assess the severity of their migraine pain one hour after the first symptoms of an attack by marking a point on a horizontal line 100 mm long. The line is marked 'No pain' at the left-hand end and 'Worst possible pain' at the right-hand end. The distance of each patient's mark from the left-hand end is subsequently measured with an mm rule, and their scores are 25 mm, 44 mm, 68 mm and 85 mm. What sort of data is this? Can you calculate the average pain of these four patients? Note that this form of measurement (using a line and getting subjects to mark it) is known as a visual analogue scale (VAS).

The baseline table

When you are reading a research report or a journal paper, you will want to know something about the participants in the study. In most published papers, the authors will provide the reader with a summary table describing the basic characteristics of the participants in the study. This will contain some basic demographic information, together with relevant clinical details. This table is called the *baseline table* or the *table of basic characteristics*. In the following three exercises, we make use of the baseline tables provided by the authors.

Exercise 1.10. Figure 1.7 contains the basic characteristics of cases and controls from a case–control study[7] into stressful life events and the risk of breast cancer in women. Identify the type of each variable in the table.

---

[7]Do not worry about the different types of study; I will discuss them in detail in Chapter 6.

Variable	Breast cancer group (n = 106)	Control group (n = 226)	p value
Age	61.6 (10.9)	51.0 (8.5)	0.000*
Social class[†] (%):			
I	10 (10)	20 (9)	
II	38 (36)	82 (36)	
III non-manual	28 (26)	72 (32)	0.094[‡]
III manual	13 (12)	24 (11)	
IV	11 (10)	21 (9)	
V	3 (3)	2 (1)	
VI	3 (3)	4 (2)	
No of children (%):			
0	15 (14)	31 (14)	
1	16 (15)	31 (13.7)	0.97
2	42 (40)	84 (37)	
≥3	32 (31)[†]	80 (35)	
Age at birth of first child	21.3 (5.6)	20.5 (4.3)	0.500*
Age at menarche	12.8 (1.4)	13.0 (1.6)	0.200*
Menopausal state (%):			
Premenopausal	14 (13)	66 (29)	
Perimenopausal	9 (9)	43 (19)	0.000[§]
Postmenopausal	83 (78)	117 (52)	
Age at menopause	47.7 (4.5)	45.6 (5.2)	0.001*
Lifetime use of oral contraceptives (%)	38	61	0.000[‡]
No of years taking oral contraceptives	3.0 (5.4)	4.2 (5.0)	0.065[§]
No of months breastfeeding	(n = 90)	(n = 195)	
	7.4 (9.9)	7.4 (12.1)	0.990*
Lifetime use of hormone replacement therapy (%)	29 (27)	78 (35)	0.193[§]
Mean years of hormone replacement therapy	1.6 (3.7)	1.9 (4.0)	0.460*
Family history of ovarian cancer (%)	8 (8)	10 (4)	0.241[§]
History of benign breast disease (%)	15 (15)	105 (47)	0.000[§]
Family history of breast cancer[¶]	16 (15)	35 (16)	0.997[§]
Units of alcohol/week (%):			
0	38 (36)	59 (26)	
0–4	26 (25)	71 (31)	0.927[‡]
5–9	20 (19)	52 (23)	
≥10	22 (21)	44 (20)	
No of cigarettes/day:			
0	83 (78.3)	170 (75.2)	
1–9	8 (7.6)	14 (6.2)	0.383[‡]
≥10	15 (14.2)	42 (18.6)	
Body mass index (kg/m²)	26.8 (5.5)	24.8 (4.2)	0.001*

*Two sample t test.
[†]Data for one case missing.
[‡]χ^2 test for trend.
[§]χ^2 test.
[¶]No data for one control.

Figure 1.7 Basic characteristics of cases and controls from a case–control study into stressful life events as risk factors for breast cancer in women. Values are mean (SD) unless stated otherwise. Source: Protheroe *et al.* (1999). Reproduced by permission of BMJ Publishing Group Ltd

Exercise 1.11. Figure 1.8 is from a cross-sectional study to determine the incidence of pregnancy-related venous thromboembolic events and their relationship to selected risk factors, such as maternal age, parity, smoking, and so on. Identify the type of each variable in the table.

Exercise 1.12. Figure 1.9 is from a study to compare two lotions, malathion and *d*-phenothrin, in the treatment of head lice in 193 schoolchildren. Ninety-five children were given malathion and 98 *d*-phenothrin. Identify the type of each variable in the table.

	Thrombosis cases ($n = 608$)	Controls ($n = 114\,940$)	OR	95%
Maternal age (y) (classification 1)				
≤19	26 (4.3)	2817 (2.5)	1.9	1.3, 2.9
20–24	125 (20.6)	23,006 (20.0)	1.1	0.9, 1.4
25–29	216 (35.5)	44,763 (38.9)	1.0	Reference
30–34	151 (24.8)	30,135 (26.2)	1.0	0.8, 1.3
≥35	90 (14.8)	14,219 (12.4)	1.3	1.0, 1.7
Maternal age (y) (classification 2)				
≤19	26 (4.3)	2817 (2.5)	1.8	1.2, 2.7
20–34	492 (80.9)	97,904 (85.2)	1.0	Reference
≥35	90 (14.8)	14,219 (12.4)	1.3	1.0, 1.6
Parity				
Para 0	304 (50.0)	47,425 (41.3)	1.8	1.5, 2.2
Para 1	142 (23.4)	40,734 (35.4)	1.0	Reference
Para 2	93 (15.3)	18,113 (15.8)	1.5	1.1, 1.9
≥Para 3	69 (11.3)	8429 (7.3)	2.4	1.8, 3.1
Missing data	0 (0)	239 (0.2)		
No. of cigarettes daily				
0	423 (69.6)	87,408 (76.0)	1.0	Reference
1–9	80 (13.2)	14,295 (12.4)	1.2	0.9, 1.5
≥10	57 (9.4)	8177 (7.1)	1.4	1.1, 1.9
Missing data	48 (7.9)	5060 (4.4)		
Multiple pregnancy				
No	593 (97.5)	113,330 (98.6)	1.0	Reference
Yes	15 (2.5)	1610 (1.4)	1.8	1.1, 3.0
Preeclampsia				
No	562 (92.4)	111,788 (97.3)	1.0	Reference
Yes	46 (7.6)	3152 (2.7)	2.9	2.1, 3.9
Cesarean delivery				
No	420 (69.1)	102,181 (88.9)	1.0	Reference
Yes	188 (30.9)	12,759 (11.1)	3.6	3.0, 4.3

Data presented as *n* (%).
OR, odds ratio; CI, confidence interval.

Figure 1.8 Table of baseline characteristics from a cross-sectional study of thrombotic risk during pregnancy. Source: Lindqvist *et al.* (1999). Reproduced by permission of Wolters Kluwer Health

Characteristic	Malathion ($n = 95$)	d-phenothrin ($n = 98$)
Age at randomisation (year)	8.6 (1.6)	8.9 (1.6)
Sex – no of children (%)		
Male	31 (33)	41 (42)
Female	64 (67)	57 (58)
Home no (mean)		
Number of rooms	3.3 (1.2)	3.3 (1.8)
Length of hair – no of children (%)*		
Long	37 (39)	20 (21)
Mid-long	23 (24)	33 (34)
Short	35 (37)	44 (46)
Colour of hair – no of children (%)		
Blond	15 (16)	18 (18)
Brown	49 (52)	55 (56)
Red	4 (4)	4 (4)
Dark	27 (28)	21 (22)
Texture of hair – no of children (%)		
Straight	67 (71)	69 (70)
Curly	19 (20)	25 (26)
Frizzy/kinky	9 (9)	4 (4)
Pruritus – no of children (%)	54 (57)	65 (66)
Excoriations – no of children (%)	25 (26)	39 (40)
Evaluation of infestation		
Live lice-no of children (%)		
0	18 (19)	24 (24)
+	45 (47)	35 (36)
++	9 (9)	15 (15)
+++	12 (13)	15 (15)
++++	11 (12)	9 (9)
Viable nits-no of children (%)*		
0	19 (20)	8 (8)
+	32 (34)	41 (45)
++	22 (23)	24 (25)
+++	18 (19)	20 (21)
++++	4 (4)	4 (4)

The two groups were similar at baseline except for a significant difference for the length of hair ($p = 0.02$; chi-square)

*One value missing in the d-phenothrin group square.

Figure 1.9   Baseline characteristics of the *Pediculus humanus capitis*-infested schoolchildren assigned to receive either malathion or *d*-phenothrin lotion. Source: Chosidow *et al.* (1994). Reproduced by permission of Elsevier

At the end of each chapter, you should look again at the chapter objectives and satisfy yourself that you have achieved them.

II

Descriptive Statistics

2

Describing data with tables

Learning objectives

When you have read this chapter, you should be able to:

- Explain what a frequency distribution is.

- Construct a frequency table from raw data.

- Construct relative frequency, cumulative frequency and relative cumulative frequency tables.

- Construct grouped frequency tables.

- Construct a cross-tabulation table.

- Explain what a contingency table is.

- Rank data.

Descriptive statistics. What can we do with raw data?

As we saw in Chapter 1, when we have a lot of raw data, for example, as in Figure 1.1 (birth-weight) or Figure 1.2 (gender), it is not easy for us to answer questions that we may have; for

Medical Statistics from Scratch: An Introduction for Health Professionals, Third Edition. David Bowers.
© 2014 John Wiley & Sons, Ltd. Published 2014 by John Wiley & Sons, Ltd.

example, the percentage of low birthweight babies or the proportion of male babies. This is because the data have not been arranged or structured in any way. If there are any interesting features in the data, they remain hidden from us. We said then that the data could not tell their story, and of course, the more the data are, the harder this becomes. Samples of many hundreds or thousands are not uncommon.

In this chapter, and the four following, we are going to describe some methods for organising and presenting the data, so that we can answer more easily the questions of interest – essentially to enable us to see what's going on. Collectively, these methods are called *descriptive statistics*. These methods are a set of procedures that we can apply to raw data, so that its principal characteristics and main features are revealed. This might include sorting the data by size, putting it into a table, presenting it as a chart, or summarising it numerically.

An important consideration in this process is the type of data you are working with. Some types of data are best described with a table, some with a chart and some perhaps with both, whereas with other types of data, a numeric summary might be more appropriate. In this chapter, we focus on organising raw data into what is known as a *frequency table*. In subsequent chapters, we will look at the use of charts, and numeric summaries. It will be easier if we take each data type in turn, starting with nominal data.

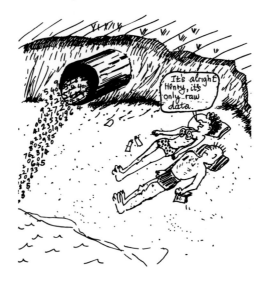

Frequency tables – nominal data

We have already seen a rudimentary frequency table in Chapter 1, with a count of male and female babies from Figure 1.2.

Male   56
Female   44

We can express this information in a more conventional form of a frequency table, as in Figure 2.1.

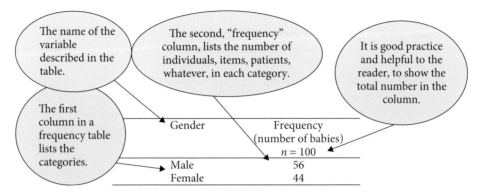

Figure 2.1   A frequency table for gender of newborn babies (raw data from Figure 1.2)

The label at the top of the first (left-hand) column indicates the variable being described in the table. The remainder of the first column is a list of the *categories* for this variable. The second (right-hand) column is the *frequency* column. Frequency is another word for 'count' and lists, in this example, the number of babies in each category, that is, males and females.

Exercise 2.1.   Using the raw data from Figure 1.3, construct a frequency table for the number of women who smoked while pregnant. Does it matter how you order the categories in column 1?

The frequency distribution

Consider another example. Figure 1.9 contains data from a nit lotion study that compared two types of treatment for nits, malathion or *d-phenothrin*, with a sample of 95 children. For each child, data were collected on nine variables, one being the child's hair colour: blonde, brown, red and dark. The frequency table (extracted from Figure 1.9) for the four colour categories is shown in Figure 2.2.

Hair colour	Frequency (number of children) $n = 95$
Brown	49
Dark	27
Blonde	15
Red	4

Figure 2.2   Frequency table showing the hair colour of each of 95 children in a study of malathion versus *d*-phenothrin for the treatment of nits

As you know, the ordering of nominal categories is arbitrary, and in this example, they are shown by the number of children in each – largest first. Notice that total frequency ($n = 95$) is shown at the top of the frequency column. You should always do this – it is helpful to any reader. Taken as a whole, Figure 2.2 tells us how the hair colour of each of the 95 children is *distributed* across the four colour categories. In other words, Figure 2.2 describes the *frequency distribution* of the hair colour data. We can see that the most common hair colour is brown and the least common red. We'll have more to say about frequency distributions later.

Relative frequency

Often of more use than the actual *number* of individuals in each category are the *percentages*. Tables with this information are called *relative* or *percentage* frequency tables. The third column of Figure 2.3 shows the percentage of children in each hair colour category.

Hair colour	Frequency (number of children) $n = 95$	Relative frequency (% of children in each category)
Brown	49	51.6
Dark	27	28.4
Blonde	15	15.8
Red	4	4.2

Figure 2.3   Relative frequency table for hair colour, showing the *percentage* of children in each hair colour category (see Figure 1.9)

Figure 2.3 tells us that over half of the children (51.6 per cent) had brown hair. This seems to be more helpful than knowing that 49 out of 95 children had brown hair.

Exercise 2.2.   Construct a relative frequency table for the smoking data shown in Figure 1.3. What percentage of women smoked while pregnant?

Exercise 2.3.   Figure 2.4 shows the frequency distribution for cause of blunt injury to limbs in 75 patients, taken from a study of the treatment of pain after limb injury. Calculate the relative frequencies. What percentage of patients had crush injuries?

Frequency tables – ordinal data

When the data in question are ordinal, we can allocate them into ordered categories. As an example, 475 psychiatric in-patients were questioned about their *level of satisfaction* with their

Cause of injury	Number of patients (n = 75)
Falls	46
Crush	20
Motor vehicle crash	6
Other	3

Figure 2.4 Frequency table showing causes of blunt injury to limbs in 75 patients, taken from a study of the treatment of pain after limb injury. Data from Rainer *et al.* (2000)

psychiatric nursing care. 'Level of satisfaction' is clearly an ordinal variable. 'Satisfaction' cannot be properly measured, and has no units, but the categories can be meaningfully ordered, as they have been ordered here. The resulting data is shown in Figure 2.5.

Satisfaction with nursing care	Number of patients (n = 475)
Very satisfied	121
Satisfied	161
Neutral	90
Dissatisfied	51
Very dissatisfied	52

Figure 2.5 Frequency table for data on level of satisfaction with nursing care by 475 psychiatric in-patients. Data from Rogers and Pilgrim (1991)

The frequency values indicate that more than half of the patients were happy with their psychiatric nursing care, 282 patients (121 + 161) out of 475. Much smaller numbers expressed dissatisfaction.

Exercise 2.4. Calculate the relative frequencies for the frequency data shown in Figure 2.5. What percentage of patients were 'very dissatisfied' with their care?

Exercise 2.5. In a study comparing two treatments for a whiplash injury, one group of patients received the usual emergency department care (normal consultation plus an advice leaflet) and the other group received 'active management' care (normal consultation plus additional help). Twelve months after the initial contact, the patients were asked to rate the benefits they felt from their treatment. The results are shown in Figure 2.6 for each group (the group with missing values has been omitted). What percentage of patients felt 'much better' in each group? What percentage felt 'much worse'? How do you think that the missing values might affect the reliability of results in general?

Self-rated benefit	Usual care group (n = 1094)	Active management group (n = 1543)
Much better	288	468
Better	297	479
Same	429	491
Worse	73	98
Much worse	7	7

Figure 2.6 Self-rated benefit by two groups of whiplash injury patients receiving different care packages, 12 months after the initial contact. Data from Lamb *et al.* (2013)

Exercise 2.6. In a randomised controlled trial of physical activity and fitness in patients with Parkinson's disease, patients were randomly assigned either to the ParkFit programme (a multifaceted behavioural change programme designed to increase physical activity levels, which included physiotherapy) or to a matched control group (physiotherapy only). The researchers compared the outcomes after two years, using the modified Hoehn and Yahr scale. This scale, with a range from 1 (least affected – unilateral involvement only) to 5 (most severely affected – wheelchair bound or bedridden unless aided), is designed to assess the degree of disability of patients with Parkinson's disease. The results are shown in Figure 2.7. (Note: this is a rare example of an ordinal scale which is not an integer). Is there a difference between the two groups in the percentage of patients with a modified Hoehn and Yahr scale score of 2?

Modified Hoehn and Yahr scale score	ParkFit group (n = 299)	Control group (n = 287)
1	7	4
1.5	7	10
2	221	223
2.5	48	36
3	16	14

Figure 2.7 Modified Hoehn and Yahr scale scores (after two years) for two groups of patients with Parkinson's disease. One group randomly assigned to a physical activity programme (ParkFit, which included physiotherapy), the other, the control group, receiving physiotherapy only. Data from van Nimwegen *et al.* (2013)

Frequency tables – metric data

We have to consider two situations here, one with discrete metric data and the other continuous. We will start with the discrete data case.

Frequency tables with discrete metric data

As we saw in Chapter 1, discrete metric data result from counting. This means that the number of possible values is *limited*; the number of cells in the human body may be very large, but it is not infinite. Parity, for example, is a discrete metric variable and is *counted* as 0, 1, 2, 3 and so on. The parity data shown in Figure 1.6, and reproduced below as Figure 2.8 (for convenience), have values that range from 0 to 10 (i.e. there are 11 different *possible* values).

If our question is, 'How many women in the sample had a parity of 0?' or 'How many a parity of 1?', we can very easily answer these questions, and similar questions, if we arrange these data into a *frequency table*. The result is shown in Figure 2.9.

0	0	2	0	0	3	3	1	0	3
0	0	0	0	1	0	3	2	3	1
2	2	3	1	10	0	1	0	1	5
1	0	1	0	0	0	0	0	0	0
2	0	0	0	2	1	0	2	2	0
1	0	0	0	0	0	1	0	0	0
0	0	2	2	3	2	2	0	3	1
0	4	0	0	2	1	0	0	0	1
3	3	0	3	0	0	6	0	1	0
2	2	1	2	4	1	0	2	1	0

Figure 2.8   Parity (number of viable pregnancies) for the mothers whose babies' birthweights are shown in Figure 1.1

Parity	Number of mothers ($n = 100$)
0	49
1	18
2	17
3	11
4	2
5	1
6	1
7	0
8	0
9	0
10	1

Figure 2.9   Frequency table for the parity of the mothers whose babies birthweights are shown in Figure 1.1

Exercise 2.7. What percentage of mothers had a parity of *either* 1 *or* 2?

Exercise 2.8. In a study comparing the safety and efficacy of biolimus-eluting (biodegradable) stents with everolimus-eluting (durable) stents, patients were randomly allocated to receive either of the two types of stents. The number of lesions, along with the corresponding number of stents per lesion, was recorded for the two groups of patients, and the data are shown in Figure 2.10. What percentage of patients in each group had lesions requiring (a) one stent and (b) two stents?

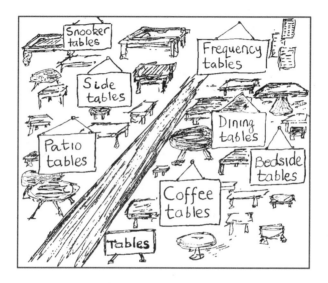

Total number of lesions	Biolimus-eluting stent ($n = 2638$ lesions)	Everolimus-eluting stent ($n = 1387$ lesions)
1 stent	1805	948
2 stents	553	300
3 stents	168	79
4 stents	53	35
5 stents	13	6
6 stents	5	0
7 stents	1	0
Unknown/0 stents	40	19

Figure 2.10 The number of lesions, along with the corresponding number of stents per lesion, for two groups of patients; one group receiving a biodegradable stent (column 2) and the other group a durable stent (column 3). Data from Smits *et al.* (2013)

Cumulative frequency

Suppose that we want to know what was the *percentage* of lesions among the patients receiving the biolimus-eluding stent that required fewer than three stents? A question like this is more easily answered if we add a percentage cumulative frequency column to the respective frequency table. The procedure, using data from Figure 2.10, is as follows:

- Step 1. Calculate the cumulative frequencies by adding up successively the values in the frequency column: 1805, 1805 + 553 = 2358, 2358 + 168 = 2526, and so on.

- Step 2. Calculate the percentage cumulative frequencies by dividing each cumulative frequency value by the total (2638) and then multiplying by 100.

The results are shown in Figure 2.11. The answer to the question, 'What was the percentage of patients receiving the biolimus-eluting stent that had lesions that required fewer than three stents?', is thus 89.38 per cent. We can also easily calculate how many patients had lesions that required three or more stents as 100 − 89.38 = 10.62%.

Total number of lesions	Frequency Biolimus-eluting stent ($n = 2638$ lesions)	Cumulative frequency	% Cumulative frequency
1 stent	1805	1805	68.42
2 stents	553	2358	89.38
3 stents	168	2526	95.75
4 stents	53	2579	97.76
5 stents	13	2592	98.26
6 stents	5	2597	98.44
7 stents	1	2598	98.48
Unknown/0 stents	40	2638	100.00

Callouts: $1805 + 553 = 2358$; $(1805 / 2638) \times 100 = 68.42$; $2358 + 168 = 2526$

Figure 2.11 Calculating cumulative and percentage cumulative frequencies for patients receiving the biolimus-eluting stent (using data in Figure 2.10)

Exercise 2.9. Use the whiplash injury data shown in Figure 2.6 to calculate the percentage cumulative frequencies for each of the two groups. Use these values to determine the total percentage of patients in the study who felt either the same, worse, or much worse in each of the two groups.

Frequency tables with continuous metric data – grouping the raw data

Constructing frequency tables for continuous metric data is often more of a problem than constructing with discrete metric data because, as we saw in Chapter 1, the number of possible values which the data can take is infinite (recall the clock-face analogy).

Organising *raw* metric continuous data (such as the birthweight data shown in Figure 1.1) into a frequency table is usually impractical because there are such a large number of possible values. Indeed, there may well be no value that occurs more than once – particularly true if the values have decimal places. This means that the corresponding frequency table is likely to have a large, and thus unhelpful, number of rows. Not of much help in uncovering any pattern in the data therefore! The most useful approach with metric continuous data is to *group* them first and then construct a frequency distribution of the grouped data. Let's see how this works.

The choice of the number of groups is arbitrary but you do not want too few groups (too much information is lost) or too many (not much more helpful than the raw data). Experience will help but as a very rough rule of thumb, no fewer than five groups and no more than 10. Of course, particular circumstances may cause these values to vary. For the first 100 values of the birthweight data in Figure 1.1, I have chosen seven groups as shown in column 1 and determined the number of birthweights in each group – these values are shown in column 2 (see Figure 2.12).

Rather dramatically, the data in Figure 1.1 is now able to reveal its message. We can see that the majority of babies had birthweights between 2500 g and 4000 g. Very few babies had birthweights outside this range. This information was not easily obtained from the raw data in Figure 1.1.

We should note that it is possible to calculate cumulative frequencies with grouped frequency data, just as it was in Figure 2.11. If we do this for the data in Figure 2.12, we get the results as shown in Figure 2.13. Because there are 100 birthweights in this sample, the arithmetic is straightforward. We see, for example, that seven per cent of babies have a birthweight <2500 g.

Birthweight (g)	Frequency (number babies) $n = 100$
1500–1999	2
2000–2499	5
2500–2999	27
3000–3499	28
3500–3999	27
4000–4499	9
4500–4999	2

Figure 2.12 A grouped frequency table for the birthweight data from Figure 1.1.

Exercise 2.10. Why does it make no sense to construct cumulative frequencies for nominal data?

Birthweight (g)	Frequency (number babies) ($n = 100$)	Cumulative frequency	% Cumulative frequency
1500 – 1999	2	2	2
2000 – 2499	5	7	7
2500 – 2999	27	34	34
3000 – 3499	28	62	62
3500 – 3999	27	89	89
4000 – 4499	9	98	98
4500 – 4999	2	100	100

Figure 2.13   Cumulative frequencies for the grouped frequency table of birthweight data in Figure 2.12 (raw data in Figure 1.1)

Exercise 2.11.   The data in Figure 2.14 is from a study to ascertain the extent of variation in the case-mix of adult admissions to intensive care units (ICUs) in Britain and Ireland and its impact on outcomes. The figure records the percentage mortality in 26 ICUs. Construct a grouped frequency table of percentage mortality. What do you observe?

ICU	1	2	3	4	5	6	7	8	9	10	11	12	13
% mortality	15.2	31.3	14.9	16.3	19.3	18.2	20.2	12.8	14.7	29.4	21.1	20.4	13.6

ICU	14	15	16	17	18	19	20	21	22	23	24	25	26
% mortality	22.4	14.0	14.3	22.8	26.7	18.9	13.7	17.7	27.2	19.3	16.1	13.5	11.2

Figure 2.14   Percentage mortality in 26 intensive care units. Data from Rowan *et al.* (1993)

Open-ended groups

One problem arises when one or two values are a long way from the general mass of the data, either much lower or much higher. These values are called *outliers*. Their presence can mean having a lot of empty or near-empty rows at one or both ends of the frequency table.

One possible solution is to use *open-ended* categories. Take as an example the parity data in Figure 2.9. We see that there are three rows with zero frequencies. The frequency table can be re-designed to display the data more economically if we use an open-ended category as shown in Figure 2.15.

Parity	Number of mothers ($n = 100$)
0	49
1	18
2	17
3	11
4	2
5	1
≥6	2

An open-ended category.

Figure 2.15 Frequency table for the parity of the mothers (see Figure 2.9) showing an open-ended category

Cross-tabulation – contingency tables

Each of the frequency tables above provides us with a description of the frequency distribution of a *single* variable. Sometimes, however, you will want to examine the association between *two* variables, within a *single* group of individuals. You can do this by putting the data into a *contingency table*, also called a table of *cross-tabulations*. In these tables, the rows represent the categories of one variable, usually an 'outcome' of some sort (e.g. a diagnosis of lung cancer – Yes or No), and the columns represent the groups within a second variable (e.g. smokers and non-smokers).

To illustrate this idea, look at Figure 2.16. This is a contingency table of the cross-tabulation of the variable 'smoked while pregnant' (Yes or No), against three categories of the variable 'birthweight': <2500 g, 2500 g – 3999 g, and ≥4000 g,[1] for a random sample of 500 newborn babies. Here, the outcome (the rows) is birthweight, and the groups (the columns) are the mothers who smoked while pregnant, and those who didn't. This table would be called a 2×2 table because there are two rows and two columns, although tables with more rows and columns are not unusual.

Exercise 2.12.   What does Figure 2.16 imply (if anything) about the effect of whether the mother smoked or not on birthweight? It might help to answer this question if the values in the cross-tabulation were expressed as percentages of the columns. Try this and see if it helps.

Exercise 2.13.   The data in Figure 2.17 is from a sample of 30 newborn babies and records their birthweights and their mothers' weight at booking. Construct a 2×2 contingency table, with columns corresponding to the mothers' weight categories of ≤60.0 kg and >60.0 kg, and rows corresponding to the birthweight categories of ≤3000 g and >3000 g. What does the table indicate about the relationship between mothers' weight and birthweight?

---

[1] For this sample of 500 babies, 2500 g corresponds to the 10th percentile and 4000 g to the 90th percentile.

		Smoked while pregnant?	
		Yes	No
Birthweight (g)	<2500	3	37
	2500 to 3999	65	353
	≥4000	9	33

Figure 2.16 Cross-tabulation of 'Smoked while pregnant?' (columns) versus three categories of birth-weight (rows). Born-in-Bradford data

Mother's weight at booking (kg)	Baby's birthweight (g)
62.0	3220
74.0	4140
54.5	2220
52.0	3540
59.5	3500
90.0	3820
110.0	3330
55.0	2840
85.0	2780
55.0	2660
52.0	2170
88.0	3340
65.0	3070
70.0	3800
81.0	3300
63.0	3380
124.0	4060
66.0	2640
55.0	2460
57.0	3460
54.0	2820
64.0	3280
91.0	3740
60.0	3000
88.0	3320
84.0	3490
100.0	3920
49.0	2460
75.0	3410
41.0	2740

Figure 2.17 The birthweights of 30 newborn babies and their mothers' weight at booking. (Born in Bradford data)

Exercise 2.14. Figure 2.18 is a 2×2 contingency table, from a study of discrimination in intimate relationships reported by people with depression. The table shows the cross-tabulation of discrimination for two groups. The columns represent those who anticipated discrimination and those who did not. The rows represent those who experienced and those who did not experience discrimination. What do the percentage figures represent? How useful are they if you want to examine any possible connection between anticipation of discrimination and experiencing it? What percentages would be more useful? What does the table suggest about a possible connection between the two variables?

Discrimination?	Anticipated ($n = 353$)	Not anticipated ($n = 510$)
Experienced	193 (22%)	156 (18%)
Not experienced	160 (19%)	354 (41%)

Figure 2.18 A 2×2 contingency table from a study of discrimination in intimate relationships reported by people with depression. Data from Lasalvia *et al.* (2013)

Ranking data

As you will see later in the book, some statistical techniques require the data to be *ranked* before any analysis takes place. Ranking means first arranging the data by size and then giving the largest value a rank of 1, the second largest value a rank of 2, and so on.[2] Any values which are the same, that is, which are *tied*, are given the *average* rank. For example, the seven values 2, 3, 5, 5, 5, 6, 8 could be ranked as 1, 2, 4=, 4=, 4=, 6, 7 because the three values of 5 have the *original* ranks of 3, 4, 5, the average of which is 4.

Exercise 2.15. The data in Figure 2.19 are the birthweights (g) for the first 25 babies in the sample in Figure 1.1. Rank them in ascending order.

2240	4110	3590	2880	2850
2660	4040	3580	1960	3550
3050	3130	2660	3150	3220
3990	4020	3040	3460	4230
4110	2780	2840	3660	3580

Figure 2.19 Birthweights for the first 25 babies in the sample

Remember to look again at the objectives at the start of the chapter and satisfy yourself that you have achieved them.

---

[2] Or you could give the smallest a rank of 1, the next smallest a rank of 2, and so on.

3

Every picture tells a story – describing data with charts

Learning objectives

When you have finished this chapter, you should be able to:

- Draw pie charts, and simple, clustered, and stacked bar charts.

- Draw histograms.

- Draw step charts and ogives.

- Draw time series charts.

- Interpret and explain what a chart reveals.

- Choose the most appropriate chart for a given data type.

Medical Statistics from Scratch: An Introduction for Health Professionals, Third Edition. David Bowers.
© 2014 John Wiley & Sons, Ltd. Published 2014 by John Wiley & Sons, Ltd.

Picture it!

In Chapters 2–6, we are 'describing' data, which means applying various statistical procedures to raw data so that any questions we might have can be more easily answered. In the previous chapter, you saw how tables can be used to do this. In this chapter, we want to turn to another approach – the chart. As my grandmother would often say, 'If you want to get ahead, get a chart!' To describe data, to see 'what's going on', an appropriate chart is almost always a good idea. A chart will often reveal previously unsuspected features of data. Which chart is appropriate depends primarily on the *type* of data you are dealing with, as well as on what particular features of it you want to explore.

In addition, a chart can often be used to illustrate or explain a complex situation for which a form of words, or a table, might be clumsy or too long. Moreover, if you are writing a report, a chart will always give you an 'impact' factor, make the page more interesting and break up blocks of possibly uninviting text. In this chapter, I am going to examine some of the charts most commonly used to describe data. We'll see which charts are appropriate for each type of data.

Charting nominal and ordinal data

The pie chart

You will all know what a pie chart is, so just a few comments here. Each segment (slice) of a pie chart should be proportional to the frequency, or more helpfully the percentage of the category it represents. As an example, the pie charts in Figure 3.1 show the incidence of burns by age, and the causes of burns, from the first of a series of papers on burns. Notice that the first segments start at 12 o'clock, which is a good practice, and helps if you are comparing two or more pie charts. Unfortunately, this paper is a little short on detail, not providing information on *where* this data relates to (the UK, the USA or global?) and *when* it was collected.

Incidentally, using the appropriate software, a good many charts can be formatted in 3D. As an example, the authors presented the pie charts in Figure 3.1 in a 3D format, as shown in Figure 3.2.

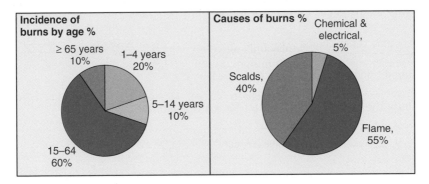

Figure 3.1 Pie charts (amended by the present author) showing the incidence of burns by age (left chart) and causes of burns (right chart). Data from Hettiaratchy and Dziewulski (2004)

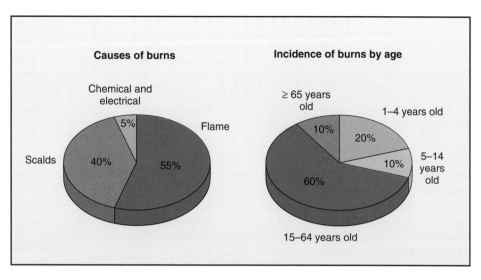

Figure 3.2 Pie charts for the burns data in Figure 3.1 as originally presented by the authors in a 3D format. Note that this book does not show different colours, so these pie charts are not as easy to interpret as they are in the original format. Source: Hettiaratchy and Dziewulski (2004). Reproduced by permission of John Wiley & Sons

Exercise 3.1. Which pie charts do you think are easier to understand, those in Figure 3.1 or those in Figure 3.2?

Some things worth noting about pie charts:

- Easy to understand.

- Can be used for either nominal or ordinal data and occasionally for discrete metric data (but for whatever data type, see the last bullet point below).

- Limited by being able to display only one variable. You will therefore need a separate pie chart for each variable you want to chart (as in Figure 3.1).

- When comparing two or more pie charts, the area of each pie chart should be proportional to its frequency.

- Pie charts expressed in percentage frequency terms can all be drawn in the same size.

- A pie chart can lose clarity if it is used to represent more than a small number of categories (four or five or thereabouts).

Exercise 3.2.   Sketch percentage pie charts (they do not have to be fantastically accurate) for self-rated benefit levels, following treatment for whiplash injury, for the usual care group and the active management group, as shown in Figure 2.6.

The simple bar chart

An alternative to pie charts for nominal or ordinal data is the *simple bar chart*. This is a chart with frequency on the vertical axis and category on the horizontal axis. The simple bar chart is appropriate if only one variable is to be shown. As an example, Figure 3.3 is a simple bar chart of the data on causes of blunt injury as shown in Figure 2.4.

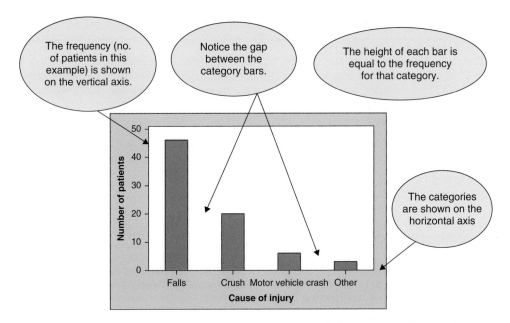

Figure 3.3   Simple bar chart for cause of blunt injury to limbs (data from Figure 2.4)

Exercise 3.3.   Draw a simple percentage bar chart of blood group for the data in column 2 of Figure 3.4 (for those patients whose kidney was *not* rejected). Data is taken from a study of kidney allograft rejection.

Exercise 3.4.   Looking at the data in Figure 3.4, which blood group seems to have the least likelihood of rejection?

Exercise 3.5.   Use the percentage values you calculated in Exercise 2.4 to sketch a simple bar chart for the satisfaction with nursing care data as shown in Figure 2.5.

Blood group	Kidney recipients without rejection ($n = 1777$)	Kidney recipients with rejection ($n = 302$)
Type A	742 (42%)	122 (40%)
Type B	176 (10%)	49 (16%)
Type O	730 (41%)	104 (34%)
Type AB	84 (5%)	27 (9%)

Figure 3.4   Blood group of patients in a study of kidney allograft rejection. Data from Lefaucheur *et al.* (2013)

The clustered bar chart

If you have more than one group and you want to compare them, you can use the *clustered bar chart*. As an example, Figure 3.5 shows the clustered bar chart for the data in Figure 3.6, from a study of long-term calcium intake and its relationship with all-cause mortality and cardiovascular mortality. The data are percentage leisure time activity for two groups of participants: the first group with a daily total intake of calcium of <600 mg/day, and the other with ≥1400 mg/day.

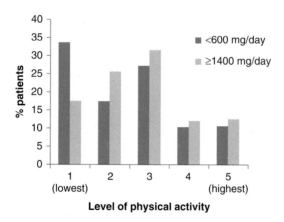

Figure 3.5   Clustered bar chart for daily calcium intake and the level of physical activity by participants (percentage of total for each group), with the level of physical activity on the category axis. On the basis of the data in Figure 3.6

Exercise 3.6.   Comment on what is revealed by the clustered bar chart in Figure 3.5.

Actually, there are two ways of presenting a clustered bar chart. Figure 3.5 shows one possibility, with the level of physical activity on the horizontal axis. This format is helpful if you want to compare the percentage of participants undertaking each level of physical activity, in each of the two levels of calcium intake.

Leisure time physical activity level*	Daily total intake of calcium (mg/day)	
	<600	≥1400
1 (lowest)	33.8	17.7
2	17.6	25.8
3	27.4	31.7
4	10.5	12.2
5 (highest)	10.8	12.7

*Leisure time physical activity during the past year, with five predefined levels ranging from one hour weekly (score 1) to more than five hours weekly (score 5).

Figure 3.6   Daily calcium intake and the level of physical activity by participants (percentage of total for each group). Data from Michaëlsson *et al.* (2013)

Alternatively, the chart could have been drawn with the two levels of calcium intake on the horizontal axis, as in Figure 3.7. This format would be more useful if you wanted to compare the percentage of participants undertaking the various levels of physical activity for each level of calcium intake. Which chart is more appropriate depends on what aspect of the data you want to investigate.

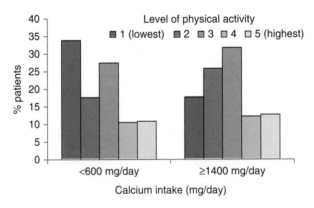

Figure 3.7   Clustered bar chart for daily calcium intake and the level of physical activity by participants (percentage of total for each group) with calcium intake on the category axis. Data from Figure 3.6

Exercise 3.7.   Draw a percentage clustered bar chart for the blood group data in Figure 3.4 using the format which tells you most efficiently which blood group is most likely to be associated with rejection.

Exercise 3.8.   The clustered bar chart in Figure 3.8 is taken from a study of low-dose combination therapy with rosiglitazone and metformin (versus placebo) to prevent type 2 diabetes mellitus and shows the outcomes of the treatment group. What does this chart indicate about the relative outcomes between the placebo and treatment groups?

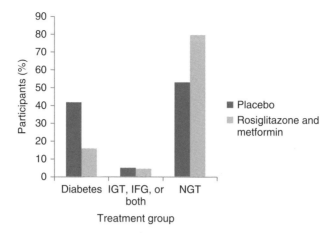

Figure 3.8 Proportion of participants who developed diabetes (Diabetes), regressed to normal glucose tolerance (NGT), or had impaired glucose tolerance (IGT) or impaired fasting glucose (IFG), or both, by treatment group, as measured by the oral glucose tolerance test. Data from Zinman *et al.* (2010)

Some things worth noting about bar charts:

- Fairly easy to understand (but see the last bullet point below).

- Can be used for either nominal or ordinal data, and occasionally for discrete metric data (but for whatever data type, see the last bullet point).

- Have the advantage over pie charts in that the *clustered* bar chart can show several groups at once, enabling direct comparisons to be made.

- Be sure to leave gaps between the category bars. This emphasises the categorical (or discrete) nature of the data.

- Bar charts are best expressed in percentage frequency terms; otherwise, comparisons can be difficult.

- A clustered bar chart can lose clarity if it is used to represent more than a small number of groups (five or six, or thereabouts).

The stacked bar chart

Figure 3.9 shows a *stacked* bar chart, with the level of calcium intake on the category (horizontal) axis, for the same data used in Figures 3.5 and 3.7. However, instead of appearing side by side, as in the clustered bar charts, the bars are now stacked on top of each other. This chart could have been formatted with levels of physical activity rather than calcium intake on the horizontal axis.

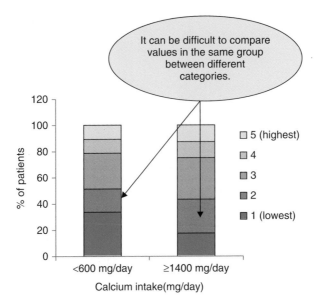

Figure 3.9 Stacked bar chart, with the level of calcium intake on the category axis, showing levels of physical activity for the same data as shown in Figures 3.5 and 3.7

Stacked bar charts are appropriate if you want to compare the percentage (or number) of subjects in each group (each level of physical activity in this example), in each category (calcium intake in this example). You can probably see their drawback. It can be difficult to compare the percentages in a particular group (say, level of activity = 2) between categories. This problem is magnified if there are more than two categories on the horizontal axis. For this reason, stacked bar charts are not seen as often as clustered bar charts.

Exercise 3.9. The stacked bar chart in Figure 3.10 shows weight loss from an obesity study. Participants were randomly allocated to one of the following programmes: Weight Watchers, Slimming World, Rosemary Conley (three commercial programmes); Size-Down (a group weight-loss programme), a nurse-led one-to-one support in general practice, one-to-one support by a pharmacist (three NHS primary care-led weight reduction programmes). A final group was allowed to choose whichever programme they wished (the Choice group). The chart shows the percentage of participants who attended each of the seven weight-loss programmes. What does the chart indicate about attendance at each of the programmes?

Exercise 3.10. Draw a percentage stacked bar chart for the self-rated post-whiplash data as shown in Figure 2.6.

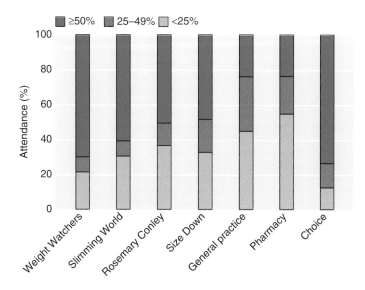

Figure 3.10 Stacked bar chart from a study to compare percentage attendance at a range of commercial versus primary care-led weight reduction programmes, with a minimum intervention control group for weight loss in obesity. Source: Jolly *et al.* (2011). Reproduced by permission of BMJ Publishing Group Ltd

Charting discrete metric data

We can use bar charts to graph discrete metric data in the same way as with ordinal data. For example, Figure 3.11 shows the parity of 100 mothers,[1] and it is reproduced here from

Parity	Number of mothers ($n = 100$)
0	49
1	18
2	17
3	11
4	2
5	1
6	1
7	0
8	0
9	0
10	1

Figure 3.11 The parity of the mothers whose babies birthweights are shown in Figure 1.1 (see also Figure 2.9)

---

[1] Data from the Born in Bradford study.

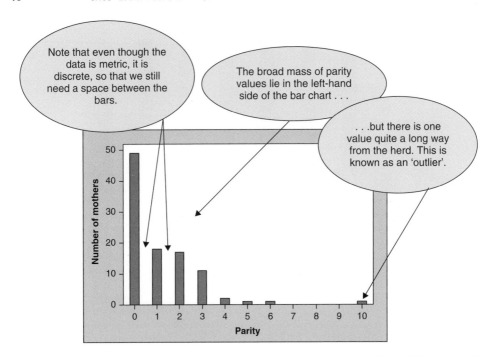

Figure 3.12   A simple bar chart for the parity data shown in Figure 3.11, showing a high-value outlier

Figure 2.9 for convenience. A simple bar chart for this metric discrete data is shown in Figure 3.12. Notice the presence of a rather unusual value for one woman with a parity of 10. Values a long way from the broad mass of the data are known as *outliers*.

Exercise 3.11.   Comment on what the bar chart in Figure 3.12 indicates about parity. Which method of presenting the parity data do you think the most effective at conveying the information, Figure 3.11 or Figure 3.12?

Charting continuous metric data

The histogram

As you have seen, a continuous metric variable can take a very large number of values, so it is usually impractical to plot them without first grouping the values. The *grouped* data is plotted using a *frequency histogram*, which has frequency plotted on the vertical axis and group size on the horizontal axis.

A histogram looks like a bar chart but without any gaps between adjacent bars. This empha-sises the continuous nature of the underlying variable. If the groups in the frequency table are all of the same width, then the heights of the bars in the histogram will be proportional to

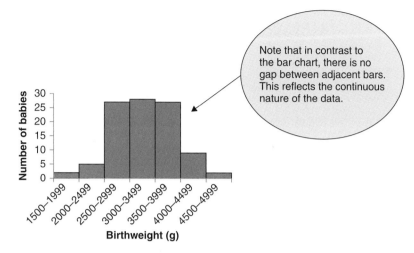

Figure 3.13 A histogram for the grouped birthweight data in Figure 3.14

Birthweight (g)	Frequency (number babies) ($n = 100$)
1500–1999	2
2000–2499	5
2500–2999	27
3000–3499	28
3500–3999	27
4000–4499	9
4500–4999	2

Figure 3.14 A grouped frequency table for the first 100 birthweights in Figure 1.1

their frequency. As an example, Figure 3.13 is a histogram of the grouped birthweight data in Figure 3.14 (reproduced for convenience from Figure 2.12).

Exercise 3.12. The data in Figure 3.15 shows the weight (kg) at booking of the mothers of the first 30 babies whose birthweights are shown in Figure 1.1. Group this data and draw a histogram of the grouped data. What does this show about mothers' weights?

Exercise 3.13. The grouped age data in Figure 3.16 is from a study to identify predictive factors for suicide, and shows the age distribution by sex of 974 subjects who attempted suicide (unsuccessfully) and those among them who were later successful. Sketch separate histograms of age for the percentage of *male* attempters and male later succeeders (omit the categories 'Living alone' and 'Employed'). Comment on what the charts show.

64	105	50	61	63	50
84	60	56	79	48	60
50	55	50	63	80	54
120	74	60	71	43	55
78	95	46	90	47	63

Figure 3.15 The weight (kg) at booking, of the mothers of the first 30 babies whose birthweights are shown in Figure 1.1

	No. (%) attempting suicide		No. (%) later successful	
	Men ($n = 412$)	Women ($n = 562$)	Men ($n = 48$)	Women ($n = 55$)
Age (years)				
15–24	57 (13.8)	80 (14.2)	3 (6.3)	3 (5.5)
25–34	131 (31.8)	132 (23.5)	10 (20.8)	12 (21.8)
35–44	103 (25.0)	146 (26.0)	16 (33.3)	16 (29.1)
45–54	62 (15.0)	90 (16.0)	11 (22.9)	9 (16.4)
55–64	38 (9.2)	58 (10.3)	4 (8.3)	4 (7.3)
65–74	18 (4.4)	43 (7.7)	3 (6.3)	8 (14.5)
75–84	1 (0.2)	11 (2.0)	0	2 (3.6)
>85	2 (0.5)	2 (0.4)	1 (2.1)	1 (1.8)
Living alone	96 (23.3)	85 (15.1)	17 (35.4)	14 (25.5)
Employed	139 (33.7)	185 (32.9)	14 (29.2)	13 (23.6)

Figure 3.16 Grouped age data from a follow-up cohort study to identify predictive factors for suicide. Data from Nordentoft *et al.* (1993)

One limitation of the histogram is that it can represent only one variable at a time (as in the case of the pie chart), and this can make comparisons between two histograms difficult because if you try to plot more than one histogram on the same axes, invariably parts of one chart will overlap the other.

The box (and whisker) plot

Figure 3.17 shows an example of what is known as a *box plot*, or more precisely, a box and whisker plot. This form of chart can be used with either ordinal data (with a decent number of data values) or metric data, but it is more common with the latter, as in this example, which shows sperm concentration among survivors of childhood cancer and a control (non-cancer) group.

The bottom and top of the box mark what are called the 25th and 75th *percentiles*, respectively. The 25th percentile is the value below which 25 per cent of the values in the sample lie (and thus 75 per cent exceed this value) – about 50×10^6/ml for the control group. The 75th percentile is the value above which 25 per cent of the sample values lie (and 75 per cent below) – about 120×10^6/ml. The line across the inside of the box (not necessarily in the

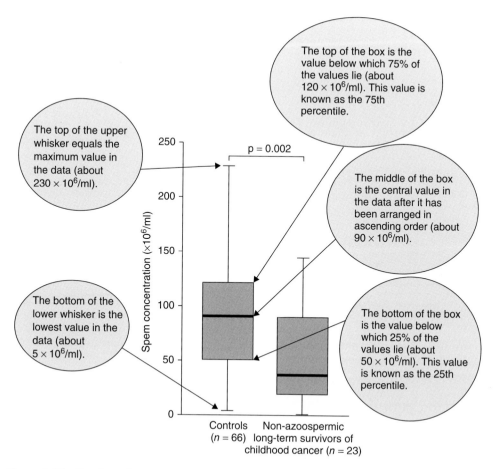

Figure 3.17   Boxplots of sperm concentration in non-azoospermic long-term survivors of childhood cancer and in non-cancer controls. From a study of semen quality and spermatozoal DNA integrity in survivors of childhood cancer. Source: Thomson *et al.* (2002). Reproduced by permission of Elsevier

middle) marks the value which divides the sample into two equal numbers of values – 50 per cent below this value and 50 per cent above it, about 85×10^6/ml here, is the 50th percentile. The bottom and top of each whisker mark the smallest and the largest values in the sample, respectively. We will have more to say about boxplots in Chapter 6, once we have discussed measures of location and spread.

Exercise 3.14.   The box plots in Figure 3.18 are from a study of iodine concentration in UK schoolgirls. Comment on what is revealed by these plots. The dots which extend above the upper whiskers are large-value outliers. There are a lot of them in this case! Different computer programs have different rules for defining outliers.

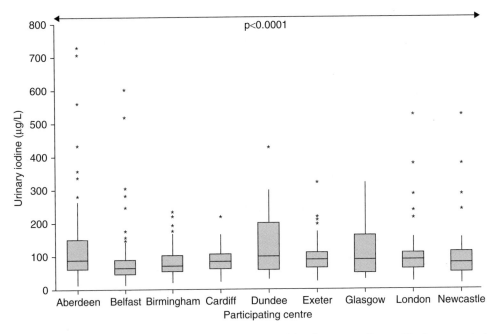

Figure 3.18   Box plots of urinary iodine according to participating centre. Source: Vanderpump *et al.* (2011). Reproduced by permission of Elsevier

Charting cumulative data

The cumulative frequency curve with discrete metric data

Cumulative frequency can be plotted for ordinal cumulative data but is more often used with metric data so that's what we'll concentrate on. The approach for discrete and continuous metric data is a little different – we will start with the discrete data case. The cumulative frequency chart with discrete data is known as the *step chart*, for which the most frequent application is with survival analysis, which you will encounter in Chapter 19. Here, I will just introduce the method fairly briefly.

Figure 3.19 shows percentage cumulative frequency for the number of lesions among patients with a biodegradable stent. The corresponding percentage step chart (you can see why it is called so) is shown in Figure 3.20. Hopefully, the chart is fairly easy to understand, but basically, each time there is an increase in cumulative percentage, the step chart steps up by the amount of that increase.

The cumulative frequency curve with continuous metric data

With *continuous* metric data, which is assumed to be a smooth *continuum* of values, you can chart cumulative frequency with a correspondingly smooth curve, known as a *cumulative*

Number of lesions	Number of patients with biodegradable stent ($n = 1229$)	% cumulative number of patients
1	903 (73.5%)	73.5
2	253 (20.6%)	94.1
3	61 (5.0%)	99.1
>3	12 (1.0%)	100.0*

*Allowing for small rounding error

Figure 3.19 Percentage cumulative number of lesions among patients with a biodegradable stent. From a study to investigate the effects, in terms of stent thrombosis, of a biodegradable stent compared to a durable stent. Data from Christiansen *et al.* (2013)

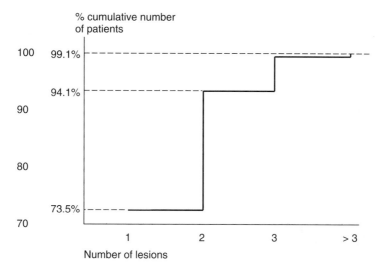

Figure 3.20 Step chart of cumulative percentage number of patients according to the number of lesions

frequency curve or an *ogive.*[2] As an example, Figure 3.21 is a cumulative frequency curve from a study of the relative efficacy of paclitaxel-eluting balloons, paclitaxel-eluting stents, and balloon angioplasty, in the management of restenosis in patients who have received a drug-eluting stent 6–8 months previously.

The curves show the cumulative frequency of the diameter stenosis (per cent) for each of the three treatments. The diameter stenosis (per cent) is a measure of how much the vessel has narrowed following the insertion of the stent – the higher the percentage is, the worse will be

[2]The 'g' in ogive is pronounced as the j in 'jive'.

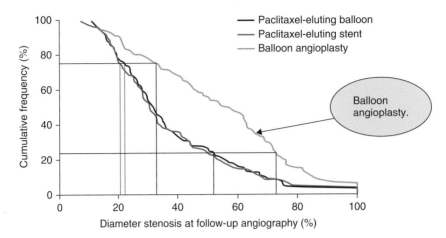

Figure 3.21 A cumulative frequency curve of diameter stenosis, from a study of the relative efficacy of paclitaxel-eluting balloons, paclitaxel-eluting stents and balloon angioplasty in the management of restenosis in patients who have previously received a drug-eluting stent. Source: Byrne *et al.* (2013). Reproduced by permission of Elsevier

the result. As you can see, balloon angioplasty (top curve) gave the worst result: 25 per cent of these patients had a diameter stenosis of about 72 per cent or more, when compared to only about 50 per cent or more for those with either paclitaxel-eluting balloons or paclitaxel-eluting stents, and 75 per cent of balloon angioplasty patients had a diameter stenosis of about 32% or more when compared to about 22% or more for patients with either paclitaxel-eluting balloons or paclitaxel-eluting stents.

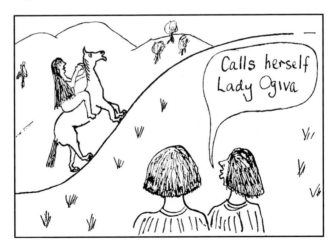

Exercise 3.15.   What does Figure 3.21 indicate about the approximate levels of diameter stenosis for each of the three treatments experienced by 50 per cent of the patients?

Exercise 3.16. Calculate percentage cumulative frequencies for the mothers' weight data shown in Figure 3.15 and draw the percentage cumulative frequency curve. Half of the mothers weighed what weight (or more)? Note: If you are drawing this by hand, you should plot each cumulative frequency value against the *lower* boundary of its corresponding group. To plot the origin point, you have to imagine a fictitious group below your lowest group, whose cumulative frequency is 0. The largest (uppermost) cumulative frequency value should be plotted against the *upper* boundary of its group.

Charting time-based data – the time series chart

If the data you have collected are from measurements made at regular intervals of time (minutes, weeks, etc.), you can present the data with a *time series chart*. Usually, these charts are used with metric data but may also be appropriate for ordinal data. Time is always plotted on the horizontal axis and data values on the vertical axis.

As an example, Figure 3.22 shows the rate of knee replacement for men and women in the UK between 1991 and 2006. This chart is pretty much self-explanatory, but we can notice an acceleration in the rate from about 2000 onwards.

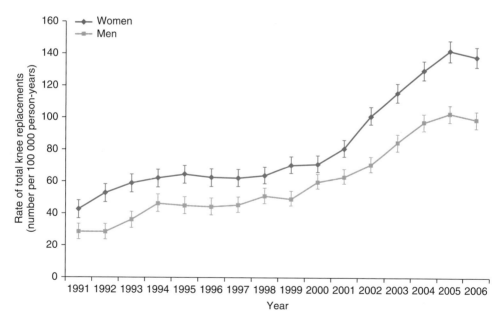

Figure 3.22   Rates of total knee replacement in the UK, 1991–2006. Note: the short vertical bars represent the 95% confidence intervals, which we will discuss in Chapter 9. Source: Carr *et al.* (2012). Reproduced by permission of Elsevier

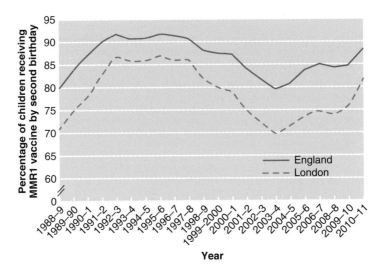

Figure 3.23   Annual uptake of MMR1 for England and London, 1988–2010 (note that the y-axis effectively starts at 60). Data source: Health Protection Agency. Source: Cockman *et al.* (2011). Reproduced by permission of BMJ Publishing Group Ltd

Exercise 3.17.   Figure 3.23 is a time series chart showing (separately for England and London) the percentage of children receiving the MMR1 vaccine between 1988 and 1989 and between 2010 and 2011. Comment on what the chart reveals. Note: Andrew Wakefield's discredited paper on a possible link between MMR and autism was published in 1998.

Figure 3.24 may help you to decide on the most appropriate chart for any given type of data.

Data type	Pie chart	Bar chart	Histogram (if data grouped)	Box plot	Step chart	Cumulative frequency curve
Nominal	Yes	Yes	No	No	No	No
Ordinal	Yes*	Yes	No	Yes	Yes	Yes
Metric discrete	Yes*	Yes*	No	Yes	Yes	Yes
Metric continuous	No	No	Yes	Yes	Yes	Yes

*If number of values is small.

Figure 3.24   Which chart is appropriate for which type of data?

4

Describing data from its shape

Learning objectives

When you have finished this chapter, you should be able to:

- Explain what is meant by the 'shape' of a frequency distribution.

- Sketch and explain negatively skewed, symmetric, and positively skewed distributions.

- Sketch and explain a bimodal distribution.

- Describe the approximate shape of a frequency distribution from a frequency table or chart.

- Sketch and describe a Normal distribution.

The shape of things to come

A quick recap of where we have got to:

- In Chapter 1, we saw that variables come in different flavours. I indicated then that the type of variable, as well as how its data are distributed (its 'shape', if you like), would influence which method of analysis is appropriate for that data.

Medical Statistics from Scratch: An Introduction for Health Professionals, Third Edition. David Bowers.
© 2014 John Wiley & Sons, Ltd. Published 2014 by John Wiley & Sons, Ltd.

- In Chapter 2, we saw how we can 'describe' raw data by putting it into a tabular form, thereby making it easier for us to answer any questions we might have and letting the data tell its story.

- In Chapter 3, we continued with this descriptive statistics approach by seeing how data can be put into one of several types of chart, once again making it easier for us to answer questions.

In this chapter, we examine what we mean when we talk about the 'shape' of a set of data. This is not a 'descriptive statistics' method as such, but the discussion will give us the vocabulary, the 'words', we need when we want to describe the way data is distributed. Later in the book, we will see how we need to consider shape when choosing a method of analysis.
By 'shape' I mean:

- Are the values fairly *evenly spread* throughout, from small through to large? This would be described as a *uniform* distribution.

- Are most of the values concentrated towards the bottom of the range (smaller values) with progressively fewer and fewer larger values? This is a *right* or *positively skewed* distribution. In other words, there is a long *tail to the right* (in the positive direction).

- Or are the values concentrated towards the top of the range (larger values), with progressively fewer and fewer smaller values? This is a *left* or *negatively skewed* distribution. That is, a long tail to the left (in the negative direction).

- Do most of the values clump together around *one* particular value, with progressively fewer and fewer values both below and above this value? This is a *symmetric* or *mound-shaped* distribution.

- Do most of the values clump around *two* or more particular values? This is a *bimodal* or *multimodal* distribution.

One simple way to assess the shape of a frequency distribution is to plot a bar chart or a histogram. Here are some examples of the shapes described earlier.

Negative skew[1]

An example of negative skew is shown by the histogram in Figure 4.1 (although the authors have drawn their histogram more like a bar chart, with gaps between adjacent bars). This shows the age distribution of 2454 patients with acute pulmonary embolism; the data is drawn

---

[1] *Skewness* is the primary measure used to describe the asymmetry of frequency distributions, and many computer programs will calculate a skewness *coefficient* for you. This can vary from −1 (strong negative skew) to +1 (strong positive skew). Values of zero or close to it, indicate lower levels of skew, but do *not* necessarily mean that the distribution is symmetric.

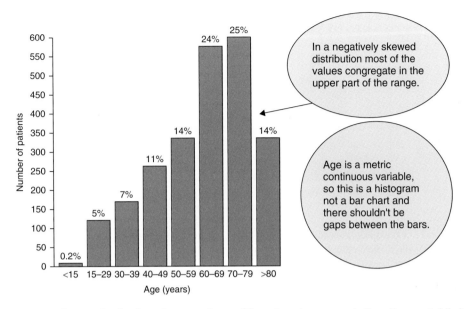

Figure 4.1 The age distribution of 2454 patients with acute pulmonary embolism. Source: Goldhaber *et al.* (1999). Reproduced by permission of Elsevier

from 52 hospitals in seven countries. You can see that most values lie towards the top end of the range, with progressively fewer lower values; in other words, this distribution is *negatively skewed*. Notice that the authors have attached percentage values to the top of each bar, which can be helpful.

Exercise 4.1. In Figure 4.1, which age group has (a) the highest number of patients? and (b) the lowest number?

Positive skew

Figure 4.2 is an example of positive skew, taken from a study of the association between pregnancy weight gain and birthweight, and shows weight gain by mothers. Notice the long tail to the right and the high-value outlier at about 45 kg.

Exercise 4.2. What sort of skew does the simple bar chart of data in Figure 3.12 have?

Exercise 4.3. The histogram in Figure 4.3 shows the birthweights of 500 babies.[2] How would you describe the shape of this distribution?

---

[2] Data from the Born in Bradford study.

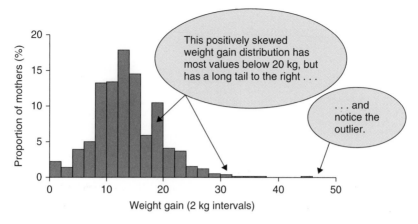

Figure 4.2 A positively skewed histogram showing weight gain by mothers from a study of the association between pregnancy weight gain and birthweight. Source: Ludwig and Currie (2010). Reproduced by permission of Elsevier

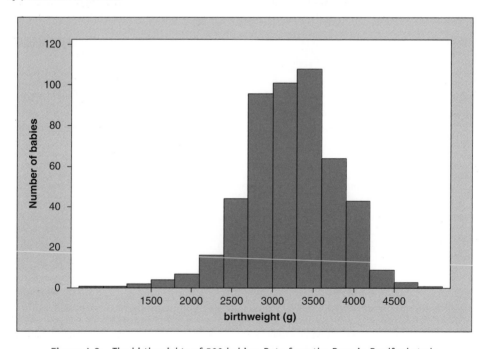

Figure 4.3 The birthweights of 500 babies. Data from the Born in Bradford study

Exercise 4.4. Plot a histogram for the percentage number of illnesses data as shown in Figure 4.4, taken from a study to determine the accuracy of a clinical decision rule (the traffic light system developed by the National Institute for Health and Clinical Excellence (NICE)) for detecting three common serious bacterial infections (urinary tract infection, pneumonia and bacteraemia) in young febrile children. What shape is the distribution?

Age (months)	Number of illnesses (%)
<3	4.7
3–5	5.9
6–11	19.0
12–23	30.8
24–35	18.1
36–47	12.5
48–60	9.0

Figure 4.4 The percentage number of illnesses among children in a study to determine the accuracy of a clinical decision rule for detecting serious bacterial infections. Data from De *et al.* (2013)

Symmetric or mound-shaped distributions

Figure 4.5 illustrates a symmetric distribution – in this case, birthweight. Notice the equal-sized (and relatively long, in this example) tails to the left and right of the central values.

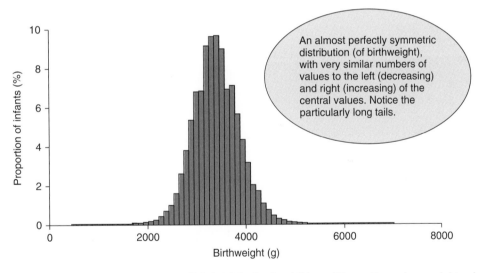

An almost perfectly symmetric distribution (of birthweight), with very similar numbers of values to the left (decreasing) and right (increasing) of the central values. Notice the particularly long tails.

Figure 4.5 A symmetric distribution of birthweight for the children of the mothers whose weight gain is shown in Figure 4.2. From the same study of the association between pregnancy weight gain and birthweight. Source: Ludwig and Currie (2010). Reproduced by permission of Elsevier

Exercise 4.5. What would you guess is the average birthweight for the data in Figure 4.5? What do you think accounts for the long tails on each side of the distribution?

> **Exercise 4.6.** Comment (by eyeballing the frequency distributions) on the shapes of the age distributions shown by the data in Figure 3.17 for male and female suicide attempters and later succeeders.

Normal-ness – the Normal distribution

There is one particular symmetric bell-shaped distribution, known as the *Normal distribution*, which has a special place in the heart of statisticians.[3] Many human clinical features are distributed Normally, and the Normal distribution has a very important role to play in what is to come later in this book. A Normal distribution is characterised by having a perfectly symmetrical shape, although in practice, never quite perfect (we should be so lucky!).

We have already seen a Normal distribution – that in Figure 4.5 for birthweights. A second example is shown in Figure 4.6. This shows the distribution of the cord platelet count (10^9/L) in 4382 Finnish infants, from a study of the prevalence and causes of thrombocytopaenia[4] in

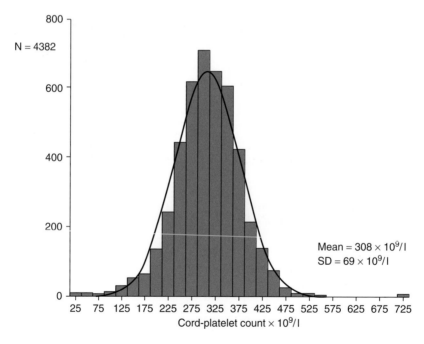

Figure 4.6 Cord platelet counts from 4382 full-term infants showed Normal distribution. Source: Sainio *et al.* (2000). Reproduced by permission of Wolters Kluwer Health

---

[3]Note the capitalised, 'N', to distinguish this statistical usage from that of the word 'normal' meaning usual, ordinary, etc.
[4]Thrombocytopenia is deemed to exist when the cord platelet count is less than 150×10^9/L. It is a risk factor for intraventricular haemorrhage and contributes to the high neurological morbidity in infants affected.

full-term infants. The authors have superimposed a Normal curve on the histogram. But, even without the help of this curve, you can see that the distribution has the typical bell-shaped symmetric distribution – in fact it is pretty well as Normal as it gets with real data. By the way, we will deal with what is meant by Mean and SD, shown on the right of the histogram, in Chapter 5.

Exercise 4.7.   (a) What is the approximate range of the cord platelet counts in Figure 4.6 and (b) what is the approximate cord platelet count of most infants?

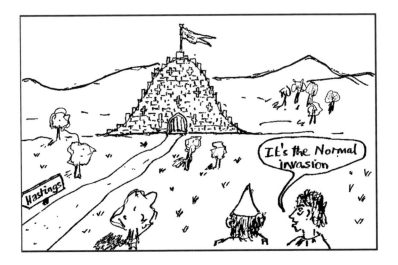

Although the Normal distribution is one of the most important in a health context, you may also encounter the *binomial* and *Poisson* distributions. As an example of the binomial distribution, suppose you need to select a sample of 20 patients from a very large list of patients that contains *equal* numbers of males and females. The chance of choosing a male patient is thus 1 in 2. Provided that the probability of picking a male patient each time remains fixed at 1 in 2, the binomial equation will tell you the probability of getting any given number of males (or females), in your 20 selected patients. For example, the probability of getting eight males in a sample of 20 patients is 0.1201 – about 12 chances in a 100.

The Poisson distribution is appropriate for calculating chance or probability when events occur in a seemingly random and unpredictable fashion. It describes the probability of a given number of events occurring in a fixed period of time. For example, suppose that the average number of children with burns arriving at an Emergency Department in any given 24-hour period is 12. Then, the Poisson equation indicates that the probability of one child with burns arriving in the next hour is 30 in 100, the probability of two arriving is about 7 in 100 and so on. Interesting as these distributions are, unfortunately we do not have the room to discuss them in any further detail. Maybe next time!

Bimodal distributions

A bimodal distribution is one with two distinct humps. These distributions are less common than the shapes described earlier and are sometimes the result of two separate distributions, which have not been disentangled. Figure 4.7 shows a bimodal distribution of the birthweights of Mexican-American and non-Hispanic babies taken from a study into why there are relatively few low-weight births among Mexican-Americans, despite their socioeconomic disadvantages.

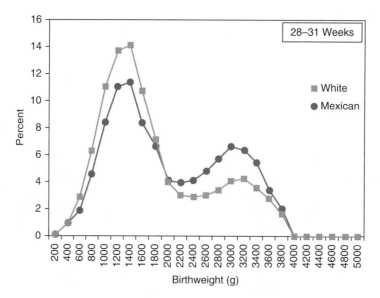

Figure 4.7 Bimodal distribution of birthweights of Mexican-American and non-Hispanic white pre-term babies at 28–31 weeks of gestation. Source: Buekens *et al.* (1999). Reproduced by permission of John Wiley & Sons

The authors suggest that this, 'bimodal distribution strongly suggests misclassification of gestational age, and this finding was seen more often for the Mexican-American babies. While errors concerning gestational age occur for only a small portion of all births, they can make up a large fraction of pre-term births'.

Determining skew from a box plot

We can get some idea of the skewness of a distribution by looking at its box plot. Look again at Figure 3.18, the box plot of sperm concentrations for a group of survivors of childhood cancer and a group of controls. If we rotate this box plot through 90 degrees, as shown in

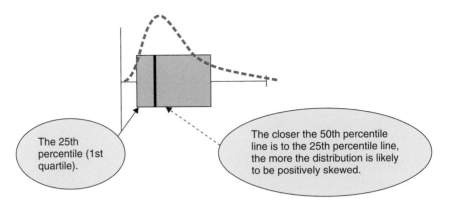

Figure 4.8   Boxplot of sperm concentration in non-azoospermic long-term survivors of childhood cancer, rotated through 90 degrees (from Figure 3.18)

Figure 4.8, it will help in our explanation. Let's isolate the box plot for the survivors. What do you see?

You will notice first that the 50th percentile value (the thick line across the inside of the box) is closer to the 25th percentile value (the left-hand end of the box), than it is to the 75th percentile value (the right-hand end of the box). Second, the whisker on the left of the box (showing the minimum value) is much shorter than that on the right-hand side of the box (showing the maximum value). The only distributional shape that will fit this geometry is one with a positive skew, as you can see.

If we do the same thing with the box plot for the control group, in which the 50th percentile is much more towards the middle of the box, we see (in Figure 4.9) that the corresponding distributional shape is more symmetrical but still with a long tail to the right.

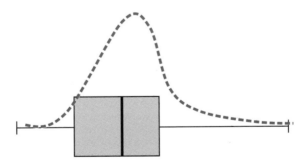

Figure 4.9   Boxplot of sperm concentration in controls, rotated through 90 degrees

In short, when we examine a box plot in its normal configuration (i.e. vertical), then if the 50th percentile bar is closer to the 25th percentile (the bottom of the box), than it is to the

75th percentile (the top of the box), the distribution is most likely to be positively skewed. (Conversely, if the 50th percentile bar is closer to the 75th percentile, then the distribution is more likely to be negatively skewed.)

To sum up so far. You have seen that you can describe the principal features of a set of data using tables and charts. A description of the shape of the distribution is also an important part of the picture. In the next chapter, you will meet a way of describing data using *numeric summary values*.

5

Numbers R us

Part I. Percentages, proportions and measures of location

Learning objectives

When you have finished this chapter, you should be able to:

- Explain what a summary measure of location is. Show that you understand the meaning of and the difference between the mode, the median, and the mean.

- Calculate the mode, median, and mean for a set of values.

- Demonstrate that you understand the role of data type and distributional shape in choosing the most appropriate measure of location.

- Explain what a percentile is and calculate any given percentile value.

- Draw a boxplot using values for the median, interquartile range, and the minimum and maximum.

Preamble

You collect data so that you can answer questions. 'What is the prevalence of asthma in children?' 'Is drug A better than drug B?' 'What are the risk factors for stillbirth?' and so on. To help

---

Medical Statistics from Scratch: An Introduction for Health Professionals, Third Edition. David Bowers.
© 2014 John Wiley & Sons, Ltd. Published 2014 by John Wiley & Sons, Ltd.

you do this, you can arrange the raw data into a tabular form or chart it (and examine its shape). These two procedures are particularly useful if you are making a presentation. In addition, you will almost always want to summarise the data *numerically*. There are three ways we can do this:

- First, most simply, for each categorical variable, provide the numbers involved in each category, along with the percentage (or proportion) values.

- Second, (for ordinal and metric data) find a value around which the data congregate or cluster. This value is known as a *summary measure of location* (or *central tendency*).

- Third, find a value that measures the degree to which the data are (or are not) spread out. This value is called a *summary measure of spread* (or *dispersion*).

When you know these values, you can then compare different sets of data *quantitatively*. Moreover, the latter two *summary statistics* (as they are called) form a crucial bridge between the sample data and the characteristics of the population from which the sample was taken (we will begin to saunter across this bridge in Chapter 7).

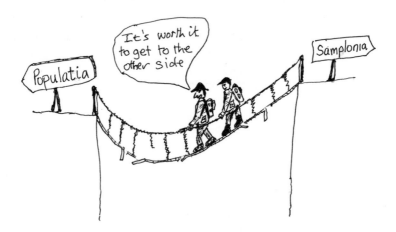

In this chapter, we look first at very basic stuff – counting numbers and expressing them in a percentage form. Then, we discuss the first of the summary measures – measures of location. In the next chapter, I will then examine the second of the summary measures – measures of spread or dispersion.

Numbers, percentages, and proportions

One of the simplest things that you can do with raw data is count it. For example, count the number of women and men, or the number of individuals with a particular blood group, or, the number of individuals with Stage II cancer, or the number of newborn babies with an Apgar score of 6 or less.[1] When you present the results of an investigation, you will almost certainly want to provide the reader (or audience) with this basic information, usually in the form of a baseline table – as we saw in Chapter 1. If you look back at Figures 1.7, 1.8 and 1.9, you will see that the authors of each of these three baseline tables have provided (where appropriate) both numbers and percentages (percentages usually in brackets after the number) in the various categories of each variable.

As a further example, Figure 5.1 is a table of the baseline characteristics of the participants in a study to investigate whether the insertion of a cervical pessary in women with a short cervix reduces the rate of early pre-term delivery. The female participants in the study were randomly allocated either to the group receiving the pessary (the cervical pessary group) or to the group not receiving a pessary (the expectant management group). As you can see, the values (percentage) are given for each of the nine categorical variables (see table footnote).

Exercise 5.1.   What percentage of women in each group in Figure 5.1 smoked during pregnancy?

Exercise 5.2.   The data in Figure 5.2 are taken from a study of duration of breastfeeding and arterial distensibility leading to cardiovascular disease. The table describes the basic characteristics of two groups; 149 participants who were bottle-fed as infants, and 182 who were breastfed. What proportion (and percentage) of men were (a) breastfed, and (b) bottle-fed?

Handling percentages – for those of us who might need a reminder

Sometimes, it is difficult to remember quite simple stuff, which you did some time ago. I think percentage calculations can often fall into this category, so here is a reminder of some typical problems which I hope will jog your memories (if you need it of course).

(a) Suppose that we have the following annual mortality figures for some procedure:

$$2011 = 12 \text{ deaths}$$

$$2012 = 16 \text{ deaths}$$

$$2013 = 14 \text{ deaths}$$

---

[1] The Apgar score is a measure of the well-being of a newborn baby, and it ranges from 0 to 10 (low scores, bad; high scores, good).

The number and percentage in each category.

	Cervical pessary group (n = 190)	Expectant management group (n = 190)
Maternal age (years)	30·3 (5·1)	29·6 (5·4)
Body-mass index (kg/m²)	24·9 (4·6)	24·5 (4·3)
Obstetrical history		
Nulliparous	94 (49%)	96 (51%)
Parous with no previous preterm births	75 (39%)	74 (39%)
Parous with at least one previous preterm birth	21 (11%)	20 (11%)
Cigarette smoking during pregnancy	37 (??%)	38 (??%)
Ethnic origin (self reported)		
White	107 (56%)	110 (58%)
Latin American	58 (31%)	56 (29%)
Other	25 (13%)	24 (13%)
Gestational age at randomisation (weeks)	22·2 (0·9)	22·4 (0·9)
Cervical length at randomisation (mm)	19·0 (4·6)	19·0 (4·9)
Funnelling at randomisation (yes)	81 (43%)	85 (45%)
Sludge at randomisation (yes)	5 (3%)	4 (2%)

Data are number (%) or mean (SD).

Figure 5.1 Baseline characteristics of participants in the cervical pessary and expectant management groups. I have omitted the percentages for cigarette smoking in pregnancy (see Exercise 5.1). Data from Goya *et al.* (2012)

What is the percentage *increase* in mortality from 2011 to 2012?

Answer = the difference between the two years divided by the number in the starting (base) year, multiplied by 100

$$= \left[\frac{(16-12)}{12}\right] \times 100 = \left[\frac{4}{12}\right] \times 100 = 0.3333 \times 100 = 33.3 \text{ per cent}$$

Similarly, the percentage *decrease* from 2012 to 2013 (2012 is now the base year):

$$= \left[\frac{(16-14)}{16}\right] \times 100 = \left[\frac{2}{16}\right] \times 100 = 0.1250 \times 100 = 12.5 \text{ per cent}$$

(b) Hospital A has 16 intensive care deaths in a three-month period. Hospital B has 20 deaths in the same period.

Variable	Breast fed		Bottle fed		p value for difference between groups
No of participants (men/women)	149	(67/82)	182	(93/89)	–
Age (years)	23	(20 to 28)	23	(20 to 27)	0.07
Height (cm)	170	(10)	168	(9)	0.03
Weight (kg)	70.4	(14.5)	68.7	(13.1)	0.28
Body mass index (kg/m²)	24.2	(4.1)	24.3	(3.7)	0.83
Length of breast feeding (months)	3.33	(0 to 18)	–		–
Resting arterial diameter (mm)	3.32	(0.59)	3.28	(0.59)	0.45
Distensibility coefficient (mm/Hg⁻¹)	0.133	(0.07)	0.140	(0.08)	0.38
Cholesterol (mmol/l)	4.43	(0.99)	4.61	(1.01)	0.11
LDL cholesterol (mmol/l)	2.71	(0.88)	2.90	(0.93)	0.07
HDL cholesterol (mmol/l)	1.18	(0.25)	1.18	(0.31)	0.96
Systolic blood pressure (mm Hg)	128	(14)	128	(14)	0.93
Diastolic blood pressure (mm Hg)	70	(9)	71	(8)	0.31
Smoking history (No (%)):					
Smokers	49	(33)	64	(35)	
Former smokers	25	(17)	22	(12)	0.78
Non-smokers	75	(50)	96	(53)	
No (%) in social class:					
I	12	(8)	13	(7)	
II	36	(24)	33	(18)	
IIINM	51	(34)	62	(34)	
IIIM	24	(16)	36	(20)	0.19
IV	22	(15)	33	(18)	
V	4	(3)	5	(3)	

Values are mean (SD or range) unless stated otherwise.
LDL, low density lipoprotein; HDL, high density lipoprotein

Figure 5.2 Basic characteristics of two groups of individuals, breastfed and bottle-fed, from a study of duration of breastfeeding and arterial distensibility leading to cardiovascular disease. Source: Leeson *et al.* (2001). Reproduced by permission of BMJ Publishing Group Ltd

How many *more* deaths (in percentage terms) does Hospital B have than Hospital A?

Answer = difference in number of deaths divided by the number of deaths in

Hospital A, multiplied by 100

$$= \left[\frac{(20 - 16)}{16} \right] \times 100 = \left[\frac{4}{16} \right] \times 100 = 0.25 \times 100$$

$= 25$ per cent more deaths.

How many *fewer* deaths (in percentage terms) does Hospital A have than Hospital B?

Answer = difference in number of deaths divided by the number of deaths in

Hospital B, multiplied by 100

$$= \left[\frac{(20 - 16)}{20}\right] \times 100 = \left[\frac{4}{20}\right] \times 100 = 0.20 \times 100$$

$$= 20 \text{ per cent fewer deaths.}$$

(c) The number of individuals attending an Emergency Department during the month of December 2012 increased by 20 per cent to 10 080 during December 2013. How many attendances were there in 2012?

Number of attendances in 2013 = number in 2012 × 1.20 = 10 080

So number in 2012 = 10 080/1.2 = 8400

(d) In a sample of 36 children, 8 have asthma. The proportion of children in the sample with asthma is:

$$\frac{8}{36} = 0.2222$$

To express this proportion as a percentage, just multiply by 100. So the percentage of children with asthma is:

$$0.2222 \times 100 = 22.22 \text{ per cent.}$$

(e) Twenty per cent of a sample of 180 children have eczema. How many children have eczema?
The number of children with eczema = 180 × 0.20 = 36

(f) The proportion of a sample of 600 children with asthma is 0.015. How many children have asthma?

The number of children with asthma = 0.015 × 600 = 9

Summary measures of location

With nominal data, we can provide readers with the numbers involved and a percentage (or a proportion) value – as we have seen earlier. With ordinal and metric data, we can do this but go further and provide a *summary measure of location*. This is a value around which most of the data seem to congregate or centre. In descriptive statistics, we use three main measures of location: the mode, the median, and the mean. As you will see, the choice of the most appropriate measure depends crucially on the type of data involved. We see in this chapter which measure(s) you can most appropriately use with which type of data. We'll start with the mode.

The mode

The *mode*, or *modal value*, is the value in the data with the highest frequency (i.e. occurs the most often). In this sense, the mode is a measure of *common-ness* or *typical-ness*. For example, the Apgar scores of 22 infants with neonatal encephalopathy are shown in Figure 5.3.

The modal Apgar score is 8as this value occurred more than any other value (six times).

Exercise 5.3. The delivery method for the same 22 babies in Figure 5.3 is shown in Figure 5.4. What is the modal delivery method?

When the data are grouped, the group with the highest number (the highest frequency) is the modal *category*. As an example, the modal category for Smoking history in Figure 5.2 is Smokers, among both breastfed and bottle-fed participants (49 and 64, respectively). The modal category for Social Class is IIINM in both groups (51 and 62).

---

0 3 4 3 8 7 5 7 9 5 3 5 6 1 8 5 8 8 8 0 8 5

Figure 5.3   The Apgar scores of 22 infants with neonatal encephalopathy

---

1. Spontaneous vaginal delivery
2. Spontaneous vaginal delivery
3. Elective Cesarean Section
4. Spontaneous vaginal delivery
5. Emergency Cesarean Section
6. Emergency Cesarean Section
7. Spontaneous vaginal delivery
8. Emergency Cesarean Section
9. Emergency Cesarean Section
10. Spontaneous vaginal delivery
11. Spontaneous vaginal delivery
12. Vacuum-assisted vaginal delivery
13. Emergency Cesarean Section
14. Emergency Cesarean Section
15. Forceps
16. Spontaneous vaginal delivery
17. Emergency Cesarean Section
18. Spontaneous vaginal delivery
19. Emergency Cesarean Section
20. Forceps
21. Vacuum-assisted vaginal delivery
22. Forceps

Figure 5.4   The delivery mode of the same 22 babies as shown in Figure 5.3

As a descriptive measure, the mode has a few shortcomings:

- There may be more than one mode.

- It is not usually useful with metric continuous data, where no two values may be the same – imagine trying to find the modal birthweight from the data in Figure 1.1. (Actually there are three modes, each with nine values: 2840 g, 3200 g and 3300 g). It is much easier though, to find the modal *category* from grouped data, such as that for birthweight in Figure 3.14.

- The mode is not useful with discrete metric data, when the number of values is large.

The mode does, however, have the virtue of being relatively easy to determine.

Exercise 5.4.   Determine the modal category for: (a) Social class, for both cases and controls, in the stress and breast cancer study shown in Figure 1.7, (b) the level of satisfaction with nursing care, from the data shown in Figure 2.5, (c) the self-rated benefit scores in each group shown in Figure 2.6, and (d) modal parity shown in Figure 2.9.

The median

If we arrange the data in ascending order of size, the *median* is the middle value. Thus, half of the values will be equal to or less than the median value and half equal to or greater than it. The median is therefore a measure of *central-ness*.

As an example of the calculation of the median, suppose that you had the following data on age (in ascending order of years), for five individuals:

30 31 **32** 33 35

The middle value is 32, so the median age for these five people is 32 years.

If you have an *even* number of values, the median is the average of the two values on either sides of the 'middle'. So for example, with six individuals aged: 30 31 32 33 35 50, the median is half-way between the two 'middle' values, 32 and 33, that is, 32.5. Notice that the median does not have to be equal to any of the values.

Some properties of the median:

- It discards a lot of information because it ignores most of the values, apart from those in the centre of the distribution.

- It is not much affected by skewness in the distribution, or by outliers, and is therefore a *stable* measure.

- It is not easy to determine (by hand) unless the sample has been ordered first.

Exercise 5.5. Why does it not make any sense to try and determine the median method of delivery from the data in Figure 5.4?

Exercise 5.6. What is the median of the Apgar score data given in Figure 5.3?

There is another, quite easy, way of determining the value of the median, which will also come in useful a bit later on. If you have n values arranged in ascending order, then:

the median is the value in the $\frac{1}{2}(n+1)^{th}$ position

So, for example, if the ages of six people are: 30 31 32 33 35 50, then $n = 6$, and therefore:

The median is the value in the position : $\frac{1}{2}(n+1) = \frac{1}{2} \times (6+1)$

$= \frac{1}{2} \times 7$, that is, in the 3.5th position.

In other words, it is the value half way between the 3rd value of 32 and the 4th value of 33, or 32.5 years, which is the same result as we have got before.

Incidentally, the median birthweight for the data in Figure 1.1 is 3200.0 g.

Exercise 5.7. (a) Determine the median percentage mortality of the 26 ICUs in Figure 2.14. (b) From the data in Figure 3.17, determine which age group contains the median age for (i) men and (ii) women, both for those attempting suicide and for later successful suicides. (c) What are the median categories for the levels of self-rated benefit for each group in Figure 2.6?

The mean

The *mean*, or the arithmetic mean to give it its full name (there are other types of mean), is more commonly known as the average. So to determine the value of the mean, we add values together and divide this total by the number of values (as you know!). A few things about the mean:

- It uses all of the information in the data set – every value is included.

- Because of this, it is affected by skewness in the distribution and by outliers.

- As a consequence, the mean, on occasion, might be unrepresentative of the general mass of the data.

- It cannot be used with ordinal data (recall from Chapter 1 that ordinal data are not real numbers, so they cannot be added or divided).

Exercise 5.8. Comment on the likely relative sizes of the mean and median in the distributions of: (a) age, (b) weight gain and (c) birthweight, shown in the histograms in Figures 4.1, 4.2 and 4.5, respectively.

Exercise 5.9. Determine the mean percentage mortality among the 26 ICUs in Figure 2.14 and compare with the median value you determined in Exercise 5.5.

Exercise 5.10. The histogram of red blood cell thioguanine nucleotide concentration (RBCTNC), in *pmol/8×10^8 red blood cells*, in 49 children, shown in Figure 5.5, is from a study into the potential causes of high incidence of secondary brain tumours in children after radiotherapy. (a) Using the information in the figure, calculate median and mean RBCTNC for the 49 children. (b) Remove the two outlier values of 3300, and re-calculate the mean and median. Compare and comment on the two sets of results.

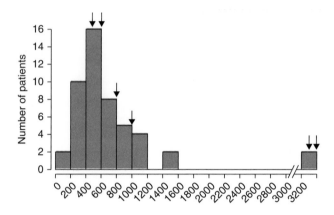

Figure 5.5   Frequency of maximum red blood cell thioguanine nucleotide concentrations before cranial radiotherapy. Arrows show values for six patients who went on to develop secondary malignant brain tumours. Source: Relling *et al.* (1999). Reproduced by permission of Elsevier

Percentiles

Percentiles are the values which divide an ordered set of data into 100 equal-sized groups. As an illustration, suppose that you have birthweights of 1200 infants, which you have put in ascending order. If you identify the birthweight that has 1 per cent (i.e. 12) of the birthweight values below it and 99 per cent (1188) above it, then this value is the *1st percentile*. Similarly, the birthweight which has 2 per cent of the birthweight values below it, and 98 per cent above it is the 2nd percentile. You could repeat this process until you reached the 99th percentile, which would have 99 per cent (1188) of birthweight values below it and only 1 per cent above it. Notice that this makes the median the *50th percentile* as it divides the data values into two equal halves, 50 per cent above the median and 50 per cent below.

Calculating a percentile value

How do you determine any particular percentile value? Take the example of the 30 birthweights shown in Figure 2.17, which we reproduce in Figure 5.6, but now in an ascending order, along with their position in the order:

Baby's birthweight (g) $n = 30$	Baby's birthweight (g) in ascending order $n = 30$	Position of each value ascending
3220	2170	1
4140	2220	2
2220	2460	3
3540	2460	4
3500	2640	5
3820	2660	6
3330	2740	7
2840	2780	8
2780	2820	9
2660	2840	10
2170	3000	11
3340	3070	12
3070	3220	13
3800	3280	14
3300	3300	15
3380	3320	16
4060	3330	17
2640	3340	18
2460	3380	19
3460	3410	20
2820	3460	21
3280	3490	22
3740	3500	23
3000	3540	24
3320	3740	25
3490	3800	26
3920	3820	27
2460	3920	28
3410	4060	29
2740	4140	30

Figure 5.6 The 30 birthweights from Figure 2.17 but now shown also in ascending order, along with their position in the order

The pth percentile is the value in the $(p/100) \times (n+1)$th position.

For example, the 20th percentile (i.e. $p = 20$), is the value in the $[(20/100) \times (n+1)]$th position.

With the 30 birthweight values, $n = 30$ and the 20th percentile is therefore the value in the:

$$\frac{20}{100} \times (30 + 1)\text{th position, which is the } 0.2 \times 31\text{st value} = 6.2\text{th position.}$$

The 6th value is 2660 g and the 7th value is 2740 g, a difference of 80 g, so the 20th percentile is:

$$2660\,g \text{ plus } 0.2 \text{ of } 80\,g, \text{ which is } 2660\,g + 0.2 \times 80\,g = 2660\,g + 16g = 2676\,g.$$

You might be thinking this all seems a bit messy, but a computer will perform these calculations effortlessly and instantly. As well as percentiles, you might also encounter *deciles*, which sub-divide the data values into 10, not 100, equal divisions, and *quintiles*, which sub-divide the values into five equal-sized groups. Collectively, percentiles, deciles and quintiles, are called *n-tiles*.

Exercise 5.11. Use the method described earlier (or some other more cunning method!) to calculate the 25th, 50th and 75th percentiles, for the birthweight data shown in Figure 5.6 and interpret your results.

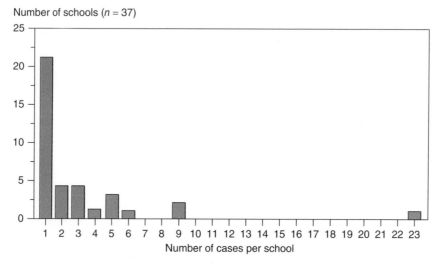

Figure 5.7 The distribution of the number of measles cases in 37 schools, Jefferson County, Kentucky. Source: Prevots *et al.* (1997). Reproduced by permission of John Wiley and Sons

		Summary measure of location	
Type of variable	Mode	Median	Mean
Nominal	Yes	No	No
Ordinal	Yes	Yes	No
Metric discrete	Yes	Yes, if distribution is markedly skewed	Yes
Metric continuous	No	Yes, if distribution is markedly skewed	Yes

Figure 5.8 A guide to choosing an appropriate measure of location

What is the most appropriate measure of location?

How do you choose the most appropriate measure of location for some given set of data? The main things to remember are that the mean *cannot* be used with ordinal data (because they are not real numbers), and the median can be used for both ordinal and metric data (particularly when the latter is skewed). As noted by the authors of a study to evaluate whether a multifaceted behavioural change programme increases physical activities in individuals with Parkinson's disease:

> Because the physical activity level was skewed, we present medians and interquartile ranges and did analyses after logarithmic transformation.
>
> *van Nimwegen (2013)*

(We will deal with the interquartile range in the next chapter). As an illustration of the last point, see Figure 5.7, which shows the distribution of the number of measles cases in 37 schools. Not only is this distribution positively skewed but it also has a single high-value outlier. The median number of measles cases is 1, but the mean number is 2.91, almost three times as many! The problem is that the long positive tail, along with the outlier, is dragging the mean to the right. In this case, the median value of 1 seems to be more representative of the data than the mean. I have summarised the choice of a measure of location in Figure 5.8.

6

Measures of spread

Learning objectives

When you have read this chapter, you should be able to:

- Explain what a summary measure of spread is, show that you understand the difference between and can calculate: the range, the interquartile range and the standard deviation.

- Estimate the median and the interquartile range from a cumulative frequency curve.

- Use values for the quartiles and the maximum and minimum values to draw a boxplot.

- Explain what the area properties of the Normal distribution are.

- Outline the idea of transformation and how it can be used.

- Demonstrate that you understand the role of data type and distributional shape in choosing the most appropriate measure of spread.

Medical Statistics from Scratch: An Introduction for Health Professionals, Third Edition. David Bowers.
© 2014 John Wiley & Sons, Ltd. Published 2014 by John Wiley & Sons, Ltd.

Preamble

We saw in the previous chapter that there are two important summary measures in the descriptive statistics armoury. One of these was a measure of location and the other is a *measure of spread* or *dispersion*. There are three main measures of spread in common use: the range, the interquartile range (IQR) and the standard deviation. As you will see, the type of data being described will influence which measure of spread is the most appropriate.

The range

The *range* is the distance from the smallest value to the largest. The range is not particularly affected by skewness but is sensitive to the addition or removal of an outlier value. As an example, the range of the 30 birthweights shown in Figure 5.6 is (2170.0 to 4140.0) g. The range is best written like this, rather than as the single-valued difference, that is, as 1970 g (in this example), which is much less informative. Another example of the use of the range is shown in Figure 6.5.

> **Exercise 6.1.** What is the range of the Apgar scores in Figure 5.3?

The interquartile range (IQR)

One solution to the problem of the sensitivity of the range to outliers is to chop a quarter (25 per cent) of the values off both ends of the distribution (which removes any troublesome outliers) and then measure the range of the remaining values.

- The value which cuts off the bottom 25 per cent of values is known as the *first quartile* and denoted *Q1*.

- The value which cuts off the top 25 per cent of values is known as the *third quartile* and denoted *Q3*.

The IQR is then written as (Q1 − Q3).
The IQR is not affected by outliers but it can be affected by distributions, which are markedly skewed. It does not use all of the information in the data set as it ignores the bottom and top quarters of values.
With the birthweight data in Figure 1.1: Q1 = 2840 g and Q3 = 3580 g. Therefore:

$$\text{interquartile range} = (2840 \text{ to } 3580)\,\text{g}.$$

In other words, the middle 50 per cent of infants by weight weighed between 2840 g and 3580 g.

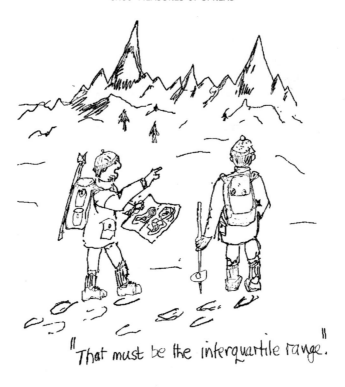

"That must be the interquartile range".

As an illustration of the use of the median and IQR, Figure 6.1 is from a study to compare the basic characteristics of individuals with and without Barrett's oesophagus, for the two groups: those with circumferential lengths of the affected segment of ≥1 cm and ≥2 cm, respectively. So, for example, among those with an affected oesophagus length of ≥1 cm, the median age is 64.0 years with an IQR of (59.0 to 67.0) years. This means that 25 per cent of this group were aged 59 or less and 25 per cent aged 67 or more.

Exercise 6.2.   From Figure 6.1, interpret the median and IQR values for smoking (pack years) among those in the ≥2 cm group, with and without Barrett's oesophagus.

Exercise 6.3.   What is the IQR for the birthweight data shown in Figure 5.6? (You have already calculated the 25th and 75th percentiles in Exercise 5.11).

Estimating the median and interquartile range from the cumulative frequency curve

You can, if necessary, estimate the median and the IQR from the percentage cumulative frequency curve. Figure 6.2 shows the percentage cumulative frequency curve for the birthweight data shown in Figure 1.1.

The median and IQR values for various baseline characteristics, among patients with a circumferential length of affected segment ≥ 1 cm, in individuals with Barrett's oesophagus . . .

. . . and among those without.

Characteristics	Circumferential length ≥1 cm			Circumferential length ≥2 cm		
	Barrett's oesophagus (n = 15)	No Barrett's oesophagus (n = 486)	p value	Barrett's oesophagus (n = 10)	No Barrett's oesophagus (n = 491)	p value
Male to female ratio	1.5:1	0.84:1	0.26	1.75:1	0.84:1	0.36
Age	64.0 (59.0 to 67.0)	62.0 (56.0 to 66.0)	0.18	63.5 (58.7 to 66.2)	62.0 (56.0 to 66.0)	0.39
Body mass index	31.6 (27.5 to 33.5)	29.4 (26.2 to 32.9)	0.55	31.6 (27.8 to 33.5)	29.4 (26.2 to 32.9)	0.59
Waist to hip ratio	0.95 (0.86 to 0.99)	0.91 (0.85 to 0.96)	0.16	0.96 (0.89 to 1.02)	0.91 (0.85 to 0.96)	0.06
Smoking (pack years)	8.0 (0.0 to 31.4)	0.4 (0.0 to 19.5)	0.30	23.0 (3.0 to 31.0)	0.3 (0.0 to 19.2)	0.03
Alcohol consumption (units/week)	4.0 (2.0 to 10.0)	6.0 (1.0 to 14.0)	0.24	2.0 (0.0 to 10.0)	6.0 (1.0 to 14.0)	0.09
Symptoms (GERD score)	4.0 (2.0 to 6.0)	4.0 (2.0 to 6.5)	0.67	4.0 (2.0 to 6.0)	4.0 (1.7 to 6.1)	0.99
Acid suppressants* (%)	73.3	66.2	0.36	80.0	66.2	0.26

GERD, The Gastro-oesophageal Reflux Disease impact scale: a patient management tool for primary care.
*Proton pump inhibitors or H₂ receptor antagonists, or both.

Figure 6.1 Use of median and interquartile range values to compare the basic characteristics of patients with and without Barrett's oesophagus, stratified by the circumferential length cut-off point of the affected segment: ≥1 cm and ≥2 cm. Data from Kadri et al. (2010)

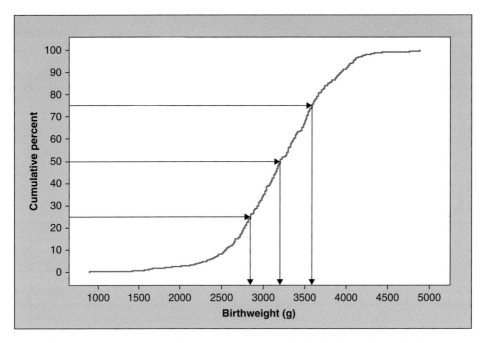

Figure 6.2   The percentage cumulative frequency curve for the birthweight data in Figure 1.1

If you draw horizontal lines from the values 25 per cent, 50 per cent and 75 per cent, respectively, on the vertical axis, to the percentage cumulative frequency curve and then down to the birthweight (horizontal) axis, the points of intersection on the birthweight axis approximate values for Q1, Q2 (the median), and Q3, of 2800 g, 3200 g and 3600 g, respectively. Thus, if you happen to have a percentage cumulative curve handy, these approximations can be helpful.

Exercise 6.4.   Using Figure 6.2, (a) what birthweight defines the first decile? (b) What percentage of babies weighed more than 4000 g?

Exercise 6.5.   For the control group, estimate the median and the IQR for total blood cholesterol from the percentage cumulative frequency curve shown in Figure 6.3.

The discussion on measures of spread continues on the following pages, but now I want to expand the discussion of boxplots (first mentioned in Chapter 3).

The boxplot (also known as the box and whisker plot)

Now that we have discussed the median and IQR, we can return to the boxplot. What I could not say then (because we hadn't dealt with them at that time) was that the boxplot is a graphical representation of the quartile values.

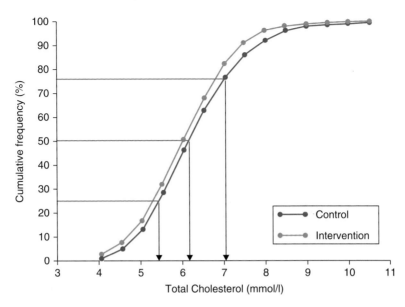

Figure 6.3 Cumulative frequency curves of total cholesterol concentration in control and intervention groups. From a study of the effectiveness of health checks conducted by nurses in primary care: final results of the OXCHECK study. Source: Imperial Cancer Fund OXCHECK Study Group (1995). Reproduced by permission of BMJ Publishing Group Ltd

Boxplots are usually plotted with values on the vertical axis. Like the pie chart, the boxplot can only represent one variable at a time, but a reasonable number of boxplots can be set along-side each other for comparison purposes. To illustrate this idea, see the boxplots shown in Figure 6.4. These boxplots are taken from a study of the effect of participatory intervention with women's groups on birth outcomes and maternal depression in India, and show neonatal mortality rates (deaths per thousand live births), for three years after the start of the study. The three boxplots on the left are for the control area (no participatory intervention) and those on the right are for the intervention area. As a matter of interest, we can see that in the intervention area, the median infant mortality rate falls over the three-year period, whereas as that for the control rises.

Let's look at the second boxplot from the left – the neonatal mortality rates in Year 2 for the control area (no intervention):

- The bottom end of the lower 'whisker' (the line sticking out of the bottom of the box), corresponds to the minimum value – about 10 deaths per 1000 live births.

- The bottom of the box is the 1st quartile value, Q1, with a value of about 45 deaths per 1000 live births. So for about 25 per cent of the live births, the neonatal mortality rate was less than about 45 per 1000.

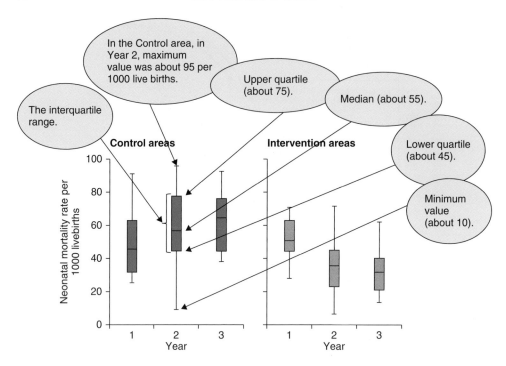

Figure 6.4 These boxplots of neonatal mortality rates are taken from a study of the effect of participatory intervention with women's groups, on birth outcomes and maternal depression in India. They show neonatal mortality rates in control areas and intervention areas, for each of the three years following the start of the intervention. Source: Tripathy *et al.* (2010). Reproduced by permission of Elsevier

- The line across the inside of the box (it won't always be across the middle of the box unless the distribution is symmetrical), is the median, Q2, with a value of about 55 deaths per 1000 live births. So for about half (50 per cent) of the live births, the neonatal mortality rate was less than 55 per 1000 and for half it was greater than about 55 per 1000.

- The top of the box is the third quartile Q3. So for about 25 per cent of the live births the neonatal mortality rate was more than about 75 per 1000.

- The top end of the upper whisker is the 'maximum' neonatal rate – about 95 per 1000 live births.

Exercise 6.6.   Sketch the boxplot for the birthweight data shown in Figure 5.6 using the values you calculated in Exercise 5.11. What can you glean from the boxplot about the shape of the distribution of the birthweights?

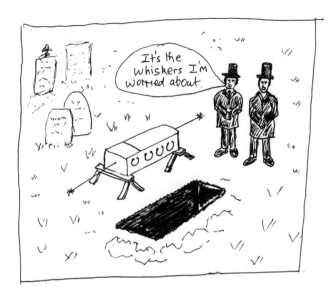

Standard deviation

The limitation of IQR as a summary measure of spread is that (like the median) it doesn't use all of the information in the data, as it omits the top and bottom quarter of values. An alternative approach gives us what is known as the *standard deviation*, or SD. The advantage of the standard deviation is that, unlike the IQR, it uses all of the information in the data. But remember that it can only be used with metric data. The standard deviation can be thought of as a measure of the *average distance of the data values from their collective mean*. If the data are widely spread, the average distance of the values from their mean will clearly be large. If the values are narrowly spread, the average distance will be small.

To see how this works, let's calculate, step by step, the standard deviation of the following five (i.e. $n = 5$) diastolic blood pressure values (mmHg)[1]:

$$100 \quad 60 \quad 80 \quad 70 \quad 110$$

Step 1. Calculate the mean:

$$\frac{(100 + 60 + 80 + 70 + 110)}{5} = 84\,\text{mmHg}$$

---

[1] This is a very tedious procedure. If you have an SD key on your calculator, use that. In practice, you would use a computer!

Step 2. Subtract this mean from each of the values, to give the *difference* values:

$$(100 - 84) = 16$$
$$(60 - 84) = -24$$
$$(80 - 84) = -4$$
$$(70 - 84) = -14$$
$$(110 - 84) = 26$$

Step 3. In theory, we can find the average distance of these five difference values from the mean of 84 by adding them and then dividing by five. Unfortunately, the sum is 0! and always will be, whatever numbers we start with because the even and odd values always cancel out. What to do?

    Well, we can employ what appears to be a fiddle. If we square each difference value, this will get rid of these pesky negative values (recall that a minus times a minus is a plus). Then, we can find the average of these squared values and finally take the square root. After all, we don't want blood pressures in mmHg^2.

    So, by squaring the difference values, summing them (to get what is called the *sum of squares*) and then dividing by 5, we get the average:

$$\frac{(16^2 + -24^2 + -4^2 + -14^2 + 26^2)}{5} = \frac{(256 + 576 + 16 + 196 + 676)}{5} = \frac{1720}{5} = 344$$

Step 4. So finally (you might think), take the square root of this value to get from mmHg^2 to mmHg. This is the standard deviation – sort of:

$$\text{Standard deviation (sort of)} = \text{Square root of } 344 = 18.5 \, \text{mmHg}$$

So the above five values of diastolic blood pressure are on an average of 18.5 from the mean of 84 mmHg.

    Well not quite.

Step 5. For rather technical reasons, which we do not need to go into, this final value (of 18.5 in this example) is always a little too small. We need to correct it by dividing the sum of squares not by $n = 5$, but by $(n - 1)$, that is, $5 - 1$ (in this example) $= 4$.

    This gives:

$$\frac{1720}{4} = 430$$

$$\text{Square root of } 430 = 20.7 \, \text{mmHg}$$

So the standard deviation is 20.7 mmHg.

Phew!!! Not something you will want to do by hand too often.

But the basic concept, that *the standard deviation can be thought of as a measure of the average distance of the data values from their collective mean*, is worth remembering.

Exercise 6.7. In Figure 4.6, the authors tell us that the mean cord platelet count is $308 \times 10^9/l$ and the standard deviation is $69 \times 10^9/l$ (notice that the two measures have the same units).[2] Explain what this value for the standard deviation means.

An illustration of the use of the mean and standard deviation as summary measures is shown in Figures 5.1 and 5.2. For convenience, I have reproduced an abbreviated version of Figure 5.2 (labelled Figure 6.5). The footnote to the table tells us that the values shown are either mean and SD or mean and range. It is not clear why the authors have used two different measures of spread. So you can see that the average distance of the weight values is about 14.5 kg from the sample mean of 70.4 kg. Similarly, the diastolic blood pressure values are, on average, about 9 mmHg from the mean of 70 mmHg.

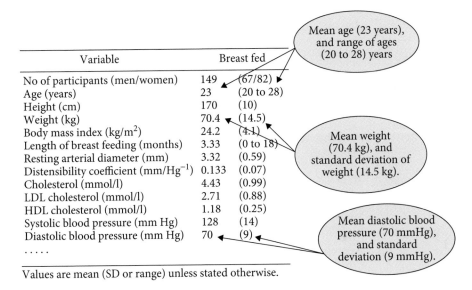

Variable	Breast fed	
No of participants (men/women)	149	(67/82)
Age (years)	23	(20 to 28)
Height (cm)	170	(10)
Weight (kg)	70.4	(14.5)
Body mass index (kg/m²)	24.2	(4.1)
Length of breast feeding (months)	3.33	(0 to 18)
Resting arterial diameter (mm)	3.32	(0.59)
Distensibility coefficient (mm/Hg⁻¹)	0.133	(0.07)
Cholesterol (mmol/l)	4.43	(0.99)
LDL cholesterol (mmol/l)	2.71	(0.88)
HDL cholesterol (mmol/l)	1.18	(0.25)
Systolic blood pressure (mm Hg)	128	(14)
Diastolic blood pressure (mm Hg)	70	(9)
. . . . .		

Mean age (23 years), and range of ages (20 to 28) years

Mean weight (70.4 kg), and standard deviation of weight (14.5 kg).

Mean diastolic blood pressure (70 mmHg), and standard deviation (9 mmHg).

Values are mean (SD or range) unless stated otherwise.

Figure 6.5 An abbreviated version of Figure 5.2, showing the first 13 rows for the Breast Fed group only. From a study of duration of breastfeeding and arterial distensibility leading to cardiovascular disease. Source: Leeson *et al.* (2001). Reproduced by permission of BMJ Publishing Group Ltd

Exercise 6.8. Look at Figure 6.5. Relatively speaking, which is further, on average, from their respective means: the LDL cholesterol values or the HDL cholesterol values? Hint: one possible approach would be to divide each standard deviation by its mean. This gives a measure known as the *coefficient of variation*. Try it and see what you think.

---

[2] 10^9 means 1 000 000 000

So which measures of spread are appropriate when?

- With ordinal data, use either the range or the IQR. The standard deviation is not appropriate because of the non-numeric nature of ordinal data.

- With metric data, use either the standard deviation, which uses all of the information in the data, or the IQR. The latter if the distribution is skewed, and/or you have already selected the median as your preferred measure of location.

- Do not mix-and-match measures – standard deviation goes with the mean and IQR with the median.

Figure 6.6 may help you to choose an appropriate measure of spread.

Type of variable	Summary measure of spread		
	Range	Interquartile range	Standard deviation
Nominal	No	No	No
Ordinal	Yes	Yes	No
Metric	Yes	Yes, if skewed	Yes

Figure 6.6 Choosing an appropriate measure of spread

Standard deviation and the Normal distribution

If you are working with metric data that is distributed Normally, the standard deviation can be used to explore the *area properties of the Normal distribution*. These area properties are illustrated in Figure 6.7 for the histogram of birthweight data for a random sample of 500 babies.[3] A Normal curve is superimposed on this histogram using Minitab, which also calculates these birthweights to have a mean of 3209 g and a standard deviation of 564.4 g.

The area properties are as follows:

- About 68 per cent of the birthweight values in the sample lie within one standard deviation on either side of the mean.

In this example, this is from (3209 g − 564.4 g) to (3209 g + 564.4 g), or from 2644.6 g to 3773.4 g.

- About 95 per cent of the birthweights will lie within two standard deviations on either side of the mean.

---

[3] From the Born in Bradford study.

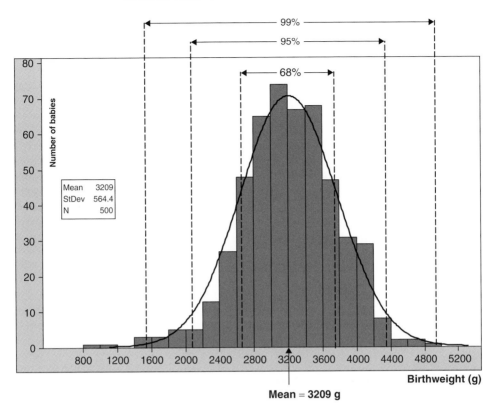

Figure 6.7 A symmetric distribution of birthweight for 500 babies, showing the area properties of the Normal distribution. From the Born in Bradford study

In this example, this is from (3209 g − 1128.8 g) to (3209 g + 1128.8 g) or from 2080.2 g to 4337.8 g.

- About 99 per cent of the birthweights will lie within three standard deviations on either side of the mean.

In this example, this is from (3209 g − 1693.2 g) to (3209 g + 1693.2 g) or from 1515.8 g to 4902.2 g.

So, if you have some data that you know is Normally distributed and you also know the values of the mean and the standard deviation, then you can make statements such as, 'I know that 95 per cent of the values must lie between so-and-so and so-and-so.'

To illustrate the usefulness of the Normal area properties, look again at the histogram of the cord platelet count for 4382 infants shown in Figure 4.6, which appears to be reasonably Normal and has a mean of $308 \times 10^9/l$, and a standard deviation of $69 \times 10^9/l$. You can therefore say that about two-thirds (67 per cent) of the 4382 infants, that is, 2936 infants, had a cord platelet count between $308 − 69$ and $308 + 69$, which is between 239 and $377 \times 10^9/l$.

Exercise 6.9.   Assume that the weight among breastfed men in Figure 6.5 is Normally distributed. If this is true, what percentage of men weigh: (a) less than about 41 kg? and (b) more than about 114 kg?

Exercise 6.10.   Figure 6.8 is from a study of the effectiveness of lisinopril as a pro-phylactic for acute migraine, in which one group of patients was given lisinopril and a second group a placebo. Outcome measures included 'Hours with headache', 'Days with headache' and 'Days with migraine' (all three of which are metric continuous variables) for which the mean and standard deviation (in brackets) for both groups are shown. (a) Can any of these variables be Normally distributed? Explain your answer. (b) What do you think about the use of the mean and standard deviation for the measures in the bottom half of the table?

	Lisinopril	Placebo	Mean % reduction (95% CI)
Primary efficacy parameter			
Hours with headache	129 (125)	162 (142)	20 (5 to 36)
Days with headache	19.7 (14)	23.7 (11)	17 (5 to 30)
Days with migraine	14.5 (11)	18.5 (10)	21 (9 to 34)
Secondary efficacy parameter			
Headache severity index	297 (325)	370 (310)	20 (3 to 37)
Triptan doses	15.7 (15)	20.2 (17)	22 (7 to 38)
Doses of analgesics	14.5 (23)	16.2 (20)	11 (−16 to 37)
Days with sick leave	2.30 (4.32)	2.09 (2.50)	−10 (−64 to 37)
Bodily pain*	63.7 (29)	53.8 (23)	−18 (−35 to −1)
General health*	73.6 (20)	74.1 (21)	1 (−6 to 7)
Vitality*	61.1 (24)	58.2 (21)	−5 (−18 to 8)
Social functioning*	81.4 (25)	79.5 (23)	−2 (−11 to 6)

*From SF-36.

Figure 6.8   Output measures from a study of the effectiveness of lisinopril as a prophylactic for acute migraine. Figures are means (SD). Source: Schrader *et al.* (2001). Reproduced by permission of BMJ Publishing Group Ltd

Transforming data

Later in the book, you will meet some procedures that require the data to be Normally dis-tributed. But what if it isn't? Happily some non-Normal data can be *transformed* to make the distribution more Normal (or at least more Normal than it was to start with). I think it will be convenient to deal with this now, while we are on the subject of the Normal distribution, although we won't need it until we get to Part V. The most popular approach is to take the *log*

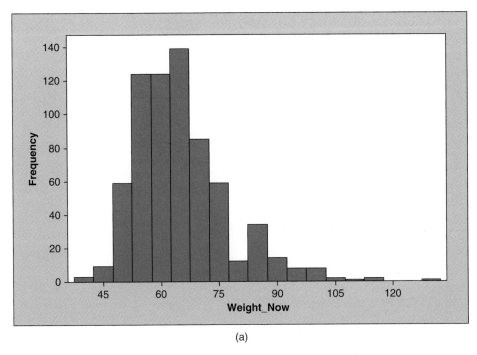

(a)

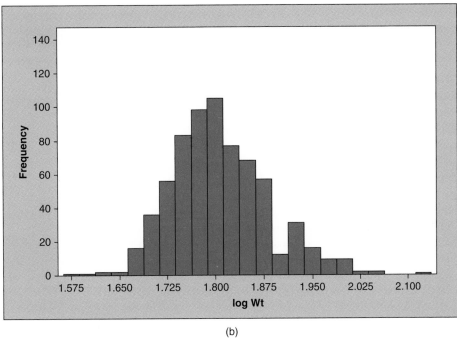

(b)

Figure 6.9   The effect of applying a $\log_{10}$ transformation on the shape of the distribution of the weight of 685 women in a diet and health study

of the data (to base 10), first because it works more often than other procedures and second because the back-transformation (i.e. anti-logging the results at the end of the analysis) can be meaningfully interpreted.

Here are some comments on transformation by authors of three research papers:

> The distribution of baseline ulcer area and baseline ulcer duration was highly skewed, so we used the logarithm of baseline ulcer area and ulcer duration in the subsequent analysis.
>
> *Watson* et al. *(2011)*

> Because the physical activity level was skewed, we present medians and interquartile ranges, and did analysis after logarithmic transformation.
>
> *Van Nimwegen* et al. *(2013)*

> We used a square-root transformation of the outcome to improve normality …
>
> *Gebre* et al. *(2013)*

Finally, as a comment on the use of different methods of location and spread according to the type of variable and on the use of transformation, here is a quote from a paper on the relationship between physical activity and fat mass in 12–14-year-old children:

> Means and standard deviations were calculated for continuous variables that approximated a normal distribution. Medians and interquartile ranges were calculated for skewed variables (physical activity, fat mass). Log fat mass was used throughout subsequent analyses, because of its skewed distribution. Although both physical activity variables showed some skewness, these variables were not log transformed in order to facilitate comparisons with our previously reported cross sectional analysis.
>
> *Riddoch* et al.*(2009)*

As an example of transformation, Figure 6.9 shows histograms for the original and transformed data on the weight (kg) of 685 women in a diet and health cohort study.[4] The original data is positively skewed, Figure 6.9a. If we transform the data by taking $\log_{10}$, you can see that the transformed data has a more Normal-ish shape, Figure 6.9b.

Incidentally, if you want to compare two distributions for whatever reason, the log transformation usually makes their spreads more equal, if they were not so to start with. This is quite a useful property of transformation as we will see in Chapter 14.

In Part II, I discussed ways of looking at sample data – with tables, with charts, from its shape, and with numeric summary measures. Collectively, these various procedures are known as *descriptive statistics*. I have said nothing so far about how we might collect the data to which we can apply the methods of descriptive statistics. I will deal with this in Chapter 8. In the next chapter, we leave descriptive statistics to discuss a very important topic in health statistics – the problem of confounding.

---

[4]This data was kindly supplied by Professor Janet Cade of Leeds University Medical School.

III

The Confounding Problem

7

Confounding – like the poor, (nearly) always with us

<hr>

Learning objectives

When you have finished this chapter you should be able to:

- Explain what confounding is.

- Summarise briefly the possible consequences of confounding.

- Outline how confounding might be detected.

- Describe possible ways of overcoming confounding, including restriction, matching, randomisation, stratification, and adjustment methods.

<hr>

Preamble

This is quite a short chapter but deals with a very important concept in health statistics. Whenever you are investigating the possible relationship between two (or more) variables, you will need to take into account the possible (more likely the probable) existence of *confounding*. Confounding can be a major problem, which if not dealt with can lead you to draw misleading or plainly wrong conclusions.

Medical Statistics from Scratch: An Introduction for Health Professionals, Third Edition. David Bowers.
© 2014 John Wiley & Sons, Ltd. Published 2014 by John Wiley & Sons, Ltd.

What is confounding?

Let me give you a simple illustration of this concept. Suppose that you are studying the possible causes of myocardial infarctions in men. You notice that men with grey (or greying) hair have a higher incidence of myocardial infarctions than men with non-grey hair. You might conclude that having grey hair is the probable cause of myocardial infarctions. This idea is illustrated in Figure 7.1. But you would have to be a half-wit to entertain this idea for more than a millisecond!

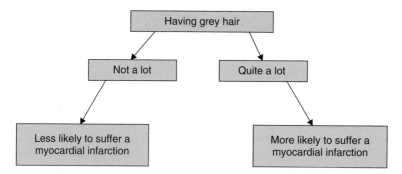

Figure 7.1 What is the exposure or risk factor for myocardial infarction? You might conclude that having grey hair is a likely cause

It is true that on the whole, men experiencing myocardial infarctions will tend to have more grey hair than men not having myocardial infarctions, but in your bones you feel that the amount of grey hair (which is known as the *exposure* variable or the risk factor) is not likely to be the critical risk factor. When you think about it, a much more likely candidate is *age*. In this example, age is a confounding variable (usually just called a *confounder*) – it confuses or *confounds* the relationship. We are being led up the garden path in our conclusions about the role of grey hair in causing myocardial infarctions by the confounding effect of age. To be a confounder, a variable:

- must be *associated* (causally or not) with the exposure of interest (e.g. grey hair).

- must be *causally related* to the outcome (myocardial infarction).

- must not be a part of the exposure–outcome causal pathway.

When we say that a variable is *associated* with another variable, we mean that both variables tend to increase or decrease together. We are *not* saying that increases (or decreases) in one variable CAUSE increases or decreases in the other variable directly. However, when we say a variable is *causally related* to another variable, we mean that changes (increases or decreases) in one variable do CAUSE changes in the other variable. (I will have a lot more to say on association in Chapter 19 and causality in Chapter 21). In this example, we are saying that age and grey hair are associated (they may be causally related but they don't have to be related to satisfy the above first requirement for confounding). But we *are* saying that increases in age *cause* increases in the incidence of myocardial infarctions. This satisfies the above second requirement for age to be a confounder.

Finally, to satisfy the third requirement, there is unlikely to be a causal pathway linking having grey hair (the exposure) to age and then to the outcome (myocardial infarctions), as having grey hair is not the cause of ageing.

Therefore, for age to be a confounder, it has to be both:

- causally related to the outcome variable (myocardial infarctions) – which it is; as men get older, they have a high incidence of myocardial infarctions.

- *and* associated with the exposure variable (grey hair) – which it is; as men get older, their hair (generally) gets greyer.

So, age has a link with both of the other two variables. This idea is illustrated in Figure 7.2.

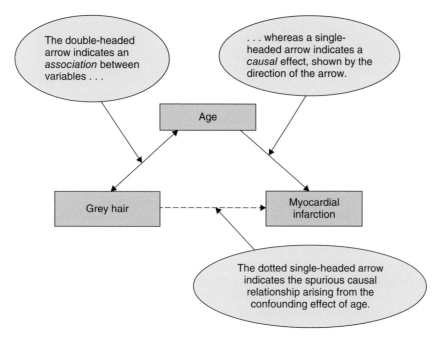

Figure 7.2 A more likely relationship. It is increasing age that increases the frequency of myocardial infarction (and at the same time is associated with hair becoming grey). Age is the confounding variable here – it is causing us to make an erroneous conclusion about the role of grey hair in myocardial infarctions

As an example from practice, researchers noticed that mothers who smoke more (while pregnant) have fewer Down syndrome babies than mothers who smoke less (or do not smoke at all) (Chi-Ling *et al.* 1999). So at first glance, smoking less seems to be a risk factor for Down syndrome. It would appear that if a mother wants to reduce the risk of having a baby with Down syndrome she should smoke a lot! See Figure 7.3.

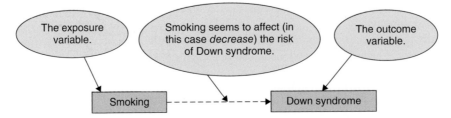

Figure 7.3   At first glance, the data seems to suggest that women who smoke while pregnant are less likely to have a Down syndrome baby

What is happening, however, is that younger mothers have fewer Down syndrome babies but smoke more, whereas older mothers have more Down syndrome babies but smoke less. Thus, the apparent connection between smoking and Down syndrome babies is a mirage. It disappears when we take age into account. So age is confusing the relationship between smoking and Down syndrome, that is, age is a *confounder*. The linkages are shown in Figure 7.4.

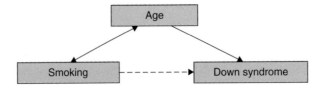

Figure 7.4   The relationship shown in Figure 7.3 is spurious, caused by the confounding effects of age. This is a more credible explanation, with age as a confounder

Notice (Figure 7.4) that age satisfies the dual relationship criteria. Age is related to *both* exposure variables – smoking – and *also* has an association with having a Down syndrome baby. In this example, the presence of the confounding variable (age) leads us to believe, wrongly, that there is a direct causal relationship between smoking and Down syndrome.

In fact, there are two types of confounding: *positive confounding*, which can lead to the effect of the exposure variable being inflated, and *negative confounding*, which can lead to the effect of the exposure variable being under-estimated.

It is worth noting that age is commonly found to be a confounder, as is gender. When we allow for the effects of possible confounders, we are said to be *adjusting* for confounders. Results which are based on unadjusted data are said to be unadjusted or *crude* results.

Exercise 7.1.   Suppose that you believe that obesity (BMI > 30) is a likely risk factor for myocardial infarction.[1] However, you also believe that hypertension may confound this

---

[1] Body mass index, used to measure obesity, is equal to a person's weight (kg) divided by their height squared (m²). A BMI of between 20 and 25 is considered 'normal' and 25 and 30 indicates a degree of obesity. Higher scores indicate greater levels of obesity.

relationship. (a) What is the exposure variable here? (b) What is the outcome variable? (c) Sketch a diagram (along the lines of Figure 7.4) to illustrate the links between the three variables. (d) Explain how the confounding variable satisfies the three criteria for a confounder.

Detecting confounding

Potential confounding variables may be identified from the research literature, or from your own research experience or from your colleagues. Alternatively, a particular variable might look like an eminently plausible candidate. For example, if you were researching the causes of low birthweight babies and you had good reasons to believe that smoking during pregnancy was the prime causal risk factor, then you might feel that potential confounders would probably include the baby's sex, maternal age, gestational age, parity, mother's education level, socioeconomic status, and maybe a few more. You would want to adjust for these variables at some point in your study – probably at the data analysis stage.

To show that a variable is actually a confounder requires an evaluation of the difference between the comparative risk of an outcome when the confounder is controlled for (adjusted for) and when it is not. For example, if in your study of low birthweight, you compared the proportion of low birthweight babies among women who smoked while pregnant with the proportion among women who did not smoke, first not adjusting for say, socioeconomic status, and then adjusting for socioeconomic status, then if the relative proportions are the same in both cases (adjusting and not adjusting), then you can reasonably conclude that socioeconomic status is not a confounder. We will meet up with this concept in Chapter 12 when we discuss ratios.

If confounding is such a problem, what can we do about it?

There are a number of ways of dealing with the potential for confounding among the variables (we can refer to it as *controlling* for confounding). Some methods we can pursue at the design stage and some at the data analysis stage.

At the design stage, we can use:

- restriction

- matching

- randomisation

At the data analysis stage, we can use:

- stratification

- adjustment

We will come across all of these methods later in the book; however, as a taster of restriction, matching, and stratification, consider the following scenario. Suppose that you are investigating the causes of stillbirths. You study several thousand births and notice that mothers who were obese (BMI > 30) had a higher proportion of stillbirths than women who were not obese. You might conclude therefore that obesity in the mother is a risk factor for stillbirth. But when you look more closely at the data you also notice that the proportion of women who smoked while pregnant in the stillbirth group was twice as high as that among women not having a stillbirth. Maybe smoking is a confounder? Now what?

Using restriction

First, we could exclude from our study all women who smoked. This method of dealing with confounding is known as *restriction*. It would mean that if we do find a relationship between BMI and stillbirth, it can have nothing to do with smoking, because we haven't got any smokers! The limitation of this approach is that because a portion of the sample is excluded, it may be difficult to generalise the results of the study to a wider population.

Using matching

Second, we could deliberately select our sample so that the proportion of smokers among the stillbirth group was the same as the proportion of smokers among the non-stillbirth mothers. This approach to confounding is called *matching*. This would mean that if we find a relationship between BMI and stillbirth, it can have nothing to do with smoking, because the proportion of smokers in each group is the same. This method is largely confined to case–control studies, which we will deal with in the next chapter.

We will encounter the idea of matching a number of times in the following chapters but now seems to be a convenient time to say a few more words about the idea before we end this chapter. Matching is a process of making a number of selected features in two separate groups similar. There are two types of matching.

Frequency matching. In this type of matching, samples are selected so that the *proportions* of relevant characteristics in two groups are broadly similar. For example, the proportion of males, smokers, those aged over 50, an ethnic minority, and so on.

One-to-one matching. The first group is selected using an appropriate sampling procedure (we will discuss sampling methods in Chapter 10). A second group is selected so that each individual in the second group is of the same age, gender, degree of illness, occupation, and so on as that of an individual in the first group.

Using stratification

Third, suppose that we examine the data even more closely and notice that the proportion of stillborn babies is lower in social classes I, II and III (non-manual) and higher in social classes III (manual), IV and V. Maybe social class is a confounder? We could deal with this possibility by dividing our sample into two, namely, the higher social classes: groups I, II and III (non-manual), and the lower social classes: groups III, IV and V. We now consider the relationship between obesity and stillbirths again but this time for each social class group separately. If the relative proportions of stillbirths are different for the two social class groups, then this implies that social class is a confounding variable. This method of dealing with confounding is called *stratification*. It involves dividing the sample into strata or groups on the basis of the levels of some criterion of interest.

A problem with this method is that although the original sample may be plenty big enough, the more the sample is stratified, the smaller each stratum becomes, and it may thus become less easy to detect any significant differences in outcome in these smaller strata.

Using adjustment

Adjustment, one of the most widely used methods of dealing with confounding, is applied at the analysis stage. We will discuss it in the context of modelling using regression, the methods described in Chapters 21 and 22. However, potential confounding variables *must* be identified at the beginning of the study and the relevant data collected.

Using randomisation

This is perhaps the ideal way of dealing with confounders as it embraces both known and unknown confounding variables. We will discuss randomisation in Chapter 9 but briefly it involves the random allocation of participants in the study into separate groups. For example, in an investigation of the efficacy of a new drug for controlling nausea associated with chemotherapy, participants would be randomly assigned to either the treatment group (the new drug) or the placebo group.

In the next chapter, we will discuss how to design a study and we will meet confounding again.

Exercise 7.2. Suppose that you are investigating the possible link between sudden infant death syndrome (SID) and the sleeping arrangement for the baby: in the same bed as that of the parents, in a separate bed in the same room, and in a separate bed in a different room. You think that smoking by one or both parents and social class may also be contributory factors. Explain how you would deal with the possible confounding influences of these two variables at the design stage.

Exercise 7.3. (a) List the possible ways of dealing with confounding. (b) Which of these methods can be applied at the design stage? (c) What are the drawbacks of the restriction and stratification methods? (d) What do we need to do at the beginning of the study if we are going to control for confounding by using adjustment?

IV

Design and Data

8

Research design – Part I: Observational study designs

'I did it my way' and now I wish I hadn't! Finding an appropriate study design

---

Learning objectives

When you have finished this chapter, you should be able to:

- Explain the difference between observational and experimental studies.

- Briefly describe the main features of case reports and case series.

- Briefly describe the main features of cross-sectional, cohort, and case–control studies.

- Outline the advantages and limitations of each type of study design.

- Explain how confounding might be dealt with in observational study designs.

Medical Statistics from Scratch: An Introduction for Health Professionals, Third Edition. David Bowers.
© 2014 John Wiley & Sons, Ltd. Published 2014 by John Wiley & Sons, Ltd.

Preamble

We have now dealt with (but definitely *not* forgotten!) descriptive statistics – the various ways in which we can uncover the principal characteristics of our sample data. We have also examined the idea of confounding – a very important concept. We can now sit back for a few moments, have an espresso, enjoy the sunshine and think about what we need to do next. Remember this is all about answering a question, such as 'Is drug A better than drug B in the treatment of hypertension?', 'What are the risk factors for stillbirth?', 'What is the best treatment for sore throat?'

   We are going to use our sample data to help us answer our questions. But how should we go about doing this? What is the best way to structure our analysis? There may be a number of alternative methods to choose from. These different methods are called *study designs*. (Note that I am going to assume, for now, that we have already selected an appropriate sample of individuals. In Chapter 10, we discuss the issue of sample selection in detail).

   The research question itself will, to some extent, indicate which study design we should use to answer it. Below are a few typical research questions, along with some likely methods (designs). We will deal with each approach in detail shortly.

Question: 'What proportion of women smoked during pregnancy?'
Method: Interview some women who have recently given birth and ask them whether they smoked while pregnant. This is a *cross-sectional* study design.
Question: 'Are the babies of women who smoked during pregnancy more likely to be stillborn than the babies of women who did not smoke?'
Method: Measure the proportion of stillbirths among the babies of women who smoked while pregnant and the proportion of stillbirths among the babies of women who did not smoke. Compare these proportions. This could either be a *case–control* study – we would choose a group of women who had smoked while pregnant – these would be the cases and a group of women who had not smoked – these would form the control or the comparison group. Then, we would determine the proportion of stillbirths in each group and compare. Or it could be a *cohort* study. We would select a group of women of child-bearing age and follow them up for a number of years. After they give birth, we can ask all mothers (those with both live births and stillbirths) whether they smoked while pregnant.
Question: 'Is the new drug A more efficient than an existing drug B for treating hypertension?'
Method: Select a group of individuals with hypertension. Allocate them (randomly) to receive either drug A or drug B. Measure the average blood pressure of the individuals in each group. Give the individuals in each group the assigned drug for some suitable interval of time. Measure the average blood pressure of the individuals in each group at the end of the study. Compare changes in average blood pressures. This is a *randomised controlled trial*.

The above is just an outline of the possible alternatives when we choose a study design. Now, I want to discuss each type of design in more detail.

Hey ho! Hey ho! It's off to work we go

Study design embraces issues such as:

- What is the research question?

- Which variables do we need to measure – what data do we need to collect to answer the research question?

- Which is our main *outcome variable* (the variable we are most interested in)?

- Are we going to make some form of clinical intervention or simply observe (and measure)?

- Do we need a comparison group?

- At what stage are we going to ask questions or take measurements? Before, during, after, etc.?

- How long will the study take? What will it cost? And so on.

Study design is a systematic way of dealing with these issues and offers a good-practice guide, which is applicable in almost all research situations.

Types of study

Study design is divided into two main types:

Observational studies and *experimental* studies.

Other terms that we may come across include *prospective* studies, *retrospective* studies, and *longitudinal* studies. I will explain these other terms along the way. Figure 8.1 illustrates the study design portfolio.

Broadly speaking, an *observational* study is one in which researchers *actively* observe the participants involved, perhaps asking questions, or taking some measurements, or looking at clinical records, but they *do not* control, change or affect in any way, the selection, treatment or care of the participants. An *experimental* study, on the other hand, does involve some sort of *active* intervention with the participants: selection, treatment, aftercare, and so on. In this chapter, I discuss observational study design. In the next chapter, I will discuss experimental study design.

> **Exercise 8.1.** What is the fundamental difference between an observational study and an experimental study?

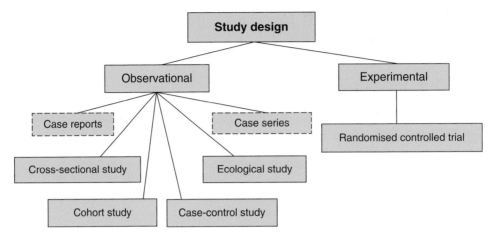

Figure 8.1   The portfolio of study designs. Note the broad division between observational study designs and experimental study designs. I have added *case reports* and *case series* to this array, although they are not really study designs in the same way as the others

Observational studies

There are three principal types of observational study, to which I have added (below) the *case report* and the *case series*. Neither of these involve 'design' as such, and the participants are not chosen by some sampling method. The participants arise 'out of the blue' as it were – they are there because their clinical circumstance was interesting enough to catch the eye of a health professional for some reason. Nonetheless, they are important enough to include in our discussion. The five approaches are as follows:

- case reports

- case series

- cross-sectional studies

- cohort studies

- case–control studies

Case reports

A *case report* is the simplest of all observational studies. It does not arise as a result of a research question, but may well suggest one. It will usually consist of an account of some clinical situation that the author thinks might interest journal readers, perhaps because of the unusual circumstances or unexpected outcome.

For example, a series of case reports led to the possibility that the drug orlistat (used to treat obesity) might be associated with an increased risk of serious liver damage. The US Food and

Drug Administration first issued a warning about a possible link between orlistat and liver injury in 2009, based on an analysis of 32 *case reports* received between 1999 and 2008.

The analysis of individual case reports often cannot provide reliable conclusions about causality, and a range of population-based studies are usually needed to help inform decisions about, in this case, the likely risks and benefits of orlistat. A meta-analysis of clinical trial data involving around 10 000 patients found no evidence that orlistat was associated with increases in selected variables of liver function and concluded that there was no strong evidence to determine a causal association.

Case series studies

A health professional may see a series of patients (cases) with similar but unusual symptoms or outcomes, find something interesting and write it up as a study. This is a *case series*. Once again, case series do not always arise as a result of a specific research question but may suggest such a question.

For example, the series of case reports (see previous section) which suggested the possibility that the drug orlistat might be a risk factor for serious liver injury, led researchers to investigate this possibility by means of a case series study, whose objective was to measure the association between orlistat and acute liver injury. The research was carried out using 94 695 patients receiving orlistat and registered in the UK Clinical Practice Research Datalink and linked with the Hospital Episode Statistics data, between 1999 and 2011. Incidentally, the analysis showed no evidence of an increased risk of liver injury during treatment with orlistat. Douglas *et al.* (2013).

In the same way, a new variant CJD was also first suspected from an unusual series of deaths of young people in the UK from an apparent dementia-like illness, a disease normally associated with the elderly.

Case series studies often point to a need for further investigations as was the case in each one of the quoted examples above.

Cross-sectional studies

While, in case series, 'participants' arise out of the blue as it were, a cross-sectional study aims to take a 'snapshot' of some situation at some particular point in time.[1] Researchers deliberately decide to collect an appropriate sample of individuals whom they can then study. Typically, data on one or more variables is collected *only once* from each participant. (We'll see how they might do this in the next chapter). These individuals will often be those who are already in touch with the health service in some way, or they may be drawn from the general population, or from case registers or patient records. There are two broad types of cross-sectional study, *descriptive* and *analytic*.

Descriptive cross-sectional studies

In the descriptive cross-sectional study, research will often focus on determining a prevalence or incidence of some condition. For example, the proportion of schoolchildren with iron

---

[1]In practice, this 'point' in time may in fact be a short-ish *period* of time.

deficiency, or the number of new shingles cases in those aged 70 or more. Other recent cross-sectional descriptive studies have had the following objectives:

- are children younger than 18 years still using sunbeds after the ban introduced in England in April 2011.

- to determine the place of death of individuals with dementia (hospital, home, etc.).

- to investigate the changes in energy content in fast food restaurants following the introduction of calorie labelling.

- to measure patient satisfaction, safety, and quality of hospital care in 1105 hospitals in 12 European countries, and in the US, by measuring the views of 131 318 patients and 61 168 nurses.

It can be noticed from the above examples that no attempt is made to examine the possible associations between variables by making comparisons between groups.

Confounding in descriptive cross-sectional studies

Confounding problems do not often arise in descriptive cross-sectional studies, particularly those which aim to determine a prevalence. However, where more than one variable is measured, there will be a potential for confounding. For example, in the patient satisfaction study described earlier, the authors reported adjusting for several possible confounding variables – particularly the composition of the nurse workforce: age, sex, employment status (full-time or part-time) and speciality; and similar adjustments were made for differences in the structural characteristics of hospitals. These adjustments were made at the analysis stage for which the authors used regression analysis (which you will meet in Chapters 21 and 22). Adjustment at the analysis stage with the use of regression models is common.

> **Exercise 8.2.**   Give two examples of the possible use of the descriptive cross-sectional design in a clinical setting.

Analytic cross-sectional studies

The *analytic* cross-sectional study design will attempt to address more complex situations than the descriptive cross-sectional design discussed earlier. Potential linkages between variables will be investigated and comparisons made between *two* or *more variables* among *groups* of individuals. Recent cross-sectional analytic studies have had the following objectives:

- To examine, in new refugees, associations between mental health outcomes and social determinants, including among the latter the ability to understand English, frequency of contact with relatives, satisfaction with accommodation, employment, money management and so on.

- To establish the impact of age and sex on primary preventive treatment for cardiovascular disease in primary care. Variables measured included patient demographics (age, sex, ethnicity), cardiovascular disease risk factors (blood pressure, cholesterol, smoking) and prescriptions for drugs to lower blood pressure and cholesterol concentration.

- To determine the trend in the association between socioeconomic status and sex, and median age of death from cystic fibrosis, over the past 50 years. Data were collected from national statistics sources each year from 1959 to 2000.

Note that in the last example, the cross-sectional analysis is carried out several times – actually each year between 1959 and 2008. There is therefore a considerable amount of extra work required when compared with the conventional one-off cross-sectional analysis. When the cross-sectional analysis involves taking a number of measurements over some period of time, it may be called a cross-sectional *longitudinal* analysis.

It is important to note that in cross-sectional studies, even though we might determine that there is an association between variables, we cannot determine the direction of any potential causality. Put more simply, we cannot say which variable is the cause and which the effect. In other words, if we were doing a cross-sectional analysis involving age, sex, obesity and diabetes and we find an association between diabetes and obesity, we cannot say whether obesity leads to diabetes or diabetes leads to obesity. The reason for this shortcoming of the cross-sectional design is that measurements are taken (e.g. on obesity and diabetes) *at the same time*. To be able to identify the direction of any causal effect, we need to refer to the study designs discussed in the following sections.

To illustrate the idea of analytic cross-sectional study in more detail, the following is an extract from a study carried out in 1993 on 2542 rural Chinese participants to determine the relationship between body mass index and cardiovascular disease (explained in the 1st paragraph below). The population of this region of China was about 6 million, and the 2542 individuals included in the sample were selected using a two-stage sampling process, as explained in the 2nd paragraph. Each participant was then interviewed and the necessary measurements were taken (3rd paragraph).

> A total of 2542 participants aged 20–70 years from a rural area of Anqing, China, participated in a cross-sectional survey, and 1610 provided blood samples in 1993. Mean BMI (kg/m^2) was 20.7 for men and 20.9 for women …
>
> … These participants were selected from 20 townships in four counties based on a two-stage sampling approach. The sampling unit is a village in the first stage and a nuclear family in the second stage, based on the following criteria: 1) both parents are alive; and 2) there are at least two children in the family. We limited the analysis to 2542 participants aged 20 years or older from 776 families …
>
> … Trained interviewers administered questionnaires to gather information on each participant's date of birth, occupation, education level, current cigarette smoking, and alcohol use … measurements, including height and weight, were taken using standard protocols, with participants not wearing shoes or outer-wear. BMI was calculated as weight (kg)/height (m^2). Blood pressure measurements were obtained by trained nurses after participants had been seated for 10 minutes by using a mercury manometer and appropriately sized cuffs, according to standard protocols.
>
> *Hu* et al. *(2000)*

Note that there is no intervention by the researchers into any aspect of the participants' care or treatment – the observers only take measurements, ask some questions, or study records. The results from the above study showed that participants in the sample with higher body mass index values were also likely to have higher blood pressures.

Confounding in analytic cross-sectional studies

There is a greater possibility for confounding in analytic cross-sectional models than in simple descriptive designs. For example, in the BMI–cardiovascular disease study described earlier, the researchers controlled for the following possible confounders: age, sex, education levels, occupation, current smoking, and alcohol use. Once again, adjustment for the confounders was made at the analysis stage, for which the authors used regression analysis (see Chapters 21 and 22). As explained earlier, adjustment for confounders at the analysis stage, using regression models, is common.

Incidentally, after controlling for the confounders, the authors of the paper reported that:

> We observed strong positive associations between body mass and blood pressure and hypertension in this very lean rural Chinese population. We also observed an inverse association of BMI with HDL cholesterol levels and direct associations with total cholesterol/HDL cholesterol ratio, fasting glucose, and triglyceride levels.

To sum up, cross-sectional studies:

- take only one measurement from one or more variables from each participant at one moment of time

- can be used to investigate a link between two or more variables but *not* the *direction* of any causal relationship. The Anqing study does not reveal whether a higher body mass index leads to higher blood pressure (e.g. more strain on the heart) or whether higher blood pressure lead to higher body mass index (maybe higher blood pressure increases appetite and/or reduces the inclination to exercise), it simply establishes some sort of association

- are not particularly helpful if the condition being investigated is rare. If, for example, only 0.1 per cent of a population has some particular illness, then a very large sample would be needed to provide any reliable results. Too small a sample might lead you to conclude that nobody in the population had the disease!

Cross-sectional studies that aim to uncover attitudes, opinions or behaviours, are often referred to as *surveys*. For example, the views of clinical staff towards having patients' relatives in Emergency Department trauma rooms.

Exercise 8.3. (a) Name two of the principal shortcomings of the analytic cross-sectional design. (b) Give two examples of the possible use of analytic cross-sectional design in a clinical setting.

From here to eternity – cohort studies

The main objective of a cohort study is to identify the *risk factors* (exposures) that lead to a particular *outcome*; for example, smoking and lung cancer, or obesity and stillbirth, or calcium intake and cardiovascular mortality, and so on. The principal structure of a cohort study is that a group of individuals, free from disease, is selected at random from:

- the general population, for example, all women residing in Manchester

- a particular population, for example, all call-centre workers

- a clinical setting, for example, those attending a headache clinic

  Then:

- At the start of the study, those participants who are exposed to some suspected risk factors (say high levels of calcium intake) are identified (as are, of course, those who are not exposed). The whole group is followed up forward over a period of time and the participants monitored. Occurrences of the outcome under consideration (say cardiovascular mortality) are recorded.

- At the end of the study, a comparison is made between groups exposed and not exposed to the risk factor in terms of the relative number of outcomes of interest, for example, the proportion of cardiovascular deaths in each group.

- A reasoned conclusion is drawn about the relationship between the outcome of interest and the exposure to the suspected risk factor.

  The cohort study (which may also be referred to as a *follow-up* or *longitudinal* study) can be either:

- *prospective* – participants are followed up forward from the present

- or *retrospective* – participants are followed up forward from some date in the past, sometimes to the present, sometimes for some shorter period of time. Retrospective cohort studies will usually make use of historical sources – medical records or registry data

The design of the cohort study means that we can say something about the direction of any possible relationship. This is because the exposure (in healthy individuals) comes *before* the outcome (the occurrence of the disease). So for example, healthy individuals regularly take calcium supplements over a period of time and, eventually, some will experience cardiovascular mortality. Obviously, the cardiovascular mortality can't be causing the high calcium intake. But it could be the other way round.

An example of a (well-known) prospective cohort study is that conducted by Doll and Hill (1956) who were able to establish a possible connection between mortality and cigarette smoking. They recruited about 60 per cent of the doctors in the UK, determined their age and smoking status (among other things), and then followed them up over the ensuing years, recording deaths as they arose. Very quickly the data began to show significantly higher mortality among doctors who smoked.

An example of a retrospective cohort study – an investigation into the relationship between weight during infancy and the prevalence of coronary heart disease (CHD) in adult life – used a sample of 290 men born between 1911 and 1930 and residing in Hertfordshire, whose birth-weights and weights at one year were on record. In 1994, various measurements were made on the 290 men, including the presence or absence of CHD. So 'forward' here means from each birth year between 1911 and 1930 up to 1994.

The researchers found that 42 men had CHD, a prevalence of 14 per cent, $(42/290) \times 100$. Weight at *birth* was not influential on adult CHD. However, men who weighed 18 lbs (8.2 kg) or less, *at one year*, had almost twice the risk of CHD as that of men who weighed more than 18 lbs. This, of course, is only the sample evidence. Whether this finding applies to the population of *all* men born in Hertfordshire during this period, or today, or indeed in the UK, depends on how representative this sample is of either of these populations.

Figure 8.2 shows this cohort study expressed as a contingency table (see Chapter 2). The participants are grouped according to their exposure or non-exposure to the risk factor (in this case weighing 18 lbs or less at one year is taken to be the risk factor), and these groups form the columns of the table. The rows identify the presence or otherwise of the *outcome*, CHD. Clearly, this design does suggest (but certainly does not prove) a cause and an effect – low weight at one year seems to lead to CHD in adult life.

Exercise 8.4.   Figure 8.3 is taken from a prospective cohort study of risk factors for stillbirth. The figure shows the data for stillbirths among smokers (including passive smokers) and non-smokers. (a) What does 'prospective' mean in this context? (b) What is the risk factor here? (c) What do the results seem to indicate about a possible relation-ship between the two variables? In Chapters 21 and 22, you will see how you can answer this question more definitely.

Exercise 8.5.   Figure 8.4 is taken from a retrospective cohort study (1990–2005) to examine the effect of systolic and diastolic blood pressure achieved in the first year of treatment, on all-cause mortality in patients newly diagnosed with type 2 diabetes, with and without established cardiovascular disease. (a) What does 'retrospective' mean in this context? (b) What is the risk factor here? (c) What do the results seem to indicate about a possible relationship between the two variables?

Cohort studies have the following favourable features:

- Several outcomes (diseases) can be studied for exposure to the same risk factor.

- The time-order is clear so a relationship between exposure and outcome can be established (i.e. if one exists).

- The design suits itself to *rare* exposures.

- Less potential for bias compared to case – control studies (see below).

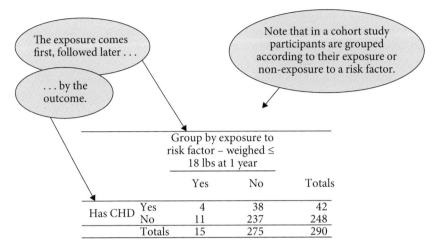

Figure 8.2 The cohort study of weight at one year and its effect on the presence of CHD in adult life, expressed in the form of a contingency table. Notice that in a cohort study, the participants are selected according to whether they have been exposed to the supposed risk factor. Data from Fall (1995)

		Smoker or passive smoker?	
		Yes ($n = 32\,864$)	No ($n = 52\,639$)
Stillbirth?	Yes	167	166
	No	32\,697	52\,473

Figure 8.3 The number of stillbirths among a cohort of mothers who smoked (or were passive smokers), taken from a prospective cohort study. Data from Gardosi (2013)

Died in study period (1990–2005)?	Patient had cardiovascular disease at baseline?	
	Yes ($n = 12379$)	No ($n = 113\,713$)
Yes	3535	21960
No	8844	91753

Figure 8.4 The number of deaths among patients newly diagnosed with type 2 diabetes, with and without cardiovascular disease. From a retrospective cohort study (from 1990 to 2005). Data from Vamos et al. (2012)

But cohort studies suffer shortcomings, for example:

- Selection of appropriate participants may cause difficulties. If participants are chosen using a convenience sample, for example, attendees at a clinic, then the outcomes for these individuals may be different from those in the general population.

- If the condition is rare in the population, that is, if it has a low prevalence, it may require a very large cohort to capture enough cases to make the exercise worthwhile. This makes cohort studies liable to be expensive.

- The participants will have to be followed up for a long time, possibly many years, before any worthwhile results are obtained. This can be expensive as well as frustrating and not good if a quick answer is needed.

- The long time period allows for considerable losses as participants drop out for a variety of reasons – they move away, they die from other non-related causes and so on. To add to the problem, the drop-out rate may differ between the exposed and non-exposed groups. This drop-out problem can lead to biased results and is the principal drawback of cohort studies.

- Over a long period, a significant proportion of the participants may change their habits – for example, quit smoking or take up regular exercise. However, this problem can be monitored with frequent checks of the state of the cohort.

- The possibility for confounding (is discussed in the following a few paragraphs).

Finally, note again that the selection of the groups in the cohort design is based on *whether individuals have or have not been exposed to the risk factor*; for example, weighing 18 lbs or less at one year, smoking while pregnant, or whatever.

Confounding in the cohort study design

Consider the following illustration of confounding in cohort studies. Researchers investigating the possible link between depressant medication (the exposure variable) and several adverse outcomes in a cohort of older people with depression, used 60 746 patients from a primary care research database. The authors of the study recognised the need to adjust for possible confounding variables (and how!). I have slightly abbreviated their comments:

> Confounding variables
> The potential confounding variables included in the analysis were age at study entry date; sex (male, female); year of diagnosis of depression; previous recorded diagnosis of depression before age 65; severity of index diagnosis of depression (categorised as mild, moderate, or severe); deprivation, based on Townsend deprivation score for the patient's postcode, categorised into fifths; smoking status (non-smoker, ex-smoker, current smoker); comorbidities at baseline (coronary heart disease, diabetes, hypertension, stroke/transient ischaemic attack, cancer, dementia, epilepsy/seizures, Parkinson's disease, hypothyroidism, obsessive-compulsive disorder; use of other drugs at baseline (statins, non-steroidal anti-inflammatory drugs, antipsychotics, lithium, aspirin, antihypertensive drugs, anticonvulsants, hypnotics/anxiolytics); and previous falls before baseline (for the analysis of fracture).
>
> *Coupland (2011)*

The authors concluded:

This observational study found significant associations between use of antidepressant drugs and several severe adverse outcomes in people aged 65 and older with depression.

Once again, the adjustment for confounding was made at the analysis stage using regression models (Chapters 21 and 22).

Back to the future – case–control studies

A number of limitations of the cohort design are addressed by the *case–control* design, although it is itself far from perfect, as you will see. In a cohort study, a group of participants is followed up to see if they develop an outcome (a condition) of interest. In contrast, in a case–control study, the groups are selected on the basis of having or not having the outcome of interest. The objective is the same in both types of study – can the outcome of interest be related to the candidate risk factor? The structure of a case–control study is as follows:

- Two groups of participants are selected. One group (called the *cases*) will have the condition of interest (e.g. depression or hypertension), the other will not have (these are the *controls*).

- The controls are selected to be as similar as possible (e.g. age, gender, occupation, stage of illness, etc.).

- The past exposure of individuals in both groups to the suspected risk factor is then ascertained. This may be by personal interview, from existing records or from physical measurements and laboratory tests. Because the case–control design deals with exposure in the past, case–control studies are sometimes referred to as *retrospective* studies.

- A reasoned conclusion is then drawn about the relationship between the outcome in question and exposure to the suspected risk factor.

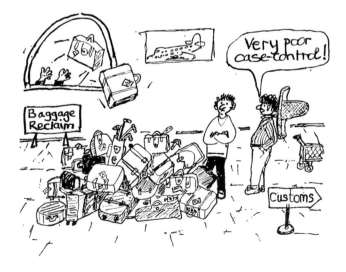

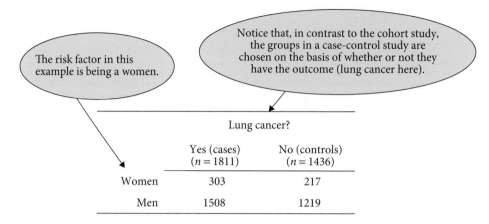

Figure 8.5 Table from a case–control study of lung cancer and gender. This table refers to former and current smokers (and does not include those who had never smoked). Data from De Matteis *et al.* (2013)

The general structure of the case–control design is shown in Figure 8.5, taken from an investigation of whether female smokers are more likely to contract lung cancer than male smokers. Notice that, in contrast to the cohort study (where groups are chosen on the basis of exposure to a risk factor), in a case–control study the groups are chosen on the basis of whether they have the output of interest or not (in this example, lung cancer), and are or have been exposed to the risk factor (being a woman in this example, so fairly obvious!). Commenting on their selection of participants, the authors reported that:

> The EAGLE Study[2] included 2,100 incident lung cancer cases (448 women and 1,652 men) and 2,120 population controls (500 women and 1,620 men). The subjects were enrolled in April 2002–June 2005 in 216 municipalities (including the cities of Milan, Monza, Brescia, Pavia, and Varese) in Lombardy, the most developed and populated (over 9 million inhabitants) region of Italy. Subjects were 35–79 years of age at diagnosis (cases) or at sampling/enrollment (controls). Response rates (participants/eligible subjects) were 86.6% (cases) and 72.4% (controls).
>
> Cases were persons with newly diagnosed primary cancer of the trachea, bronchus, or lung, of any stage and morphology, verified by means of tissue pathology (67.0%), cytology (28.0%), or review of clinical records (5.0%). They were recruited in 13 hospitals which cover over 80% of the lung cancer cases from the study area. Controls were randomly sampled from population databases of the area, frequency-matched to cases by residence (5 areas), sex, and age (5-year categories), and contacted through family physicians.

---

[2]The Eagle study is a population-based case–control study, the Environment and Genetics in Lung Cancer Etiology (EAGLE) Study (Lombardy, Italy, 2002–2005).

After several additional modifications to their analysis (e.g. including those who had never smoked, adjusting for depth of inhalation, and so on), the authors conclude:

> In conclusion, our findings do not support the controversial hypothesis that women have a higher relative risk of lung cancer than men from the same amount of tobacco exposure. Thus, as far as lung cancer is concerned, equally vigorous health policy interventions should continue to focus on eliminating smoking in both sexes.

Confounding in the case–control study design

Matching controls with cases is an inherent characteristic of case–control studies. This means that any variables that are matched between the two groups are controlled for, that is, cannot be confounders. Typically, age and gender will usually feature large in the matching process. Researchers may well add other variables to these two when they are matching cases and controls if they feel they will be significant confounders. In the lung cancer study shown in Figure 8.5, we have seen that controls were frequency-matched to cases by residence locality, sex and age (see the text above the figure). Further adjusting for confounders (education, passive smoking, and degree of nicotine dependence) was undertaken at the analysis stage by means of regression methods (Chapters 21 and 22, again!). Despite this the authors added:

> Generally speaking it becomes increasingly difficult to find matching controls for the cases the greater the number of matching variables. As a consequence, in practice cases and controls are not usually matched on more than three variables.

Bear in mind that variables on which the participants are matched cannot be used to shed any light on the relationship between outcome and risk. For example, if we are interested in coffee as a possible risk factor for people with pancreatic cancer (the cases), we should certainly not match cases with controls so that *both* groups drink a lot of coffee.

It was the outcome from a case–control study by Doll and Hill that led them to conduct the later cohort study described earlier. Before I discuss the case–control design in detail, there are a couple of important ideas to be dealt with first.

Exercise 8.6.   Figure 8.6 is taken from a case–control study of the role of caffeinated stimulants in the risk of crashes by long-distance lorry drivers in New South Wales, Australia (numbers and percentages). (a) How are the groups chosen? (b) What is the risk factor? (c) What variables would you choose to match cases and controls? (d) Do you think the data suggests any connection between the use of caffeinated stimulants and the risk of crashing? (In Chapter 21, you will see how you can answer this question more definitely).

	Involved in crash	
	Yes Cases ($n = 530$)	No Controls ($n = 517$)
Uses caffeinated stimulant:		
Yes	162 (30.6)	290 (56.1)
No	368 (69.4)	227 (43.9)

Figure 8.6   Structure of a case–control study. Associations between use of stimulant substances and crashes in long-distance commercial vehicle drivers who were recently involved in crash (cases) and control drivers who had not had crashed in previous 12 months. Figures are numbers (percentage) of participants. Data from Sharwood *et al.* (2013)

Another example of a case–control study

Figure 8.7 is from a frequency-matched case–control study to determine the possible connection between lifelong exercise and stroke. The researchers selected 125 cases with stroke and 198 controls, broadly matched by age and sex. Notice that the numbers of cases and controls need not be the same (and usually are not). All participants (or their relatives if necessary) were interviewed and asked about their history of regular vigorous exercise at various times in the past. Figure 8.7 shows the results for those participants who had and had not taken exercise between the ages of 15 and 25.

		Cases (stroke) ($n = 125$)	Controls (healthy) ($n = 198$)
Exercise undertaken	Yes	55	130
when aged 15–25	No	70	68

Figure 8.7   Outcome from an exercise and stroke case–control study for those participants who had and who had not exercised between the ages of 15 and 25. Data from Shinton and Sagar (1993)

From these results, you can calculate (you will see how later) that among those who had had a stroke, the chance that they had exercised in their youth was only about half the chance that somebody without a stroke had exercised.

I should mention briefly a hybrid design, which combines elements of both cohort design and case–control design. This is the *nested case–control* design. I can best illustrate this with an example. Suppose we have a prospective cohort study to investigate the possible relationship between smoking and emphysema. When an individual develops emphysema, they become a 'case'. For each of these cases, we select one or more individuals who have not developed emphysema. These controls will often be matched with the case on variables such as age and sex. The nested case–control design is less expensive in both time and money but is slightly less efficient statistically.

Comparing cohort and case–control designs

The case–control design has a number of advantages over the cohort design:

- With a cohort study, as you saw previously, rare diseases and conditions require large samples, but with a case–control study, the availability of potential cases is much greater and the sample size can be smaller. So they are particularly suited to rare diseases.

- Case–control studies are cheaper and easier to conduct.

- Case–control studies give results much more quickly.

But at the same time, they have a number of limitations:

- Although cases will often be convenience samples, that is, selected from patients attending particular clinics, this may result in them not being similar to the wider population of individuals with the same disease. Generalisation may thus be difficult.

- Problems with the selection of suitable control participants. You want participants who, apart from not having the condition in question, are otherwise similar to the cases. But such individuals are often not easily found.

- Problems with the selection of cases. One problem is that many conditions vary in their type and nature and it is thus difficult to decide which cases should be included.

- The problem of *recall bias*. In case–control studies, you are asking people to recall events in their past. Memories are not always reliable. Moreover, cases may have a better recall of relevant past events than controls – over the years, their illness may provide more easily remembered signposts, and they have a better motive for remembering – to get better!

In regard to recall bias, the authors of the lung cancer study (see Figure 8.5) said:

> Despite our accurate individual exposure assessment, inadequate control for confounders of smoking effect as well as recall bias for smoking are possible in any retrospective study on lung cancer, but this should not be different in males and females.

Because of these various difficulties, case–control studies often provide results, which seem to conflict with the findings of other apparently similar case–control studies. For reliable conclusions, cohort studies are generally preferred but are not always a practical alternative.

Exercise 8.7.   (a) What advantages does a case–control study have over a cohort study?
(b) What are the principal shortcomings of a case–control study?

Finally, I must mention two important concepts that come out of cohort and case–control studies, respectively. From cohort studies we can get *risk ratios*; from case–control studies we can get *odds ratios*. Both of these ideas we'll meet later in the book.

Ecological studies

An *ecological study* (sometimes called a correlation study) aims to investigate the connection between one group level variable (such as per capita alcohol consumption in several regions of a country or in several countries) and a second group level variable (such as mortality from CHD in those same regions or countries). The idea of an ecological study is to make large-scale comparisons between *groups* of people. So they are *not* about individuals but about *groups* of individuals.

As an example, in a longitudinal ecological study ('longitudinal' because time is involved), researchers wanted to investigate whether the uneven rise in prosperity between 1999 and 2008 (uneven because employment and incomes, for example, improved at slower rates in some regions than in others), accounted for the observed differential increases in life expectancy in English counties. The two variables investigated were change in life expectancy in each of 324 lower tier local authorities (the main outcome variable) and change in prosperity in the same local authorities (prosperity being measured by changes in unemployment, household income, and educational attainment).

Taken from this same study, Figure 8.8 shows the results of plotting, for groups of local authorities, the increase in life expectancy (months) against increase in household income (£000 s), between 1999 and 2008, for women and men. The results showed that the life expectancy of women increased by 26 months between 1999 and 2008 and that of men by 34 months. By the way, this sort of graph is called a scatterplot. It will be discussed again in Chapter 19. Now, there's something to look forward to!

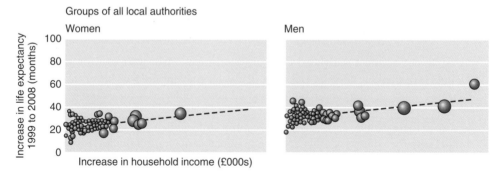

Figure 8.8 The results of plotting (for groups of local authorities) the increase in life expectancy (months) against the increase in household income (£000 s), between 1999 and 2008, for women and for men. The size of the blob is proportional to the population in the local authority. The graph (called a scatterplot) indicates that as household income increases so does life expectancy. Source: Barr *et al.* (2012). Reproduced by permission of BMJ Publishing Group Ltd

The ecological fallacy

The ecological fallacy arises from the erroneous belief that the findings from the group study can be applied to the individual. In other words, it would be wrong to assume (in the above ecological study) that just because an individual lives in a local authority region where prosperity did not improve, that that person would necessarily not experience an increase in their life expectancy. Nor can we assume that a person who has enjoyed an increase in their life expectancy necessarily lives in a region where prosperity has increased. Even in regions where prosperity *in general* did improve, there may be a considerable proportion of individuals who would not have enjoyed a rise in their living standards during the period in question.

It is because of the ecological fallacy that the ecological study is not as highly regarded as the other observational designs. This deficiency is compounded by the fact that the design is unable to deal with confounding in a convincing manner. However, ecological studies are very useful as ways of generating plausible hypotheses, which can subsequently be examined using analytic studies of one sort or another.

Exercise 8.8. (a) Outline the principal difference between an ecological study and other observational study designs. (b) What is meant by the ecological fallacy? Give an example.

9

Research design – Part II: Getting stuck in – experimental studies

Learning objectives

When you have finished this chapter you should be able to:

- Outline the general idea of clinical trials.

- Explain the concept of randomisation, and what is meant by block randomisation.

- Use random number tables to perform simple block randomisation.

- Describe what is meant by blinding and why it is used and say what is meant by a double-blind randomised controlled trial.

- Describe and compare the parallel and cross-over randomised controlled trials, along with their respective advantages and shortcomings.

- Explain intention-to-treat.

Medical Statistics from Scratch: An Introduction for Health Professionals, Third Edition. David Bowers.
© 2014 John Wiley & Sons, Ltd. Published 2014 by John Wiley & Sons, Ltd.

We can now turn to those types of design where, in contrast to observational studies, the investigators are active in some aspect of the recruitment, treatment, or care (usually all of these) of the participants in the study.

Clinical trials

Clinical trials are *experiments* that compare two or more clinical treatments. I use the word 'treatment' here to mean any sort of clinical intervention, from kind words to new drugs. Many whole books have been written that deal solely with clinical trials, and in one chapter I can only touch briefly upon some of the more important aspects of this design.

Consider the following imaginary scenario. A new drug, *Arabarb*, has been developed for treating hypertension. You want to investigate its efficacy. Here's what you need to do:

- Decide on an outcome measure – diastolic blood pressure seems to be a good candidate.

- Select a sample of individuals with hypertension. Divide them into two groups[1] in such a way that the two groups are as similar as possible. They should be similar not only for the obvious variables, such as sex and age, but also for other variables either whose existence you are aware of but can't easily measure (e.g. emotional state of mind, lifestyles, genetic differences) or whose existence you are *not* even aware of! We will see how we can do this below.

- Give the new drug, Arabarb, to the first group. This is the *treatment* group.

- Give the other group a placebo. This is the comparison or *control group*. A control group is a must. If you have only one group of people and you measure their diastolic blood pressure before and after the administration of Arabarb, you cannot conclude that any decrease in diastolic blood pressure is caused, necessarily, by Arabarb. Being in a calm, quiet clinical setting, or having someone fussing over them, might reduce diastolic blood pressure.

- At the end of the trial, compare the changes in average diastolic blood pressure in the treatment and comparison groups. Draw the appropriate conclusions.

Why do we want the treatment group and the group receiving the placebo to be as identical as possible? You will remember from Chapter 7 in our discussion on confounding, that one of the ways of dealing with the confounding problem was by matching and that this was particularly relevant in case–control studies. We also mentioned that randomisation was a way that confounding could be tackled. Well, randomisation in clinical trials is the ultimate in matching. It is like the gold standard of matching. Clearly, if the randomisation process is successful and the two groups are identical, then all variables will be matched and no confounding will be possible. And the real beauty of randomisation is that *all* the variables are matched, even the ones we do not even know about!

---

[1] Sometimes, we will want to divide our sample into three or more groups. However, to keep things simple, we will assume only two groups here.

In practice, we will not be able to produce two *completely* identical groups, so confounding can never be *completely* eliminated, but the bigger the sample size, the more probable it is that the groups will be alike. So how does randomisation work? How do we do it?

Randomisation

Randomisation means *random allocation*. We allocate each participant in the sample to either the treatment group or to the comparison group. How? One possible way would be to toss a coin for each individual in the sample – heads, they go to the treatment group and tails, to the comparison group. If the *randomisation* is successful and the original sample is large enough then the two groups should be more or less identical in the important characteristics – those which we can measure, as well as those that we cannot measure or those which we are not even aware of. The two groups will differ *only by chance*. (At base-line anyway. Participants who drop out during the course of the study may alter this balance. See intention-to-treat explained later).

This design is therefore called the *randomised controlled trial* (RCT). It is 'controlled' because we are controlling for all possible confounders. In other words, all potential confounding variables will exist in both groups more or less equally, thereby minimising (but never completely eliminating) the problem of confounding. As we noted earlier, the bigger the sample size the more effective the randomisation process will be, the more similar the groups and the less the possibility of confounding.

Of course, coin tossing is a little impractical. Instead, a table of *random numbers* can be used for the allocation process (see Appendix). Let us see how we might use this method to randomly allocate 12 patients.

You decide to allocate a participant in the trial to the treatment group (T) if the random number is *even* (we count 0 as even) and to the control group (C) if *odd*. You then need to determine a starting point in the random number table, maybe by sticking a pin in the table and identifying a start number. Suppose, to keep things simple, you start at the top of column 1 and go down the column. The first six rows contain the values: 23157, 05545, 14871, 38976, 97312, 11742. Combining these three rows and using only the first 12 values gives us the following:

The numbers	2	3	1	5	7	0	5	5	4	5	1	4
The allocations	T	C	C	C	C	T	C	C	T	C	C	T

This gives you four participants in the treatment group and eight in the control group. Problem! We want our groups to be of the same size. You can fix this with *block randomisation*.

Block randomisation

Here is how it works. You decide on a block size, blocks of four is fairly common, and write down all combinations that contain *equal* numbers of Cs and Ts. As there are six such possible combinations, you will have six blocks:

Block 1   CCTT
Block 2   CTCT
Block 3   CTTC
Block 4   TCTC
Block 5   TCCT
Block 6   TTCC

With the same random numbers as before, the first number was 2, so the first four participants are allocated according to Block 2, that is, CTCT. The next number was 3, so the next four participants are allocated as Block 3, that is, CTTC. The next number was 1, giving the allocation CCTT and so on depending on the number in the sample. We ignore numbers that we have already used (blocks already allocated) as well as, in this example, numbers greater than 6. You will end up with the allocation:

CTCT   CCTT   CTTC

which gives equal numbers, six, in both groups.

Stratification

Sometimes, you will feel it is important that certain sub-groups in the sample are adequately represented; for example, a certain ethnic group, or a group of people aged over 70. To ensure that they are not under-represented in the randomisation process, we can stratify the sample first and take a randomised sample from each stratum.

Blinding

If at all possible, you don't want the participants to know whether you are in the treatment group or the control group. This is to avoid the possibility of *response* or *placebo bias*. If a participant knows, or thinks they know, that they are getting the active drug, their psychological response to this knowledge may cause a physical, that is, a biochemical response, which conceivably might in turn affect their diastolic blood pressure. In the Arabarb trial, you could achieve this 'blinding' of the participants to their treatment, for example, by giving them all identical tablets, one containing the Arabarb and the other the placebo.

   Here is an example of the effort expended to make the placebo indistinguishable from the active ingredient. In a randomised placebo controlled trial to evaluate the efficacy of a short course of parent-initiated oral prednisolone for acute asthma in Australian children of school age, the authors reported that:

> The prednisolone solution we used was Redipred, which contains 6.72 mg/ml of the active ingredient, prednisolone sodium phosphate. The placebo solution was also manufactured by the makers of Redipred; however, the hospital pharmacist

added 0.1% quinine bisulphate to the placebo mixture to mimic the bitter taste of prednisolone. The bottles of prednisolone and placebo appeared identical.

Vuillermin et al. *(2010)*

Blinding of participants is not always possible. For example, in a study that assesses the effectiveness of adenoidectomy (removal of adenoids) in children with recurrent upper respiratory tract infection, children were randomly assigned to one of two strategies: adenoidectomy within six weeks or initial watchful waiting. It would clearly be impossible to blind the children (or their parents) to their treatment!

A further desirable precaution is also to blind the investigator to the allocation process. If the investigator does not know which participant is receiving the drug and which the placebo, their treatment of the participants will remain impartial and even-handed. Human nature being what it is, there may be an unconscious inclination to treat a patient who is known to be in the treatment group differently to the one in the control group. This effect is known as *treatment bias* and can be avoided by blinding the investigator. We can do this by entrusting a disinterested third party to obtain the random numbers and to decide on the allocation rules. Only this person will know which group any given participant is in and will not reveal this until the treatment is complete and the results collected and analysed.

Assessment bias is also overcome when the investigator is blinded. This is important when an assessment of some condition after treatment is required. For example, in trials of a drug to control agitation or anxiety, where proper *measurement* is not possible, an investigator, *knowing* that a participant got the active drug, might then judge their condition to be more improved than would an uninvolved outsider. Therefore, an uninvolved outsider should conduct the assessment process.

When both participant and investigator are blinded, we refer to the design as a *double-blind randomised controlled trial* – the gold standard among experimental designs. Without blinding, the trial is referred to as being *open*. Compared to other designs, the RCT gives the most robust and dependable results. Note that sometimes the word *masking* is used instead of blinding. The meaning is the same.

The design described above, in which two groups received identical treatment (except for the difference in drugs) throughout the period of the trial is known as a *parallel* design; this is illustrated schematically in Figure 9.1.

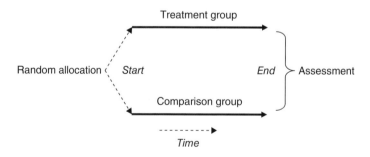

Figure 9.1   Schematic representation of parallel group trial

The cross-over randomised controlled trial

A variation on the parallel design is the *cross-over* design, shown schematically in Figure 9.2. In this design, one group gets drug A, say, for some fixed period of time, and the second group gets drug B (or placebo). Then, after a *wash-out* period to prevent the drug effect carry-over, the groups are swopped over. The group that got drug A now gets drug B and vice versa, and for the same period of time. Which group gets which treatment first is decided randomly.

As an example, the following extract describes the method used in a randomised cross-over trial of regular versus as-needed salbutamol in asthma control.

> If inclusion criteria were met at the first clinic visit, patients were enrolled in a four-week randomised crossover assessment of regular vs. as-needed salbutamol. Patients took either 2 puffs (200 mg) metered dose salbutamol from a coded inhaler or matching placebo four times daily for two weeks. On return to the clinic, diary cards were reviewed and patients assigned to receive the crossover treatment for two weeks. During both treatment arms patients carried a salbutamol inhaler for relief of episodic asthma symptoms. Thus, the placebo treatment arm constituted as-needed salbutamol.
>
> Patients were instructed to record their peak expiratory flow rate (PEFR) twice daily: in the early morning and late at night, before inhaler use. Patients also recorded in a diary the number of daytime and night-time asthma episodes suffered and the number of as-needed salbutamol puffs used for symptom relief.
>
> Data from the last eight days of each treatment period were analysed; the first six acted as an active run-in or washout period. Two investigators, blinded to the treatment assignment, examined these comparisons for each patient, and categorised each patient as: showing no difference in asthma control between treatment periods; greater control during the first treatment period; greater control during the second treatment period; or differences between treatment periods that did not indicate control to be clearly better during either.
>
> *Chapman* et al. *(1994)*

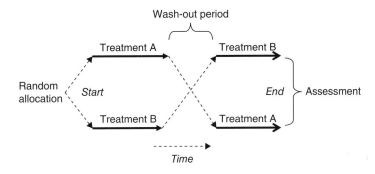

Figure 9.2   Schematic representation of cross-over group trial

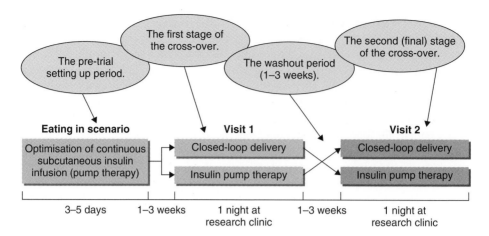

Figure 9.3   Part of a cross-over study comparing closed-loop delivery of insulin with conventional insulin pump therapy. This shows the Eating In scenario only. Source: Hovorka *et al.* (2011). Reproduced by permission of BMJ Publishing Group Ltd

As an example of the cross-over design, Figure 9.3 shows the schematic representation of a randomised cross-over trial to compare the safety and efficacy of overnight closed-loop delivery of insulin (artificial pancreas) with the conventional insulin pump therapy, in adults with type 1 diabetes.

The advantage of the cross-over design is that each participant gets both treatments and thus acts as his or her own control. 'Same-participant' matching, if you like. As a consequence of the matched-pair feature, this design requires smaller samples to achieve the same degree of efficiency. Unfortunately, there are a number of problems with this approach. Namely:

- A participant may undergo changes between the first treatment period and the second.

- The method does not work well if the drug or the treatment to be investigated requires a long time to become effective – for practical reasons cross-over trials are generally of relatively short duration (one reason is to avoid excessive drop-out).

- Despite a wash-out interval, there may still be a drug carry-over effect. If carry-over is detected, the second half of the trial has to be abandoned.

- The cross-over design is also inappropriate for conditions that can be cured – most of the participants in the active drug half of the condition might be cured by the end of the first period!

Selection of participants

Just a brief word about selection of participants for an RCT. Essentially, you want a sample of participants (and they will usually be patients of some sort) who represent a cohesive and clearly defined population. Thus, you might want to exclude participants who, although they have the condition of interest, have a complicated or a more advanced form of it, or have other significant illnesses or conditions simultaneously, or are taking drugs for another condition – indeed anything which you feel makes them untypical of the population you have in mind. If your sample is not truly representative of the population you are investigating (a problem known as *selection bias*), then any conclusions you arrive at about your target population are unlikely to be at all reliable.

As an example of participant selection and blinding procedures, the following extract is from an RCT to compare the efficacy of having midwives solely manage the care of pregnant Glasgow women with the more usual arrangements of care being shared among midwife, hospital doctors and GPs. Outcomes were the number of interventions and complications, maternal and foetal outcomes and maternal satisfaction with the care received. The first paragraph details the selection criteria, the second and third paragraphs describe the random allocation and the blinding processes, respectively.

Methods

Design and participants

The study was carried out at Glasgow Royal Maternity Hospital, a major urban teaching hospital with around 5000 deliveries per year, serving a largely disadvantaged community. Between Jan 11, 1993, and Feb 25, 1994, all women booking for routine care at hospital-based consultant clinics were screened for eligibility; the criteria were residence within the hospital's catchment area, booking for antenatal care within 16 completed weeks of pregnancy, and absence of medical or obstetric complications (based on criteria developed by members of the clinical midwifery management team in consultation with obstetricians; available from the MDU).

The women were randomly assigned equally between the two types of care without stratification. A restricted randomisation scheme (random permutated blocks of ten) by random number tables was prepared for each clinic by a clerical officer who was not involved in determining eligibility, administering care, or assessing outcome. The research team telephoned a clerical officer in a separate office for care allocation for each woman.

Women in the control group had no identifying mark on their records, and clinical staff were unaware whether a particular woman was in the control group or was not in the study. We decided not to identify control women … because of concern that the identification of the control group would prompt clinical staff to treat these women differently (i.e., the Hawthorne effect).

Turnbull et al. *(1996)*

Intention-to-treat

One problem that arises frequently in an RCT after treatment has begun, is the loss of participants, principally through drop-out (moving away, refusing further treatment, dying from non-related causes, etc.) and withdrawal for clinical reasons (perhaps they cannot tolerate adverse side effects of the treatment). Unfortunately, such losses can adversely affect the balance of the two groups achieved through the initial random allocation process.

As an example, suppose for an RCT to compare the efficacy of two drugs in treating some illness, we have randomly allocated 100 participants to receive Drug A and 100 to receive Drug B. At the end of the trial, no one has dropped out of the Drug A group, and 60 per cent of them have recovered. However, 95 of those receiving Drug B have dropped out but the remaining five have all recovered. Would we want to conclude that Drug B was better? I think not. We would want to know what happened to all of those drop-outs in group B. Why did they leave? Was it, for instance, due to adverse side effects?

In these circumstances, it is a good practice to analyse the data as if the lost participants were still in the study, as you originally intended – even if all of their measurements are not complete. This is known as *intention-to-treat* analysis. The reasoning behind this approach is pragmatic and reflects the degree of drop-out that frequently happens in clinical practice. It does, however, require that you have information on the outcome variable for all participants who were originally randomised, even if they did not complete the course of treatment in the trial. Unfortunately, this information is not always available and in many studies therefore, intention-to-treat may be more of an aspiration than a reality.

There are ways of trying to fill in the blanks by using methods to impute missing values. For example, we could use the average value of all the existing values for a particular variable, to provide us with a missing value for a dropped-out participant. Or we could use what is called the *last value carried forward* method, to fill in a missing value when sequential measurements are being taken over time (e.g in either treatment or follow-up). Unfortunately, none of the methods available are spectacularly successful, and missing values remain a problem for researchers.

Note that if researchers analyse only those participants who *complete* a trial and provide full information on outcomes, then this approach is called *per protocol* analysis. This form of analysis re-introduces the potential for confounding because participants who drop-out may upset the initial balance between groups.

Exercise 9.1.   What is the principal purpose of randomisation in clinical trials?

Exercise 9.2.   Explain how the possibility of treatment bias, assessment bias and response bias, may be overcome in the design of an RCT.

Exercise 9.3.   Using block randomisation, with blocks of four, and a random number table, allocate 40 participants into two groups, each with 20 individuals.

Exercise 9.4.   Explain the difference between a parallel design RCT and a cross-over design. What are the advantages and possible drawbacks of the latter design?

Exercise 9.5.   What is meant by intention-to-treat analysis? How does it differ from per protocol analysis?

10

Getting the participants for your study: ways of sampling

Learning objectives

When you have finished this chapter you should be able to:

- Explain the relationship between a sample, a study population and a target population.

- Explain the relationship between a sample statistic and a population parameter.

- Explain the importance of getting a representative sample.

- Explain the differences among various types of samples (random samples, convenience samples, cluster samples, etc.).

- Explain what is meant by inclusion and exclusion criteria.

Medical Statistics from Scratch: An Introduction for Health Professionals, Third Edition. David Bowers.
© 2014 John Wiley & Sons, Ltd. Published 2014 by John Wiley & Sons, Ltd.

From populations to samples – statistical inference

As you saw right at the beginning of this book, we gather data because we want to answer questions such as what causes stillbirths? What is the best treatment for hypertension? What is the prevalence of asthma in UK schoolchildren?[1]

Take the last question on asthma in schoolchildren. The seemingly obvious way to answer it would be to interview all 5 – 16-year-old children in the UK and ask them (or more likely their parents) whether they are receiving treatment for asthma. However, the population of schoolchildren in the UK is very large – around 13 million, and it would, in practice, be impossible to interview all of them. It would take too long, be too expensive and besides which, we would have to have an address for each one of them.

Let's call this whole population (the 13 million schoolchildren) the *target population*. From this target population, we can take a sample. We then assume that what is true of the sample will also be true of the target population. We intend to generalise from the sample to the target population. This process is called *statistical inference*. We are making inferences (informed guesses) about features of the population (these features are called *population parameters*) on the basis of the corresponding features (called *sample statistics*) that we discover in the sample. For example, the population proportion and the population mean are population parameters. This idea is shown schematically in Figure 10.1.

But how would we do this? In practical terms, it would still be virtually impossible to access all schoolchildren in the UK, which we would need to do before we could select our sample. It would be better, and more feasible, to take our sample from a more accessible group. For

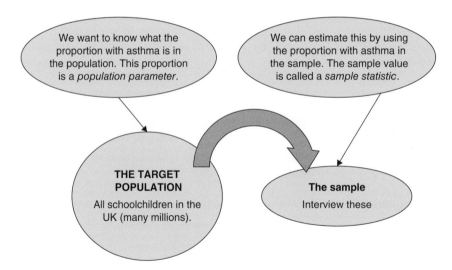

Figure 10.1 The sample and the target population. We use the value of the sample proportion with asthma to estimate the population proportion with asthma. This is called *inference*.

---

[1] Approximately 1.1 million children are receiving treatment for asthma in the UK. That is about one in 11 or just below 10 per cent.

example, all schoolchildren in Leeds, Birmingham or Glasgow, wherever you have reasonable access to potential participants. This more restricted group is called the *study population*. We hope that our study population, say all schoolchildren in Leeds, is *representative* of all schoolchildren in the whole of the UK (the target population). And in addition, that our sample, taken from our study population, is representative of the target population. This idea is illustrated in Figure 10.2.

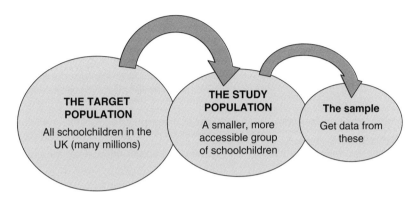

Figure 10.2   The target population, the study population and the sample. We are generalising from the sample *statistic* to the population *parameter*, the process of statistical inference. We hope that the sample is representative of the study population and that the study population is representative of the target population

In a nutshell, we are going to use the value of a sample statistic, obtained from a represntative sample, to make an informed guess as to the value of the corresponding population parameter. For example, the sample statistic might be sample mean birthweight, and the population parameter might be population mean birthweight. It is worth noting that Greek letters are used to denote population parameters, for example, μ is used to denote the population mean and Π the population proportion.

Exercise 10.1.   (a) Explain the differences between a target population, a study population and a sample. (b) Explain, with an example, why it is almost never possible to study every member of a population. (c) What is a population parameter? How can we estimate its value?

Collecting the data – types of sample

So far I have talked rather blithely about taking a sample from a population. Now, I want to talk about how we go about doing this, and how we hope to ensure that out sample is representative of the population from which it has been drawn.

Needless to say, samples are never perfect replicas of their populations; therefore, when we draw a conclusion about a population based on a sample, there will always be what is known as *sampling error*. For example, if the percentage of 5 – 16-year-old children in the UK population with asthma is 10 percent (we would not know this of course), and if a sample produces a sample percentage of 9 percent, then the difference between these two values, 1.0 per cent, is the sampling error. We can never completely eliminate sampling error as this is an inherent feature of any sample. Now to the data collection question.

The simple random sample and its offspring

The most important consideration is that any sample should be *representative* of the population from which it is taken. For example, if your population has equal numbers of male and female babies, but your sample consists of twice as many male babies as that of female babies, then any conclusions you draw are likely to be, at least, misleading. Generally, the most representative sample is a *simple random sample*. The only way that a simple random sample will differ from the population will be *due to chance* alone.

For a sample to be truly random, every member of the population must have an equal chance of being included in the sample. Unfortunately, this is rarely possible in practice as this would require a complete and an up-to-date list (name and contact details) of, for example, *every* 5–16-year-old children in the UK. Such a list is called a *sampling frame*. In practice, compiling an accurate sampling frame for any given population is hardly ever going to be feasible! Nonetheless, the simple random sample, although in practice unachievable, provides the gold standard, against which other sampling methods might be compared.

This same sampling frame problem applies also to two close relatives of simple random sampling, as you will now see.

Exercise 10.2.   What is the principal difficulty with random sampling?

The systematic random sample

With this approach, some fixed fraction of the sampling frame is selected, say every 10th or every 50th member, until a sample of the required size is obtained. For example, suppose we have a population size of 100,000 and we want a sample size of 500. The fraction required is thus:

$$\frac{100,000}{500} = 200$$

Therefore, we select every 200th person from the sampling frame. The starting point is chosen using a random number table. So if the random number is 18, we select the 218th perosn, the 418th person and so on. Provided there are no hidden patterns in the sampling frame, this method will produce samples as representative as a random sample. Trouble is – we still need a sampling frame to use this method.

The stratified random sample

In stratified sampling, the sampling frame is first broken down into strata relevant to the study, for example, men and women, or non-smokers, ex-smokers and smokers. Then, each separate stratum is sampled using a systematic sampling approach, and finally these strata samples are combined to provide the final amalgamated sample. As before, the limitation of this design is the need for a sampling frame. However, the method is often employed in conjunction with cluster sampling (see next section), which obviates the need for a sampling frame.

As an example of stratification, in a study of the effects of gestational age at birth on health outcomes at 3 and 5 years of age, respectively, the authors stratified their sample to ensure that children born to mothers in deprived areas and to ethnic minority mothers were adequately represented in the final sample. They stated:

> Stratified sampling at electoral ward level with over-sampling of ethnic minority and disadvantaged areas ensured adequate representation of these populations.
>
> *Boyle* et al. *(2012)*

The cluster sample

The cluster sampling approach overcomes the need for a comprehensive sampling frame and is used when the selection of individuals is not appropriate. In these situations, clusters of villages, communities, schools, GP practices and so on become the sampling units. Random selection from these clusters (sometimes more than once) is then performed to produce a representative sample.

For example, a programme to investigate the efficacy of a programme to improve the health of schoolchildren started with all 919 primary school classes (with 18 381 chilldren) in two regions of a country. Each class thus comprises a cluster of schoolchildren. Ninety-five of these classes satisfied the inclusion criteria. Twenty-seven of these classes were then randomly selected from the 95 classes to give a total sample of 535 children. The researchers then randomised these classes to treatment (additional physical activity) or control groups.

As an example from practice, in a programme whose objective was to see if a monetary incentive to head teachers was effective in reducing the levels of anaemia in schoolchildern in China, the authors described their method as follows:

> Through a canvass survey, we first created a sampling universe of all primary schools in 10 nationally designated poor counties spread across two provinces with high anaemia rates – Ningxia and Qinghai. We then identified all schools having six grades (that is, "complete" primary schools) and boarding facilities. A total of 85 schools met these criteria, and we randomly selected 72 for inclusion in our study. Finally, we randomly selected half of fourth and fifth grade students in study schools (sampling 3944 students in total). Fourth and fifth grade students were chosen because they are old enough for test scores to be relevant but also young enough not to have reached puberty (at which point nutritional requirements differ more markedly from childhood and vary by sex).
>
> *Miller* et al. *(2012)*

Cluster sampling is frequently used in randomised controlled trials. For example, in the anaemia study as described earlier, the randomisation into separate treatment groups was thus described.

Sample schools were randomly assigned to a control group, with no intervention, or to one of threee treatment arms: (a) an information arm (information about anemia only), 27 schools, 1816 students; (b) a subsidy arm (information plus subsidy), 15 schools, 659 students; or (c) an incentive arm (information plus subsidy plus financial incentive), 15 schools, 743 students.

Exercise 10.3.   Explain how the cluster sample overcomes the sampling frame problem associated with random sampling.

Consecutive samples

The need for an accurate sampling frame makes random sampling impractical in any realistic clinical setting. One common alternative is to take individuals who are in current or recent contact with the clinical services, such as *consecutive* attendees at a clinic, as a sample. Alternatively, participants might be selected from a registry or clinical records database. As an example of a consecutive sample, in the study of stress as a risk factor for breast cancer (Figure 1.7), the researchers took 332 consecutive attendees as their sample for a breast lump biopsy at Leeds General Infirmary.

Alternatively, researchers may study a group of participants *in situ*, for example, in a ward or in some other setting. In the nit lotion study (Figure 1.9), researchers took as their sample all infested children from a number of Parisian primary schools, based on the high rates of infestation in those same schools the previous year.

If your sample is not a random sample, then the obvious question is, 'How representative is it of the population?' Moreover, which population are we talking about here? In the breast cancer study, if the researchers were confident that their sample of 332 women was reasonably representative of *all such women* in the Leeds area (their study population), then they would perhaps have felt justified in generalising their findings to this population and maybe to all women in the UK (a possible target population). But if they knew that the women in their sample were all from a particularly deprived (or particularly affluent) part of the city, or if some ethnic minority formed a noticeably large proportion of the women, then such a generalisation would be more risky.

Exercise 10.4.   What is the main advantage and the main disadvantage of convenience sampling?

How many participants should we have? Sample size

One obvious question arises when we are selecting a sample for our investigation. How many people do we need to recruit? This question is one that all researchers need to answer. The solution is intimately tied up with the notion of 'power' and error, as well as the type of the study we are involved with. As such, it is probably best to deal with it later in the book (see Part VI). However, I *strongly* advise anyone contemplating a research project to consult a medical statistician about the sample size issue early in the planning stage!

Inclusion and exclusion criteria

In almost all studies, we will want to decide quite carefully not only how we are going to recruit our participants and how many participants we will need but also whom we might want to include in our study and equally whom we will need to exclude. To this end, researchers decide upon a set of *inclusion* and *exclusion criteria*.

Let us take as an example, the retrospective cohort study referred to in Exercise 8.5 to examine the effect of systolic and diastolic blood pressure achieved in the first year of treatment on all-cause mortality in patients newly diagnosed with type 2 diabetes. The researchers *included*:

> All adult patients (age ≥18 years) with a new diagnosis of type 2 diabetes between 1 January 1990 and 31 December 2005, and who had been registered with participating practices for at least 12 months.

And excluded:

> … patients diagnosed under the age of 35 years who were prescribed insulin within three months of diagnosis and who were not prescribed oral hypoglycaemic agents for longer than three months, because these patients were likely to have type 1 diabetes. We also excluded patients with a diagnosis of heart failure and an echocardiogram supporting the diagnosis to avoid reverse causality, because these patients tend to have lower blood pressure levels than those without heart failure.
>
> *Vamos* et al. *(2012)*

We will come across further examples of inclusion and exclusion criteria later in the book.

Getting the data

Having decided on a sampling method, let us say you like the idea of a consecutive sample, how will you get the actual data for each of your variables? Well, you could measure, or count, observe, touch, question (face-to-face or by questionnaire), or use an established measurement scale (e.g. the Glasgow Coma Scale, the Modified Rankin Scale, or the Health Outcomes SF36 scale). Or you could use an already assembled registry data or the data previously collected by colleagues (with their permission).

If you are going to use a questionnaire, try to use an existing one or modify an existing one. *Always* pilot a new questionnaire before you use it, preferably on those who will be responding to it (service users) and on knowledgeable colleagues. Be aware of problems arising from low response rates. Try to find out if the responders are different to the non-responders. The same applies to a measurement scale. Try to use an existing scale if possible or modify one. Develop a new scale only if absolutely necessary and *always* pilot it.

V

Chance Would be a Fine Thing

11
The idea of probability

Learning objectives

When you have finished this chapter, you should be able to:

- Define probability, explain what an event is and calculate simple probabilities.

- Explain the proportional frequency approach to calculating probability.

- Explain how probability can be used with the area properties of the Normal distribution.

Preamble

Probability is a measure of the chance of getting some particular outcome of interest from some trial or '*experiment*'. For example, the experiment might be performing a biopsy on breast lump tissue, or administering a drug to a patient having a heart attack, or it might be rolling a dice. Experiments produce outcomes. For the biopsy, the outcomes will be malignant or benign. For the patient with a heart attack, the outcomes will be to survive the first 24 hours or to die within 24 hours. For rolling a dice, the outcomes will be 1 or 2 or 3 or 4 or 5 or 6. The particular

---

Medical Statistics from Scratch: An Introduction for Health Professionals, Third Edition. David Bowers.
© 2014 John Wiley & Sons, Ltd. Published 2014 by John Wiley & Sons, Ltd.

outcomes of interest might be the patient surviving, the biopsy being benign, the dice giving a 6 and so on.

Let us look at some basic ideas about probability:

- The probability of getting any particular outcome will always lie between zero and one. The smaller the probability is, the lesser is the chance of the outcome and vice versa.

- The probability of an outcome that is certain to happen is equal to one. For example, the probability that everybody dies eventually.

- The probability of an outcome that is impossible is zero. For example, throwing a seven with a normal dice.

- If an event has as much chance of happening as of not happening (like tossing a coin and getting a head), then it has a probability of $\frac{1}{2}$ or 0.5.

- If the probability of an event happening is p, then the probability of the event *not* happening is $1 - p$. So if the probability of getting a 6 when you roll a dice is 1/6 or 0.1666, then the probability of *not* getting a 6 is $1 - 0.1666 = 0.8333$. It is common to express probabilities as a decimal rather than as a fraction.

Calculating probability – proportional frequency

The probability of getting a head when you toss a coin is 1/2 or 0.5, because there are two outcomes, each equally likely. In the same way, the probability of getting a 6 when you roll a dice is 1/6 or 0.1666. These probabilities are fairly obvious. Unfortunately, situations where all the outcomes are equally likely are rare in the clinical arena. In such cases, we use what is called the *proportional frequency* approach to calculate probability. With this method, the probability of a particular outcome is equal to the proportion of times that that outcome would occur if you were to repeat the experiment a very large number of times. Thus, we say that the probability of a patient with a certain illness surviving for five years is 0.75; this is because in the past, this is the proportion that several thousand patients with this illness have survived this long.

As an example, see Figure 2.4 (reproduced here for convenience as Figure 11.1), which shows the causes of blunt injury to limbs. I have added an extra column showing the *proportional frequency* (category frequency divided by total frequency). Notice that the proportional frequencies sum to one.

Now ask the question, 'What is the probability that if you chose one of these 75 patients at random, their injury will have been caused by crushing?'. The answer is the proportional frequency for the 'crush' category, that is, 20/75 or 0.267. In other words, we can interpret proportions as equivalent to probabilities.

> **Exercise 11.1.**   Look back at Figure 2.5 showing levels of satisfaction with nursing care. Using proportional frequencies, if a patient is chosen at random from this group, what is the probability that the patient will be (a) very satisfied? and (b) very dissatisfied?

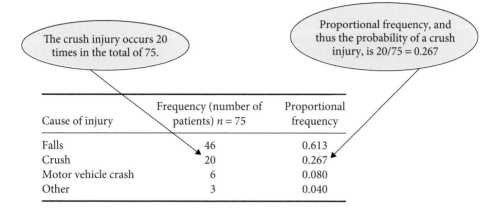

Figure 11.1   Frequency table showing causes of blunt injury to limbs in 75 patients

Two useful rules for simple probability

Rule 1. The multiplication rule for independent events

Suppose that you are interpreting biopsies performed on tissue from breast lumps. The outcome can be either benign or malignant. Past results indicate that the proportion malignant will be about 30 per cent. Assume that the figure is exactly 30 per cent. The probability that the next result will be malignant is 0.30. The probability that the result after this is malignant is also 0.30. And the next one and so on. This is because the results are independent of each other. An outcome in no way influences the result of the next outcome.

Now let's ask a different question. What is the probability that two successive outcomes will both be malignant? We can answer this question using the *multiplication rule for independent events*. This states that the probabilities of successive similar events is the product of those events. That is, we multiply the probabilities together. So the probability of two successive malignant outcomes is:

$$0.30 \times 0.30 = 0.09$$

This means that if we repeat this experiment (two biopsy results in succession) a hundred times, on nine occasions we would get two successive malignant outcomes. Similarly, if we took three biopsies, the probability that all three would be malignant is $0.30 \times 0.30 \times 0.30 = 0.027$. That is, 27 times in a 1000 tries. This rule works for any number of successive independent events.

Algebraically, if the two possible outcomes are A and B, then the probability of getting two 'A's in succession is given by:

$$P(A \text{ and } A) = P(A) \times P(A)$$

Exercise 11.2.   What is the probability of getting two successive benign results?

Rule 2. The addition rule for mutually exclusive events

Look again at Figure 3.4, which shows the blood groups of kidney recipients with and without rejection. Without rejection, the percentage blood groups of the 1777 patients were Type A = 42 per cent, Type O = 41 per cent, Type B = 10 per cent, and Type AB = 5 per cent.

Suppose that we are about to determine the blood group of an individual. The possible outcomes are A, B, O and AB, and using the proportional frequency idea and the above proportions, the probabilities are 0.42, 0.41, 0.10 and 0.05, respectively. Notice that these probabilities add up to 1.00 (allowing for some serious rounding by the authors!). In other words, a person must be in one of these blood groups.

The question is, 'What is the probability that the individual will have *either* blood group O *or* A?' We know that a person cannot be in two blood groups, so these outcomes are termed *mutually exclusive*. (Just as when we toss a coin, the outcome can be *either* a head *or* a tail – the two possible outcomes are mutually exclusive). We can answer this question using the *addition rule for mutually exclusive events*. This states that if two outcomes are mutually exclusive, then

> the probability of *either* one *or* the other occurring is the sum of the two individual probabilities.

In this case:

> Probability of being in *either* blood group O *or* blood group A = 0.42 + 0.41 = 0.83

It follows that the probability that they are in *either* blood group B *or* AB must be 1 − 0.83, that is, 0.17.

Algebraically, we can express the addition rule for two mutually exclusive events A and B as:

$$P(A \text{ or } B) = P(A) + P(B)$$

Exercise 11.3.   Referring back to Figure 2.5, what is the probability of a patient chosen at random being either satisfied or very satisfied with their nursing care?

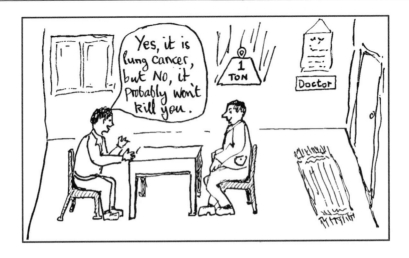

Conditional and Bayesian statistics

I can no more than briefly mention two other types of probability – *conditional probability* and *Bayesian probability*. Conditional probability is concerned with the probability of one outcome occurring given that another outcome has already occurred. For example, given that a baby has a birthweight less than 1500 g, what is the probability that its mother smoked while pregnant.

Bayesian probability deals with the idea of incorporating any *prior knowledge* that a researcher might have about a hypothesis. Bayesian statistics calculates the probability that a hypothesis is true by incorporating any new information (e.g. new data) about the hypothesis as it becomes available. Most health care professionals will unwittingly practice Bayesian statistics when confronted by a patient. They use clinical history, the existence of signs and symptoms, new information given to them by the patient, reaction (or non-reaction) to treatment and so on as prior knowledge when making (i.e. hypothesising) a diagnosis. If subsequently, new information comes in – say the result of a blood test – that can also be included in the hypothesis of what illness the patient is likely to be suffering from.

Both are important but they are more advanced topics than this book is designed to deal with. Maybe next time.

Probability distributions

Before we leave this brief examination of simple probability, I need to mention the idea of a *probability distribution* and outline three interesting probability distributions that arise in health statistics.

What is a probability distribution? It is a table or an equation that tells you the probability of each outcome when you perform some 'experiment'. For example, suppose that the experiment is rolling a dice, for which there are only six possible outcomes, with the probabilities shown in Figure 11.2. This table is thus the probability distribution for this dice rolling experiment.

Outcome X	Probability of outcome $P(X)$
1	1/6
2	1/6
3	1/6
4	1/6
5	1/6
6	1/6

Figure 11.2 Probability distribution for rolling a dice

In this example, you will notice that I have labelled the outcome from rolling the dice as X. X is a *random variable* (because it can take various values), and when a variable is the outcome from an experiment, as it is here, we call it a random variable.

The equation of the probability distribution for this dice rolling experiment is:

$$P(X) = \frac{1}{6}$$

Exercise 11.4.   (a) What is a random variable? (b) Suppose that an experiment is to toss a coin twice, write down as a table the probability distribution for the outcomes from this experiment.

Discrete versus continuous probability distributions

The probability distribution for the dice rolling experiment is a *discrete* probability distribution. Discrete because the number of possible outcomes is limited, although it may be very large. (You can revisit Chapter 1 for a reminder of the difference between discrete and continuous variables). Suppose now that our 'experiment' is to weigh a newborn baby to determine its birthweight. Here, birthweight is a *continuous* random variable (random because it is the outcome from an experiment), and continuous variables have an unlimited or infinite number of possible values. Moreover, as there are an infinite number of values, the probability of any particular value has to be zero. This means we can't show the probability distribution of a continuous random variable as a table. Instead, we have to use an equation (called a *probability density function* or pdf), which gives the probability that the continuous random variable lies between any two defined values, for example, between 2000 g and 3000 g or perhaps <1500 g.[1]

The binomial probability distribution

The first of the three probability distributions I want to mention is the *binomial* probability distribution. Suppose that we toss a coin repeatedly. We know that there are only two possible outcomes from this experiment – a head or a tail – and that the probability of each of these outcomes is 0.5 and stays at 0.5 for each toss. The random variable here is the number of heads (or the number of tails), and it has a binomial probability distribution, because it satisfies four requirements:

- There is a series of trials (we toss the coin several times).

- The trials are independent (the outcome from one trial has no effect on the output of any other trial).

- There are only two outcomes from each trial (head or tail).

- The probabilities of the outcomes remain the same for each trial (they do not of course have to be 0.5, as long as they remain constant).

---

[1] The bottom value here is 0 g.

The binomial probability distribution tells us what the probability is of getting any particular *number* of either of the two outcomes in a given number of trials and is thus a *discrete* probability distribution. For example, if we toss a coin 100 times, the binomial probability distribution will tell us the probability of getting any given number of heads (and therefore the number of tails). Because this is a discrete random variable, we can describe the probability distribution in a tabular form, as well as an equation.

As a more realistic example, about 10 per cent of babies born to lone parents in England and Wales are low birthweight (<2500 g). Let us assume that the proportion is constant at 10 per cent, that is, a probability of 0.1. There are two possible outcomes, low birthweight or not low birthweight, and the births are independent, so we can use the binomial distribution to tell us the probability of getting any given number of low birthweight babies. For example, the probability of getting eight low birthweight babies in the next 100 deliveries is 0.115.[2] And of getting 12 low birthweight babies is 0.099.

Perhaps, more useful is the *cumulative* binomial probability distribution. This gives the probability of getting a particular value for the random variable *or fewer*. For example, a given number of low birthweight babies or fewer. For example, the probability of getting eight low birthweight babies *or fewer* in the next 100 deliveries (i.e. 8, or 7, or . . . or 1 or 0) is 0.321, and for 12 or fewer the probability is 0.802. It follows that the probability of getting *more* than 12 such babies is $(1 - 0.802) = 0.198$.

Exercise 11.5.   Use a binomial calculator to determine the probability of getting: 7, 8, 9, 10, 11, 12 or 13, low birthweight babies in 100 deliveries, if the probability of this outcome is 0.1. Arrange the values in a table. Plot these probabilities (vertical axis) against number of low birthweight babies. Comment on the shape of this graph.

The Poisson probability distribution

The *Poisson probability distribution* describes the outcome of a discrete random variable. It is a count of the number of events that we can expect to occur in a given time (or less usually, in a given space). For example, the number of arrivals at an Emergency Department in a given 24-hour period or the number of stillbirths in a particular hospital in a given year. This expected value can be compared to the actual value if we have reason to believe that this is unusually low or high.

The requirements that must be satisfied for the Poisson distribution are:

- The average number of events that occur in a given time period is known.

- The events are independent.

---

[2] Type binomial calculator into a search engine (such as Google) and you will get numerous hits. I used Stattrek. There is a binomial formula, but this is a bit complicated to use and it is much, much, easier to let someone else do the work.

- The events are random.

For example, suppose that we know that the average number of stillbirths in a year in a certain hospital maternity unit averages 10 in any 12-week period. What is the probability of getting eight stillbirths in the next 12 weeks? Using a Poisson calculator, the answer is 0.113. The *cumulative* Poisson probability for eight stillbirths *or fewer* is 0.333. For 12 stillbirths or fewer, the probability is 0.792. Because this is a discrete random variable, we can describe the probability distribution in a tabular form, as well as an equation.

Exercise 11.6.   Suppose that the average number of road accident victims arriving at an Emergency Department per week averages 15. Use a Poisson calculator to determine the probability of there being 20 or more such arrivals in the next week.

The Normal probability distribution

You first met the Normal distribution in Chapter 4. The *Normal probability distribution* describes the outcomes from experiments whose output is a Normally distributed random variable. It has a smooth bell-shaped curve. The distribution is continuous, which means, as we noted earlier, that we cannot calculate the probability of any single outcome occurring (it will always be zero) but only the probability of an outcome within some interval. Many outcomes in the clinical arena are Normally distributed; for example, birthweight (Figure 4.5) and cord platelet count (Figure 4.6).

Provided we know the mean and standard deviation, we can fully describe the Normal probability distribution and determine the probability that an outcome will lie between any two specified values. In fact, you will no doubt remember what the probability is of a value lying within one, two, or three standard deviations of the mean (see Figure 6.7). There is an equation for the Normal probability distribution but it is much easier to use a Normal calculator sourced from the internet.[3]

Exercise 11.7.   Use a Normal distribution calculator and the information on cord platelet count in Figure 4.6 to determine the probability that one infant chosen at random from this sample will have a cord platelet count (a) equal to or less than $225 \times 10^9/l$, and (b) equal to or more than $425 \times 10^9/l$.

---

[3] Such as Stattrek.

12

Risk and odds

Learning objectives

When you have finished this chapter, you should be able to:

- Define and explain the idea of absolute risk and its relationship with probability.

- Calculate the absolute risk and the absolute risk reduction, of some outcome from a contingency table and interpret the result.

- Calculate and interpret the risk ratio and the reduction in the risk ratio (also known as the relative risk reduction).

- Briefly outline methods for adjusting risk ratio to take confounding into account.

- Define the number needed to treat, explain its use and calculate NNT in a simple example.

- Define and explain the idea of odds.

- Calculate odds from a case–control 2×2 table and interpret the result.

- Be able to calculate probability given the odds and vice versa.

Medical Statistics from Scratch: An Introduction for Health Professionals, Third Edition. David Bowers.
© 2014 John Wiley & Sons, Ltd. Published 2014 by John Wiley & Sons, Ltd.

- Explain what the odds ratio for some outcome is, calculate an odds ratio and interpret the result.

- Briefly outline methods for adjusting the odds ratio to take confounding into account.

- Explain why it's not possible to calculate a risk ratio in a case–control study.

Absolute risk and the absolute risk reduction

In medical statistics, we use the term *absolute risk* (sometimes just *risk*) to describe the probability of some particular outcome likely to be experienced by a group of individuals (most often patients) who are subject to some exposure (either beneficial or not). As absolute risk and probability are one and the same, this means that the absolute risk can vary between 0 (no risk – outcome will not happen) and 1 (certain risk – outcome is certain to happen). (See Chapter 11 for a reminder on probability.)

Note that:

- the value of the absolute risk for an outcome can vary from 0 to 1.

- when the risk for an outcome is greater than 0.5, the risk is *favourable* to the outcome; the outcome is *more* likely to happen than not.

- when the risk is equal to 0.5, the outcome is as likely to happen as not.

- When the risk is less than 0.5, the risk is *unfavourable* to the outcome and therefore, the outcome is *less* likely to happen than it is *to* happen.

As an example of risk, Figure 12.1 is from a study to investigate the effectiveness of supplementing the diet of pregnant women at high risk of pre-eclampsia or eclampsia, with L-arginine and antioxidant vitamins. The first row proper of the table shows the absolute risks of pre-eclampsia and eclampsia for women receiving a placebo and for those women receiving the active supplement (I will deal with the other rows of the table shortly).

As you can see the absolute risk of pre-eclampsia or eclampsia in women receiving the placebo was 0.3018, or 30.18 per cent, whereas for women receiving the supplement the absolute risk was only 0.1272 or 12.72 per cent. The L-arginine plus vitamin supplement reduced the risk by $0.3018 - 0.1272 = 0.175$ or 17.5 per cent. We call this the *absolute risk reduction*.

You might at this point ask the question, 'Could this result have occurred by chance or are we looking at a real (statistically significant) reduction in risk here?' We can answer this question by examining what are called confidence intervals, but won't deal with these until Chapter 15 (but not to keep you in suspense, the answer is 'Yes', this result is significant).

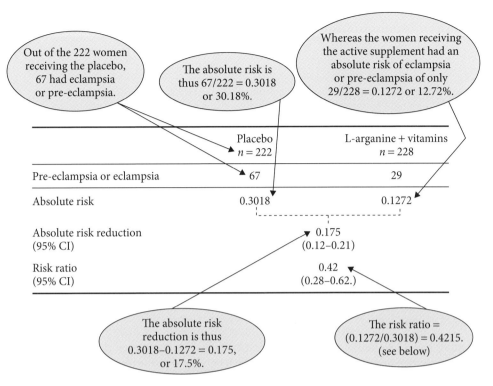

Figure 12.1 Absolute risks from a randomised controlled trial to investigate the effectiveness of supplementation during pregnancy with L-arginine and antioxidant vitamins versus a placebo on pre-eclampsia or eclampsia in a high-risk population. Data from Vadillo-Ortega *et al.* (2011)

Exercise 12.1. The contingency table in Figure 12.2 is from a study investigating the efficacy of adding zinc to the standard antibiotic treatment for infants aged between seven days and 120 days, with serious bacterial infection, in a developing country. The table shows the number of deaths among a sample of these infants who were given zinc and among those who were not given zinc (the placebo group). (a) Calculate the absolute risk of treatment failure among infants who were given zinc and among those who were given the placebo. (b) What is the absolute risk reduction?

The risk ratio

As the name implies, the risk ratio[1] is the risk of an outcome; for example, emphysema, for one group (say smokers), *compared to* the risk of emphysema for a second group (say non-smokers).

---

[1] Because it sits well with 'odds ratio', I prefer to use 'risk ratio' rather than 'relative risk', although the latter occurs more often in the literature. Where I am quoting from published research, I will use 'relative risk' if this term is used by the authors in their results.

		Zinc ($n = 332$)	Placebo ($n = 323$)
Treatment failure*	No	298	268
	Yes	34	55

*Defined as a need to change antimicrobial treatment within 7 days of randomisation, or a need for intensive care (mechanical ventilation or vasoactive drug infusion, or both), or death at any time within 21 days of randomisation.

Figure 12.2 Effect of zinc given orally as an addition to antibiotics on treatment failure in infants with serious bacterial infection. Data from Bhatnagar *et al.* (June 2012)

We call the comparison group (here it is the non-smokers) the *reference* (or *referent*) group. The risk ratio is usually associated with cohort studies.

As an example, see Figure 12.1. We see that the absolute risk of pre-eclampsia or eclampsia in the treatment group is 0.1272 and that in the placebo group is 0.3018. The ratio of these absolute risks is the risk ratio:

$$\text{risk ratio} = \left(\frac{0.1272}{0.3018}\right) = 0.4215$$

This means that those women in the treatment group receiving L-arginine and antioxidant vitamins had under half the chance (42.15 per cent) of developing pre-eclampsia or eclampsia than did women in the placebo group. Or, to put it another way, the placebo group women had $1/0.4215 = 2.37$ times the chance of getting pre-eclampsia or eclampsia than the women in the treatment group.

It is interesting to compare the absolute risk reduction of 17.5 per cent with the value for risk ratio of 42.15 per cent. The latter gives a much rosier impression of the benefits of L-arginine and antioxidant vitamins in reducing pre-eclampsia and eclampsia. For this reason, it is important to give the value for the absolute risk reduction *as well as* for the risk ratio. This reduction in risk of 17.5 per cent may not be large enough to be either cost effective or clinically worthwhile.

> **Exercise 12.2.** Following on from Exercise 12.1, calculate the risk ratio and interpret your result.

The reduction in the risk ratio (or relative risk reduction RRR)

A further useful measure in this context is the reduction in the risk ratio, perhaps, more commonly known as the *relative risk reduction* (RRR). This tells us by how much the active treatment reduces the risk of an adverse outcome in the treatment group *compared to the control* (*placebo*) *group*. In the eclampsia example as described earlier (see Figure 12.1), the value of 0.4216 for the risk ratio tells us that women who were treated with L-arginine and antioxidant vitamins had an absolute risk of pre-eclampsia and eclampsia of 0.4216 times than that of women in the placebo (control) group. In other words, the risk for those women in the treatment group was reduced by $(1 - 0.4216) = 0.5784$ compared to those treated with the placebo. This represents a relative risk reduction of 57.84 per cent. As you can see, risk ratio reduction is given by:

$$RRR = (1 - \text{relative risk}) \text{ or } (1 - \text{risk ratio})$$

The large reduction in the risk ratio (relative risk) of 57.84 per cent, in actual fact represented a comparatively small absolute change in risk (17.5 per cent, shown in Figure 12.1) as a result of the treatment.

Exercise 12.3. Following on from Exercises 12.1 and 12.2, calculate the relative risk reduction. What does this mean?

A general formula for the risk ratio

Figure 12.3 is a generalised contingency table for a cohort study. The formula for calculating the risk ratio is:

$$\text{risk ratio} = \frac{a/(a+c)}{b/(b+d)} = \frac{a\,(b+d)}{b\,(a+c)}$$

		Exposed to risk factor?		
		Yes	No	Totals
Outcome: has disease	Yes	a	b	(a+b)
	No	c	d	(c+d)
	Totals	(a+c)	(b+d)	

Figure 12.3 Generalised contingency table for risk ratio calculations in a cohort study

Reference value

Many tables that report risk ratios (or odds ratios – see later) will contain a reference category, against which the risk ratios in other categories are compared. This reference category is usually labelled 'Reference' or given the value '1'. As an example, Figure 12.4 is taken from a cohort study to assess the main factors associated with stillbirths in a multi-ethnic English maternity population.

Number needed to treat (NNT)

A very useful and intuitively appealing way of assessing the clinical (and economic) usefulness of any intervention is to calculate the *number needed to treat* or NNT. We can interpret NNT as follows:

NNT = the number of patients you would need to give the active treatment to (rather than giving them the placebo or the control group treatment) to result in one less patient experiencing the 'bad' outcome.

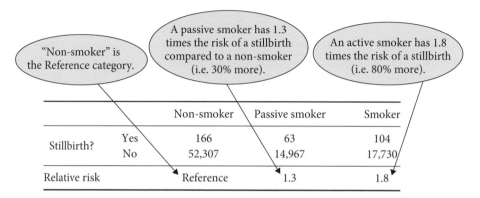

Figure 12.4 The number of stillbirths among a cohort of mothers who, while pregnant smoked, were passive smokers or were non-smokers. Taken from a prospective cohort study, showing 'Non-smoker' as the reference category (see Figure 8.3). Data from Gardosi *et al.* (2013)

NNT is easily calculated once absolute risks are known:

$$\text{NNT} = \frac{1}{\text{absolute risk reduction}}$$

In the eclampsia example described earlier, the NNT is:

$$\text{NNT} = \frac{1}{(0.3018 - 0.1272)} = \frac{1}{0.175} = 5.71$$

In other words, the treatment of six women[2] with L-arginine and antioxidant vitamins will result in one less woman experiencing pre-eclampsia or eclampsia than if the six women had received the placebo. NNT summarises this treatment effect, being a measure of the benefit of treatment with L-arginine and antioxidant vitamins compared with placebo.

Exercise 12.4. Following on from Exercises 12.1, 12.2 and 12.3, calculate NNT in each case. What does your NNT value mean?

Exercise 12.5. Figure 12.5 is from an investigation to assess the role of dutasteride in preventing the clinical progression of benign prostatic hyperplasia in asymptotic men with larger prostate. The figure contains the NNT for several individual end outcomes. Which outcome is most economically prevented? Which the least?

---

[2]Number needed to treat must be rounded up.

Outcome to be prevented	NNT
IPSS score increase ≥ 4 points	11
Acute urinary retention	16
BPH-related surgery	26
Acute urinary retention or BPH-related surgery	13
Urinary tract infection	26

Figure 12.5 Number needed to treat for various outcomes to be prevented. From a study to assess the role of dutasteride in preventing the clinical progression of benign prostatic hyperplasia in asymptotic men with larger prostate. Data from Toren *et al.* (2013)

What happens if the initial risk is small?

If the absolute risk (without treatment) is small to begin with, then the absolute risk reduction will also be small. The relative risk reduction, however, will often stay much the same and anyway will have less consequence. On top of which the NNT will be high.

I can illustrate this point with an example where the initial risk is low. The contingency table in Figure 12.6 shows the values for stillbirths and smoking while pregnant. Note that this is the same table as that shown in Figure 12.4 but the passive and active smoker categories have been amalgamated.

		Smoker or passive smoker?	
		Yes ($n = 32{,}864$)	No ($n = 52{,}639$)
Stillbirth?	Yes	167	166
	No	32 697	52 473

Figure 12.6 The number of stillbirths among a cohort of mothers who smoked (or were passive smokers), taken from a prospective cohort study (see Figure 8.3). Data from Gardosi *et al.* (2013)

We can calculate the following statistics:

- Absolute risk of stillbirth for smokers $= 167/(167 + 32697) = 0.00508$, which is very small.

- Absolute risk of stillbirth for non-smokers $= 166/(166 + 52473) = 0.00315$, which is also very small.

- Therefore, the absolute risk reduction $= 0.00193$ or 0.2 per cent, which is small.

- The risk ratio $= 0.00315/0.00508 = 0.6200$, which indicates that mothers who did not smoke while pregnant have less than two-thirds the risk of having a stillbirth than mothers who did smoke. Quite impressive it seems.

- The relative risk reduction, RRR = 1 − 0.6200 = 0.3800, which also seems quite reasonable but the absolute risk reduction shows that these figures are not quite as impressive as they might seem.

- On top of which, the number needed to treat, NNT = 1/0.00193 = 519 (rounded up), which is quite a lot of mothers to persuade not to smoke while pregnant to prevent one stillbirth, however tragic that undoubtedly would be for the mother concerned.

Confounding with the risk ratio

How can we ensure, when we calculate a risk ratio, that its value is adjusted to take into account any possible confounders? I discussed ways in which we might deal with confounding in Chapter 7, and these included some methods, which we can carry out at the design stage (e.g. matching, restrictions, and stratification) and some at the analysis stage (mainly adjustment, using regression methods). All of these methods are used with cohort studies to adjust the risk ratio, but the use of regression models is possibly the most common (see Chapters 21 and 22).

As an example of adjustment for confounders, Figure 12.7 is taken from a cohort study to investigate the frequency and risk factors for carcinogenic human papillomavirus (HPV) in 2185 sexually active young women. The adjustment for confounders in this study was achieved using regression methods. The factors adjusted for included all of those listed in the table, plus

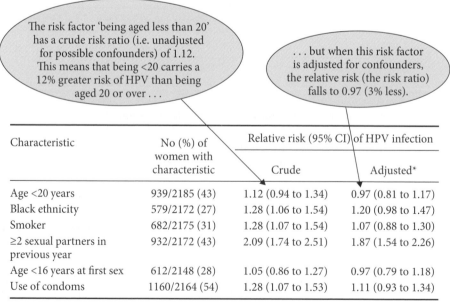

Characteristic	No (%) of women with characteristic	Relative risk (95% CI) of HPV infection	
		Crude	Adjusted*
Age <20 years	939/2185 (43)	1.12 (0.94 to 1.34)	0.97 (0.81 to 1.17)
Black ethnicity	579/2172 (27)	1.28 (1.06 to 1.54)	1.20 (0.98 to 1.47)
Smoker	682/2175 (31)	1.28 (1.07 to 1.54)	1.07 (0.88 to 1.30)
≥2 sexual partners in previous year	932/2172 (43)	2.09 (1.74 to 2.51)	1.87 (1.54 to 2.26)
Age <16 years at first sex	612/2148 (28)	1.05 (0.86 to 1.27)	0.97 (0.79 to 1.18)
Use of condoms	1160/2164 (54)	1.28 (1.07 to 1.53)	1.11 (0.93 to 1.34)

*Controlled for all significant variables from the unadjusted analysis and for age <20 and age <16 at first sex.

Figure 12.7 Risk factors for prevalent carcinogenic HPV infection ($n = 404$) in 2185 women at baseline

sexually transmitted infections (i.e. concurrent *Chlamydia trachomatis*, *Mycoplasma genitalium*, *Neisseria gonorrhoeae* or bacterial vaginosis). Note that the table includes the 95 per cent confidence intervals which I will deal with in Chapter 15.

As you can see, the difference between the crude risk ratios (relative risks in the table) and those adjusted for the various potential confounding factors differ, in some cases quite markedly. For example, young women aged <20 years old have a crude relative risk of HPV of 1.12 (12 per cent greater than those not <20 years old). But the adjusted risk ratio (relative risk) is only 0.97. We have no idea whether these values, derived from this sample of individuals, are also true of the more general population from which this sample was taken or whether it has occurred simply by chance (see Chapter 10). We need confidence intervals to answer this question – once again you will have to wait until we deal with these in Chapter 15.

Odds

We can think of the *odds* for some outcome as an alternative way of expressing probability (or risk, which we have seen is the same as probability), although it is not quite the same thing, and odds are perhaps a more difficult concept to take on board than is risk. As you have seen earlier, the probability (or risk) of a particular outcome is the number of outcomes which favour that particular outcome divided by the *total* number of outcomes. But the *odds* of a particular outcome are equal to the number of outcomes favourable to the particular outcome divided by the number of outcomes *not* favourable to the outcome.

To give a simple example, the *probability* of picking a picture card (Jack, Queen or King) from a pack of cards is 12/52 because there are 12 outcomes that favour getting a picture card[3] and 52 outcomes in total. However, the *odds* of picking a picture card is 12/40 because the number of outcomes favourable to getting a picture card is still 12, but the number of outcomes not favouring getting a picture card is 40.

Note that:

- the value of the odds for an outcome can vary from zero to infinity.

- when the odds for an outcome are less than one, the odds are *unfavourable* to the outcome; the outcome is *less* likely to happen than it is *to* happen.

- when the odds are equal to one, the outcome is as likely to happen as not.

- when the odds are greater than one, the odds are *favourable* to the outcome; the outcome is *more* likely to happen than not.

As an example, we can calculate the odds from a table such as that for the exercise and stroke case – control study as shown in Figure 12.8 (Figure 8.7 reproduced here to save you the effort of turning back many pages).

---

[3]There are 12 picture cards in a normal pack of 52 cards.

		Cases (stroke ($n = 125$))	Controls (healthy) ($n = 198$)
Exercise undertaken when	Yes	55	130
aged 15–25	No	70	68

Figure 12.8 Contingency table showing data for a sample of individuals who had or had not exercised between the ages of 15 and 25 and subsequent stroke when adult

For instance:

- Among those patients who'd *had* a stroke (the cases), 55 had exercised (been exposed to the 'risk' of exercising) and 70 had not, so the odds that those with a stroke had exercised is $55/70 = 0.7857$.

- Among those patients who *hadn't* had a stroke (the controls), 130 had exercised and 68 had not, so the odds that those who had not had a stroke had exercised is $130/68 = 1.9118$.

In other words, among those who'd had a stroke, the odds that they had exercised was 0.411 (0.7857/1.9118) – less than half the odds of those who had not had a stroke. We can conclude on the basis of this sample that exercise when young seems to confer protection against a stroke later in life. Of course we don't know if this result could have occurred just by chance or if it is *real*. We will need confidence intervals to answer this question (see Chapter 15).

Exercise 12.6.   The contingency table in Figure 12.9 is from a study exploring a possible relationship between women taking antidepressants while pregnant (some of whom were depressed and some who were not depressed[4]) and autism spectrum disorder (without intellectual disability) in their offspring. Calculate (a) the odds for depression in mothers among the cases (autism spectrum disorder), and (b) the odds among the controls. Interpret your results.

Exercise 12.7.   Figure 12.10 is from a matched case–control study into maternal smoking during pregnancy and Down syndrome (Chi-Ling *et al.* 1999). It shows the basic characteristics of mothers giving birth to babies with Down syndrome (cases) and without Down syndrome (controls). Use the information in the table to construct appropriate separate 2 × 2 contingency tables for women (a) aged under 35, and (b) aged 35 and over. In each case, calculate the odds (ignoring the Unknown category) that they had smoked during pregnancy for mothers giving birth to: (i) a Down syndrome baby, and (ii) a healthy baby. What do you conclude?

---

[4]I am not sure why someone who wasn't depressed would be taking anti-depressants.

		Number of cases (autism spectrum disorder)	Number of controls
Mother depressed during pregnancy?	Yes	7	14
	No	9	36

Figure 12.9 Contingency table showing mothers who had used antidepressant medication while pregnant, who were depressed and who were not depressed, and autistic spectrum disorder (without intellectual disability) in their offspring. Data from Rai *et al.* (2013)

		Cases (*n* = 775)	Controls (*n* = 7750)
Smoking during pregnancy?	Age < 35 years		
	Yes	112 (20.0)	1411 (20.2)
	No	421 (75.0)	5214 (74.6)
	Unknown	28 (5.0)	363 (5.2)
	Aged ≥ 35 years		
	Yes	15 (7.0)	108 (14.2)
	No	186 (86.9)	611 (80.2)
	Unknown	13 (6.1)	43 (5.6)

Figure 12.10   Basic characteristics of mothers in a case-control study of maternal smoking and Down syndrome. Data from Chi-Ling *et al.* (1999)

Why you can't calculate risk in a case–control study

For most people, the *risk* of some particular outcome, being akin to probability, makes more sense and is easier to interpret than the odds for that same outcome. That being so, maybe it would be more helpful to express the stroke/exercise result in the case–control study in Figure 12.8 as a risk rather than as odds. Unfortunately, we can't and here is why.

To calculate the risk that those with a stroke had exercised, you need to know two things: the total number who'd had a stroke and the number of those who had been exposed to the risk (of exercise). You would then divide the latter by the former. In a cohort study on the other hand, you start with healthy individuals and follow them to measure the proportion exposed to the risk factor who subsequently developed the illness. This proportion would be an estimate of the risk in the population.

However, in a case–control study, you select on the basis of whether people have some illness or condition or not. So you have one group composed of individuals who've had a stroke, and one group who have not had stroke, but *both* groups will contain individuals who were, and who were not, exposed to the risk. Moreover, you can select whatever number of cases and controls you want. You could, for example, halve the number of cases and double the number of controls. This means that the column totals, which you would otherwise need for your risk calculation, are meaningless. The result of this is that the population at risk cannot be estimated using a case–control study and so risks and risk ratios cannot be calculated. However, there is a way round this problem, as you will see shortly, when we come to calculate the odds ratio.

The link between probability and odds

The connection between probability (risk) and odds means that it is possible to derive one from another:

$$\text{risk or probablity} = \frac{\text{odds}}{(1 + \text{odds})}$$

$$\text{odds} = \frac{\text{probablity}}{1 - \text{probablity}}$$

> **Exercise 12.8.** Following on from Exercise 12.7, what is the probability that a mother chosen at random from those aged ≥ 35, will have smoked during pregnancy if they are, (a) mothers of Down syndrome babies, and (b) mothers of healthy babies?

The odds ratio

With a case–control study, you can compare the odds that those with an illness will have been exposed to the risk factor, with the odds that those who do not have the illness will have been exposed. If you divide the former by the latter, you get the *odds ratio*. In other words, an odds ratio compares the odds of acquiring the illness if exposed to the risk, with the odds of the illness if not exposed to the risk.

With Figure 12.8, you calculated the odds for the stroke and exercise study (where we are treating exercise as the risk factor) as follows:

- the odds that those with a stroke had exercised $= 55/70 = 0.7857$.

- the odds that those without a stroke had exercised $= 130/68 = 1.9118$.

- the odds ratio $= 0.7857/1.9118 = 0.4110$.

This result suggests that those with a stroke are less than half as likely to have exercised when young as the healthy controls – about 41% of the odds. It would seem that exercise is a *beneficial* 'risk' factor.

As it happens, there is a different, more useful way, of looking at the odds ratio. Let us illustrate this alternative approach with a new example. Researchers used a case–control design to investigate the odds for admission to hospital with hyperkalaemia (excessive blood potassium levels, which can be fatal) among elderly patients using spironolactone (for systolic heart failure) who were additionally prescribed either amoxicillin or trimethroprim-sulfamethoxazole (TMP-SMX) for urinary tract infection. The finger of suspicion pointed at TMP-SMX as a possible causal factor for hyperkalaemia.

Figure 12.11 shows the numbers involved in the study. The cases were patients using spironolactone plus either amoxicillin or TMP-SMX, who were admitted to hospital with hyperkalaemia. The controls were patients using spironolactone plus either amoxicillin or TMP-SMX but who were not admitted to hospital with hyperkalaemia.

Drug received	Cases (admitted with hyperkalaemia) ($n = 248$)	Controls (not admitted with hyperkalaemia) ($n = 783$)
TMP-SMX	161	162
Amoxicillin	36	325

Figure 12.11 Contingency table showing values for admission to hospital with hyperkalaemia (excessive blood potassium levels, which can be fatal) among elderly patients using spironolactone (for systolic heart failure) who were additionally prescribed either amoxicillin or trimethroprim-sulfamethoxazole (TMP-SMX). Data from Antoniou *et al.* (2011)

Odds for admission with hyperkalaemia when using TMP-SMX (rather than amoxicillin) among cases = $161/36 = 4.4722$

Odds for admission with hyperkalaemia when using TMP-SMX (rather than amoxicillin) among controls = $162/325 = 0.4985$

Thus, the odds ratio for admission with hyperkalaemia (the cases) among users of TMP-SMX compared to users of amoxicillin (the controls) was:

$$\text{Odds ratio} = \frac{4.4722}{0.4985} = 8.9720$$

So patients admitted with hyperkalaemia (the cases) had nearly nine times the odds that they had used TMP-SMX rather than amoxicillin.

Now, we come to an *alternative* way of looking at these study results. Let us face it, as health practitioners, it would be more useful if we knew the odds that a patient would develop hyperkalaemia if they were treated with SMP-TMX and not amoxicillin rather than what they might have been treated with if they have hyperkalaemia. If we know that TMP-SMX is likely to cause hyperkalaemia in patients already using spironolactone then we will not give it to them! But we would use amoxicillin instead (or some other safe antibiotic).

This alternative approach requires us to look at the contingency table 'the other way round', as you will now see.

The odds that a patient using TMP-SMX develops hyperkalaemia = $161/162 = 0.9938$

The odds that a patient using amoxicillin develops hyperkalaemia = $36/325 = 0.1108$

$$\text{So the odds ratio} = \frac{0.9939}{0.1108} = 8.9720.$$

The same result as before! So a patient using TMP-SMX has nearly nine times the odds of developing hyperkalaemia than a patient using amoxicillin. We would thus be extremely circumspect about using it. Therapeutically, this is a more useful approach. We can add that this result is statistically significant and remains so when adjusted for potential confounders (in fact, the odds increase to 12.4 times).

We can generalise the odds ratio calculation with the help of the 2×2 table shown in Figure 12.12.

The odds of exposure to the risk factor among those with the disease $= \dfrac{a}{c}$

The odds of exposure to the risk factor among the healthy controls $= \dfrac{b}{d}$

$$\text{Therefore, odds ratio} = \frac{a/c}{b/d} = \frac{ad}{bc}$$

		Cases (ill)	Controls (healthy)
Exposed	Yes	a	b
to risk?	No	c	d

Figure 12.12   Generalised 2×2 contingency table for calculation of odds ratio

Or the 'other way round':

The odds of being a case if exposed to the risk factor $= \dfrac{a}{b}$

The odds of being a control (not being a case) if exposed to the risk factor $= \dfrac{c}{d}$

$$\text{Therefore, the odds ratio} = \frac{a/b}{c/d} = \frac{ad}{bc}$$

The same result as before but therapeutically more useful.

Exercise 12.9.   Using the data in Figure 12.8, calculate the odds of having a stroke among those who had exercised compared to those who had not.

Exercise 12.10.   Use the results from Exercise 12.8 to calculate: (a) the odds ratio for smoking among the mothers of Down syndrome babies compared to mothers of healthy babies for: (i) mothers aged under 35, (ii) mothers aged 35 and over. (b) Now, do it the other way round, that is, calculate the odds ratio of a mother having a Down syndrome baby if she smoked while pregnant. (c)Interpret your results in both approaches.

Confounding with the odds ratio

How can we adjust for confounders when we calculate odds ratios? I discussed ways in which we might deal with confounding in Chapter 7, both at the design stage (e.g. matching, restriction, and stratification) and at the analysis stage (mainly adjustment, using regression methods). All of these methods can be used, but the use of logistic regression is a particularly popular method to calculate the odds ratios from case–control studies because it is a comparatively easy way of adjusting odds ratios for confounders – easier than adjusting risk ratios in a cohort study. (I will discuss logistic regression in Chapter 22).

Approximating the risk ratio from the odds ratio

I had mentioned earlier that the population at risk cannot be estimated using a case–control study, and so risks and risk ratios cannot be calculated. However, there is a happy ending. The sample odds ratio in a case–control study is an estimator of the population odds ratio, which in turn is a reasonably good estimator of the equivalent population risk ratio *but only if the illness or condition is rare*, usually taken to be less than 10 per cent. In these circumstances, this means that odds ratios can be adjusted for confounders using logistic regression and the results interpreted as adjusted risk ratios. This is a bit of a back door way of using the comparatively easy logistic regression approach for the adjustment of risk ratios for which other methods, although available, are less straightforward.

/

> **Exercise 12.11.** Using the formulae for risk ratio and odds ratio given earlier, can you show that they are approximately the same when the condition (illness) is rare?

Remember that the risk ratios and odds ratios referred to in this chapter are *sample* values. We need to know whether these values are true reflections of the situation in the corresponding populations. I will address this problem when we discuss confidence intervals for the ratios in Chapter 15.

VI

The Informed Guess – An Introduction to Confidence Intervals

13

Estimating the value of a *single* population parameter – the idea of confidence intervals

---

Learning objectives

When you have finished this chapter, you should be able to:

- Describe the sampling distribution of the sample mean and the characteristics of its distribution.

- Explain what the standard error of the sample mean is and calculate its value.

- Explain how you can use the probability properties of the Normal distribution to measure the preciseness of the sample mean as an estimator of the population mean.

- Derive an expression for the confidence interval of the population mean.

- Calculate and interpret a 95 per cent confidence interval for a population mean.

- Calculate and interpret a 95 per cent confidence interval for a population proportion.

- Explain and interpret a 95 per cent confidence interval for a population median.

Medical Statistics from Scratch: An Introduction for Health Professionals, Third Edition. David Bowers.
© 2014 John Wiley & Sons, Ltd. Published 2014 by John Wiley & Sons, Ltd.

Confidence interval estimation for a population mean

To give you an idea what a confidence interval is, suppose, contemplating a trip to Iran, you ask your travel agent, 'How hot is it at this time of year in Tehran?' She answers, 'I'm pretty certain that it's going to be between 30°C and 40°C'. She is providing you with a *confidence interval*. She is *estimating* what the the actual temperature will be, based on her knowledge and experience. And she is 'pretty certain'. This is her *level of confidence,* although you cannot be too sure exactly what this means. Does it mean she is 50 per cent sure? or 90 per cent sure? If a doctor tells a terminally ill patient that in her experience nine out of 10 patients do not survive more than a year, she can say that she is 90 per cent confident that the patient will not survive a year. The doctor is 90 per cent confident. The doctor is also making an *estimate* based on her experience and knowledge.

You saw at the beginning of Chapter 10 that we can use a sample statistic to make an informed guess, or *estimate,* of the value of the corresponding *population* parameter. For example, the sample mean birthweight for the 100 babies in Figure 1.1 is 3251.8 g, so we can estimate that the population mean birthweight of *all* infants of whom this sample is representative, will also will be *about* 3251.8 g, *plus or minus* some (hopefully) small random or sampling, error (see Chapter 10 for a reminder of sampling error). The value of the sample mean of 3251.8 g is known as the *point estimate* of the population mean. It is the *single best guess* you could make as to the value of the population mean. The crucial questions seem to be:

- How small is this 'plus or minus' bit? Can it be *quantified?*

- Can we establish how *precise* our *sample* mean birthweight is as an estimate of population mean birthweight?

- How close to the population mean can you expect any given sample mean to be?

As you can see, these are all essentially the same question, 'How big an *error* might we be making when we use the sample mean as an estimate of the population mean?' This question can be answered with what is known as a *confidence interval*, which is a numeric expression that quantifies the likely size of the sampling error. But to be able to calculate a confidence interval, we need first to introduce an important concept in statistical inference – the *standard error.*

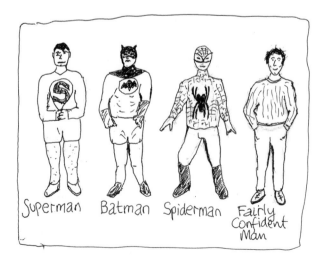

The standard error of the mean

Standard error comes with a health warning. From over 20 years of teaching medical statistics to medical students, doctors, nurses and other health professionals, I have discovered that many people find the concept difficult (not you of course!). Here goes. We can use a computer program (SPSS, Minitab, Stata, etc.) to calculate the mean birthweight of a sample of 100 babies' birthweights as shown in Figure 1.1 to be 3251.8 g. This value is our *point estimate* of the corresponding population mean. Remember, we do not actually know what the population mean is, but we hope that the value of our sample mean is close to the population mean value (it is unlikely to be exactly the same except by a remarkable coincidence).

As we noted in Chapter 10, any difference between our point estimate of 3251.8 g and the unknown population mean will be due to *sampling error*, that is, the error introduced because we are working with a sample and not the population itself. We can judge (quantify) the accuracy of our sample mean as an estimate of the population mean with the help of the value of the *standard error of the mean*, usually abbreviated to *standard error*, and we do this by using the standard error to calculate a confidence interval (which we will come to shortly). But what is the standard error?

To explain, suppose that you could take a second sample of 100 infants from the same population. This sample would produce a different value for the sample mean birthweight than the first sample (coincidentally it could be the same – possible but unlikely). And a third sample, and a fourth and so on, would each give you a different sample mean value. In fact, from any realistic population you could (*in theory*), take a huge number of different same-size samples, each of which would produce a different sample mean. Now, imagine that you took *all* possible samples of a given size from a population and calculated the sample mean for each sample, you would find that the distribution of all of these sample means:

- is Normal. This Normal-ness of the distribution of sample means is a very useful quality (to say the least); we will depend on it a lot in what is to come.

- is centred around the true population mean. In other words, the mean of all possible sample means is the same as the population mean.

This is very reassuring because it means that, *on average,* the sample mean estimates the population mean exactly. But note the 'on average'. All of the above is *completely theoretical.* You do not get to take all possible samples; in fact, you normally get to take only one. Whether its sample mean value is close to the population mean, or further away, you have no way of knowing because you do not know what the value of the population mean actually is. The good news is that your sample mean is more likely to be closer to the middle of the distribution rather than further away simply because there are are more values closer to the centre. However, the confidence interval (coming shortly!) will give you some indication of how close your sample mean is to the population mean.

Figure 13.1 illustrates the scenario mentioned earlier. This shows a hypothetical distribution of the sample means of a large number of samples taken from some population (so not *all* possible sample means but a large number anyway). It has a Normal curve superimposed upon it to give an indication of how close the distribution is to Normal (and if it was *all* possible sample means of a given size, the distribution would be perfectly Normal). The distribution is centred around the (unknown) population mean. Because the distribution is Normal, three standard errors on either side of the central value will include approximately 99 per cent of all sample

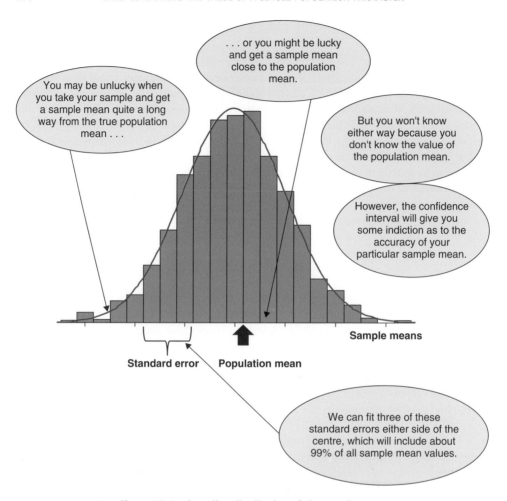

Figure 13.1 Sampling distribution of the sample mean

means (just as there are three standard deviations on either side of a Normally distributed single sample). This means that when you take a sample and calculate the sample mean, there is only a one per cent chance that your sample mean will be further than three standard errors (on either side) from the population mean.

The standard error is usually abbreviated as s.e.$(\bar{x})$, where the symbol $\bar{x}$ stands for the sample mean. Remember that the standard deviation is a measure of the spread of the data in a *single* sample, whereas the standard error is a measure of the spread in *all* (same-size) possible sample means from a population. We can *estimate* the standard error with the equation:

$$\text{s.e.}(\bar{x}) = \frac{s}{\sqrt{n}}.$$

where s is the sample standard deviation and n is the sample size. Notice that as the sample size n increases, the estimated standard error decreases. In other words, the bigger the sample, the smaller is the error in our estimate of population mean. Intuitively, this feels right.

As the distribution of sample means is Normal, we can make use of the area properties of the Normal distribution (see Figure 6.7). If the sample standard deviation is 550 g and the sample size $n = 100$, then the standard error $= (550/\sqrt{100})g = 55$ g. Because the distribution of sample means is Normal, this means that about 95 per cent of sample means will lie within plus or minus two standard errors of the population mean. That is within plus or minus 2×55 g or 110 g of the population mean. In other words, there is a pretty good chance (a probability of 0.95 in fact) that any single sample mean will be no further than 110 g from the (unknown) population mean.

The earlier discussion about taking lots of different samples from a population is entirely theoretical. In practice, as we noted previously, you will usually only get to take *one* sample from a population, the value of whose mean you will never know. To sum up, the standard error is the measure of the preciseness of the sample mean as an estimator of the population mean. *Smaller is better.* If you are comparing the precision of two different sample means as estimates of a population mean, the sample mean with the smallest standard error is likely to be the more precise.

Exercise 13.1.   A team of researchers used a cohort study to investigate the intake of vitamins E and C, and the risk of lung cancer, Yong *et al.* (1997). Nineteen years into the study, they calculated the mean (and the standard error) intake of vitamins E and C, of the individuals with and without lung cancer. These were:

Vitamin E: Lung cancer 6.03 mg (0.35 mg). Not lung cancer 6.30 mg (0.05 mg)

Vitamin C: Lung cancer 64.18 mg (5.06 mg). Not lung cancer 82.21 mg (0.80 mg).

How would you interpret these results in terms of the likely precision of each of the sample means as estimators of their respective population means?

How we use the standard error of the mean to calculate a confidence interval for a population mean

With the standard error under our belt, we can now get to grips with the *confidence interval.* Just as a reminder (think back to the holiday in Iran mentioned earlier), a confidence interval is a range of values within which you can have a certain level of confidence (invariably 95 per cent) that some population parameter (the population mean in this case) is to be found.

You have seen that we can be 95 per cent confident that any sample mean is going to be within *plus or minus two standard errors* of the population mean. With some arithmetical manipulation, we can use this fact to show that:

- we can be 95 per cent confident that the interval from the sample mean $- (2 \times$ standard error) to the sample mean $+ (2 \times$ standard error) will include the population mean.

- or in probability terms, there is a probability of 0.95 that the interval from the sample mean $- (2 \times$ standard error) to the sample mean $+ (2 \times$ standard error) will contain the population mean.

In other words, if you pick one out of all the possible sample means at random, there is a probability of 0.95 that it will lie within two standard errors of the population mean. In other words, *the 95 per cent confidence interval for the population mean* is given by the expression:

$$[\bar{x} - 2 \times \text{s.e.}(\bar{x})] \text{ to } [\bar{x} + 2 \times \text{s.e.}(\bar{x})]$$

where $\bar{x}$ is the sample mean and s.e.$(\bar{x})$ is the standard error of the sample mean (see above). Note that in practice, instead of the value 2, computers will use an appropriate value from the *t distribution*. The t distribution is similar to the Normal distribution (but slightly flatter and wider), and the similarity increases as sample size increases. In most situations, this value will be very close to 2,[1] so the above approximation is not too far out.

The above result means that you now quantify just how close a sample mean is likely to be to the population mean. A 95 per cent *confidence level* is most common, but 99 per cent confidence intervals are also used on occasion. Note that the confidence interval is sometimes said to represent a *plausible range of values* for the population parameter.

An example from practice

In the histogram in Figure 4.6, the mean cord platelet count in a sample of 4382 infants is 306×10^9/l, and the standard deviation is 69×10^9/l, so the standard error of the mean is:

$$\text{s.e.}(\bar{x}) = \frac{69 \times 10^9}{\sqrt{4382}} = 1.042 \times 10^9 \text{ per litre}$$

Therefore, the 95 per cent confidence interval for the population mean cord platelet count is:

$$(306 - 2 \times 1.042) \times 10^9 /\text{l to } (306 + 2 \times 1.042) \times 10^9 /\text{l}$$

or

$$(303.92 \text{ to } 308.08) \times 10^9 /\text{l}$$

which we can interpret as follows: we can be 95 per cent confident that the interval from 303.92×10^9/l to 308.08×10^9/l, will contain the population mean cord platelet count. Alternatively, there is a probability of 0.95 that the interval from 303.92 to 308.08 will contain the

---

[1] For example, when $n = 50$, $t = 2.009$; when $n = 100$, $t = 1.984$; when $n = 200$, $t = 1.972$ and when $n = 1000$, $t = 1.962$.

population mean value. Of course there is also a 5 per cent chance (or a 0.05 probability) that it will not!

Alternatively, we can say that the interval $(303.916 - 308.084) \times 10^9/l$ represents a *plausible range of values* for the population mean cord platelet count. The narrower the confidence interval, the more precise is the estimator. In the cord platelet example, the small width, and therefore high precision of the confidence interval, is because of the large sample. By the way, it is a good practice to put the confidence interval in brackets and to use the 'to' in the middle and not a '−' sign or a hyphen as this may be confusing if the confidence interval has a negative value.

Exercise 13.2. Use the summary age measures given in Figure 1.7 for the life events and breast cancer study to calculate the standard error and the 95 per cent confidence intervals for the population mean age of (a) the cases, and (b) the controls. Interpret your confidence intervals. What do you make of the fact that the two confidence intervals do not overlap?

An example from practice

The results shown in Figure 13.2 are from a randomised trial to evaluate the use of an integrated care scheme for asthma patients, in which care is shared between the GP and a specialist chest physician (ignore the last column for now – we will discuss the ratio of the means in Chapter 15). The treatment group patients each received this integrated care, the control group received conventional care – from their GP only. The researchers were interested in the differences between the groups, if any, in a number of outcomes shown in the figure (ignore the last column for now). The target population they have in mind is, perhaps, all asthma patients in the UK.

You can see that in the integrated care group of 296 subjects, the *sample* mean number of bronchodilators prescribed over 12 months was 10.1, with a 95 per cent confidence interval for the *population* mean of (9.2 – 11.1). So you can be 95 per cent confident that somewhere between 9.2 and 11.1 is to be found the population mean number of bronchodilators prescribed for this group. In the control group, the sample mean is 10.6 with a 95 per cent confidence interval for the population mean (9.7 – 11.7), which can be similarly interpreted.

Exercise 13.3. Interpret and compare the sample mean number of hospital admissions and their corresponding confidence intervals for the two groups in Figure 13.2.

Exercise 13.4. For the 100 birthweights shown in Figure 1.1, the mean birthweight is 3251.8 g and the standard deviation is 564.2 g. Calculate the 95 per cent confidence interval for the population mean birthweight. How would you interpret this?

Clinical outcome	Integrated care (n ≥ 296)	Conventional care (n ≥ 277)	Ratio of means
No. of bronchodilators prescribed	10.1 (9.2 to 11.1)	10.6 (9.7 to 11.7)	0.95 (0.83 to 1.09)
No. of inhaled steroids prescribed	6.4 (5.9 to 6.9)	6.5 (6.1 to 7.1)	0.98 (0.88 to 1.09)
No. of courses of oral steroids used	1.6 (1.4 to 1.8)	1.6 (1.4 to 1.9)	0.97 (0.79 to 1.20)
No. of general practice asthma consultations	2.7 (2.4 to 3.1)	2.5 (2.2 to 2.8)	1.11 (0.95 to 1.31)
No. of hospital admissions for asthma	0.15 (0.11 to 0.19)	0.11 (0.08 to 0.15)	1.31 (0.87 to 1.96)

Figure 13.2   Means and 95 per cent confidence intervals for a number of clinical outcomes over 12 months, for asthma patients. The treatment group patients received integrated care, the control group conventional GP care. Data from Grampian Asthma Study of Integrated Care (1994)

Confidence intervals as described before can also be applied to a population *percentage*, provided that the values are percentages of a metric variable (e.g. percentage mortality across a number of ICUs, see Figure 2.14). However, if the proportion in question is a response to a question such as alive or dead, malignant or benign, pre-menopausal, peri-menopausal or post-menopausal. Then the approach described below is appropriate.

Confidence interval for a population proportion

Suppose that we administer a drug to a sample of 100 patients with suspected myocardial infarction and 80 respond positively; then, the sample proportion, p, of positive responses is:

$$p = \frac{80}{100} = 0.80$$

In general, if the sample size is n and there are r positive responses, then, the *sample* proportion p, is:

$$p = \frac{r}{n}$$

We want to know what the 95 per cent confidence interval is for a *population* proportion. The sampling distribution of the sample proportion has a binomial distribution (see Chapter 11 for a brief mention of the binomial distribution) and so the approach that we need to get a confidence interval for a population proportion would be based on the binomial distribution, which is quite complicated. However, provided that the proportion is not too close to 0.1 or to 0.9, and the sample size not too small,[2] as will usually be the case, then we can use the *Normal*

---

[2] As a rule of thumb, np and $n(1 - p)$ should both exceed 5.

approximation to the binomial distribution to address this question – which makes things a lot easier. In these circumstances, the standard error of the sample proportion is:

$$\text{s.e.}(p) = \sqrt{\frac{p(1-p)}{n}}$$

where p is the sample proportion and n is sample size.

The 95 per cent confidence interval for the population proportion has a similar structure to that for the population mean and it is equal to the sample proportion plus or minus 1.96[3] standard errors:

$$[p - 1.96 \times \text{s.e.}(p)] \text{ to } [p + 1.96 \times \text{s.e.}(p)]$$

For example, as shown in Figure 1.7, 14 of the 106 women with a malignant diagnosis were pre-menopausal giving a sample proportion p of 14/106 or 0.13. The standard error of p is thus:

$$\text{s.e.}(p) = \sqrt{\frac{0.13(1-0.13)}{106}} = 0.0327$$

Therefore, the 95 per cent confidence interval for the population proportion who are pre-menopausal is:

$$(0.13 - 1.96 \times 0.0327) \text{ to } (0.13 + 1.96 \times 0.0327) = (0.0659 \text{ to } 0.1941)$$

In other words, you can be 95 per cent confident that the proportion of cases in this population who are pre-menopausal lies somewhere between 0.066 and 0.194 or between 6.6 per cent and 19.4 per cent.

Exercise 13.5.　From Figure 1.3, we can discover that the number of mothers who smoked while pregnant was 77 out of 500. Calculate the 95 per cent confidence interval for the population proportion of mothers who smoked. Comment on your result.

As a further example, Figure 13.3 shows an example of the use of 95 per cent confidence intervals with percentages. This is from a study investigating the efficacy of a recently approved drug (etanercept) as a treatment option for patients with psoriasis and active psoriatic arthritis.

The participants in this trial were suffering from psoriasis and were randomly allocated to receive etanercept *either* biweekly in a blinded randomised controlled trial, then once weekly in an open-label trial, for 12 weeks, *or* once weekly in a blinded RCT, followed by once weekly in an open-label trial. The table shows the percentage of patients achieving various ACR criteria,[4] along with 95 per cent confidence intervals, for both arms of the trial.

---

[3] When we deal with proportions, we use, not the t distribution but the z or *Standard Normal* distribution. The 95 per cent value for z is 1.96.

[4] American College of Rheumatology (ACR) Criteria. This is a scale to count the number of tender or swollen joints, with scores of ACR20, ACR50 and ACR70. For example, if 55 per cent of patients scored ACR20, then

	Etanercept 50 mg. Twice weekly then once weekly ($n = 379$)	Etanercept 50 mg Once weekly then once weekly ($n = 373$)
Participants achieving ACR response		
ACR 20 week 12	239/360 (66.4, 61.3 to 71.3)	219/360 (60.8, 55.6 to 65.9)
ACR 20 week 24	249/361 (69.0, 63.9 to 73.7)	258/360 (71.7, 66.7 to 76.3)
ACR 50 week 12	161/360 (44.7, 39.5 to 50.0)	146/360 (40.6, 35.4 to 45.8)
ACR 50 week 24	187/361 (51.8, 46.5 to 57.1)	193/360 (53.6, 48.3 to 58.9)
ACR 70 week 12	73/360 (20.3, 16.2 to 24.8)	79/360 (21.9, 17.8 to 26.6)
ACR 70 week 24	125/361 (34.6, 29.7 to 39.8)	132/360 (36.7, 31.7 to 41.9)

Figure 13.3 The table is an abbreviated extract from a study to compare the efficacy of two different etanercept regimens in the treatmentof skin manifestations of psoriasis. It shows the percentage of patients achieving American College of Rheumatology (ACR) criteria in both arms of the trial. In one arm, patients received biweekly treatment for 12 weeks with etanercept in a randomised controlled trial, followed by weekly treatment for 12 weeks in an open-label trial. In the other arm patients received *once* weekly treatment for 12 weeks in *both* periods. Data from Sterry *et al.* (2010)

Exercise 13.6. What are the point estimates of the percenatge of patients achieving ACR 20 in week 12 in each of the two groups? Which treatment regimen therefore appears to be the most successful for this criterion?

Exercise 13.7. Figure 13.4 is from a study to determine the association between the concentration of prostate specific antigen (PSA) at an age of 40–55 and the subsequent risk of prostate cancer metastasis and mortality in an unscreened population, in order to evaluate when to start screening for prostate cancer and whether rescreening could be risk stratified. The figure shows the proportion of deaths or metastases from prostate cancer captured by respective categories of increased concentrations of PSA for the same individuals at age 45–49 and 51–55. Compare the proportions and the precision of the confidence intervals for death and metastases for the highest tenth of PSA in each age group.

Estimating a confidence interval for the median of a single population

If your data is ordinal then the median rather than the mean is the appropriate measure of location (review Chapter 5 if you are not sure why). Alternatively, if your data is metric but

---

that means 55 per cent of the patients in the study achieved a 20 per cent improvement in tender or swollen joint counts as well as a 20 per cent improvement in three of the other five criteria. If a clinical trial reports that 40 per cent of patients scored ACR50, then that means 40 per cent of the patients in the study achieved a 50 per cent improvement in tender or swollen joint counts as well as 50 per cent improvement in three of the other five criteria.

	PSA concentration (µg/l)	Proportion (95% CI)	
		Deaths ($n = 245$)	Metastases ($n = 235$)
Age 45–49 at baseline screen			
Highest 10th	≥1.6	44 (34 to 53)	40 (33 to 48)
Highest quarter	≥1.06	54 (45 to 63)	51 (44 to 59)
Below median	<0.68	28 (20 to 37)	28 (22 to 35)
Age 51–55 at second screen			
Highest 10th	≥2.4	44 (32 to 56)	42 (32 to 52)
Highest quarter	≥1.4	59 (47 to 71)	56 (46 to 66)
Below median	<0.85	16 (7 to 25)	18 (10 to 26)

Figure 13.4 The proportion of deaths or metastases from prostate cancer captured by respective categories of increased concentrations of PSA at age 45–49 or 51–55. Data from Vickers *et al.* (2013)

skewed (or your sample is too small to check the distributional shape), you might also prefer the median as a more representative measure. Either way, a confidence interval will enable you to assess the likely range of values for the population median.

Calculation of a confidence interval for a single median is not as straightforward as that for a mean or a proportion. Methods, such as *bootstrapping*,[5] are available, although not overwhelmingly common in mainstream journals. As far as my knowledge goes, SPSS does not calculate a confidence interval for a single median but Minitab does and bases its calculation on the *Wilcoxon signed-rank* test[6] (I will discuss this test in Chapter 16).

As an example, Figure 13.5 shows the sample median and 95 per cent confidence interval for mothers' weight at booking, among the mothers of a sample of 500 infants from the Born in Bradford study, reproduced from Minitab and derived from the Wilcoxon signed-rank test. As you can see, the 95 per cent confidence interval for the population median mothers' weight at booking was (65.00–68.00) kg. Examples of confidence intervals for single medians are not easy to find among the more common clinical papers.

Wilcoxon Signed Rank CI: mum bkg wt					
				Confidence Interval	
	N	Median	Achieved Confidence	Lower	Upper
mum bkg wt	500	66.50	95.0	65.00	68.00

Figure 13.5 Median and 95 per cent confidence interval for mothers' weight at booking for a sample of 500 infants. Produced by Minitab using data from the Born in Bradford study (2012)

---

[5] Bootstrapping involves the repeated sampling (with replacement) of the original sample to produce a great many samples. The required statistic is computed for each sample and the results amalgamated.

[6] We will not deal with hypothesis tests until we get to Chapter 16, but the confidence intervals, which I discuss in this chapter and in the next chapter, are based on a number of such tests. The alternative would have been for me to introduce hypothesis tests before I deal with confidence intervals. However, for various pedagogic reasons I did not think this was appropriate.

	Randomised* ($n = 48$)	Declined[†] ($n = 31$)
Registered patients	7142 (4372 to 8830)	5524 (3014 to 8211)
Female doctors within a practice (%)	45.3 (10.6 to 53.5)	47.9 (32.5 to 66.5)
Postgraduate training practice		
Yes	29 (60%)	14 (50%)
No	19 (40%)	14 (50%)
Registered patients on low income (%)	32 (13 to 34)	20 (9 to 30)

Data are median (interquartile range) or n (%).
*The randomised group excludes three practices that were opted out.
[†]Three results missing for teaching practice and list size. Six missing for income, seven missing for percentage of female doctors.

Figure 13.6   Characteristics of practices randomised compared with those of practices that declined. From a study to test the effectiveness of a programme to identify victims of domestic violence in general practice. Data from Feder *et al.* (2011)

Exercise 13.8.   Figure 13.6 is taken from a cluster randomised controlled trial in the introduction to which the researchers stated:

> Most clinicians have no training about domestic violence, fail to identify patients experiencing abuse, and are uncertain about management after disclosure. We tested the effectiveness of a programme of training and support in primary health-care practices to increase identification of women experiencing domestic violence and their referral to specialist advocacy services.
>
> *Feder* et al. *(2011)*

General practices were randomly allocated to intervention (which included practice-based training sessions, a prompt within the medical record to ask about abuse and a referral pathway to a named domestic violence advocate). The table shows the characteristics of those practices that were included in the study and those that were declined. Interpret and compare the median and interquartile range values for the number of registered patients and the percentage of female doctors in the included and the declined practices. If you feel so inclined, draw boxplots of the percentage of female doctors (I know that the minimum and maximum values are missing, but the boxes are quite illuminating on their own). What is the relative skew of the two distributions?

14

Using confidence intervals to compare two population parameters

Learning objectives

When you have finished this chapter, you should be able to:

- Give some examples of situations where there is a need to estimate the difference between two population parameters.

- Briefly outline the basis for the estimation of the difference between two population means, first with two independent populations and second with two matched populations.

- Briefly outline the basis of estimation of the difference between two population medians using methods based on the Mann–Whitney test (for independent populations) and the Wilcoxon test (for matched populations).

- Interpret results from studies that estimate the difference between two population means, two proportions or two medians.

- Demonstrate an awareness of any assumptions that must be satisfied when estimating the difference between two population parameters.

Medical Statistics from Scratch: An Introduction for Health Professionals, Third Edition. David Bowers.
© 2014 John Wiley & Sons, Ltd. Published 2014 by John Wiley & Sons, Ltd.

What's the difference?

As you saw in the previous chapter, we can calculate a confidence interval for any *single* population parameter; for example, a population mean, a median and a proportion. However, a more frequent use of confidence intervals is to compare *two* population parameters to see if they are the same. For example, whether two population means or two population proportions are the same.

I will start with the difference between two population means, and we have two situations to deal with: first when the two populations are *independent* and second when they are matched or *paired* (see Chapter 5 to review matching). Let us begin with independent populations.

Comparing two *independent* population means

Suppose that the mean of one population is μ_A and of another population is μ_B. To calculate a confidence interval for the difference between two population means ($\mu_A - \mu_B$), we again, as we did with the confidence interval for a single mean in Chapter 13, use the t distribution along with the associated standard error. However, with two populations it is the standard error of *the difference between two means*. The formula for the 95 per cent confidence interval for the difference between the means of two independent populations looks like this:

$$[(\bar{x}_1 - \bar{x}_2) - 2 \times \text{s.e.}(\bar{x}_1 - \bar{x}_2)] \text{ to } [(\bar{x}_1 - \bar{x}_2) + 2 \times \text{s.e.}(\bar{x}_1 - \bar{x}_2)]$$

where $\bar{x}_1$ is the sample mean from the first population and $\bar{x}_2$ is the sample mean from the second population and s.e.$(\bar{x}_1 - \bar{x}_2)$ is the standard error of the sampling distribution of the difference in the two sample means.[1] The formula for s.e.$(\bar{x}_1 - \bar{x}_2)$ is a bit too complex for us to deal with here, and in any case you will not be calculating it by hand.

To use a t distribution-based confidence interval for the difference in the two independent population means, we need to satisfy the following three requirements:

- Data for both populations must be *metric*. As you know from Chapter 5, the mean is only appropriate with metric data anyway.

- The distribution of the relevant variable in *each* population must be reasonably *Normal*. You can check this assumption from the sample data using a histogram, although with small sample sizes this can be difficult.

- The population standard deviations of the two variables concerned should be *approximately* the same, but this requirement becomes less important as sample sizes get larger. You can check this by examining the values of the two sample standard deviations.[2]

What do we do if these requirements are not met? We will deal with this later in this chapter when we discuss the Mann–Whitney procedure.

---

[1] Note that a computer will use a value from the t distribution rather than the value 2 (see Chapter 13 for a note on this).
[2] This condition is usually stated in terms of the two *variances* being approximately the same. Variance is standard deviation squared.

An example using birthweights

Suppose that your question is, for the babies in the Born in Bradford study, 'Is there any difference in the mean birthweight between babies born to mothers who smoked while pregnant and babies whose mothers did not smoke?' We first need to establish if these two populations (smokers and non-smokers) satisfy the three criteria.

- First: the two populations are independent because all of the participants started out in the same group in this cohort study, and smoking status was only determined subsequently.

- Second: both distributions appear to be approximately Normal if the shapes of the two histograms are anything to go by (see Figure 14.1, produced using Minitab).

- Third: the spreads of the two populations appear to be similar, judging by the values of the two sample standard deviations, which Minitab calulates as 552 g (smokers) and 567 g (non-smokers), respectively.

Therefore, we can use the method based on the *t* distribution. Minitab produces the results as shown in Figure 14.2. You can see that the difference in *sample* means is 33.3 g, but bear in mind that just because the two sample means are not the same (and they invariably are not), it doesn't

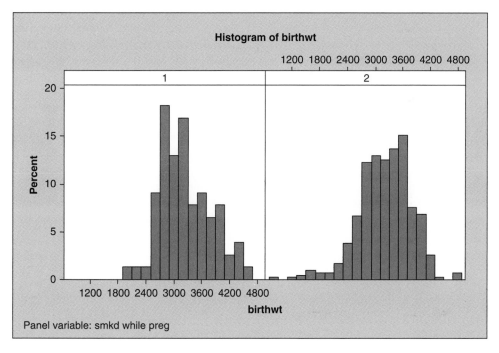

Figure 14.1 Histograms of birthweight for babies born to mothers who smoked while pregnant (left-hand panel) and those who did not. The distributions are both approximately Normal – Normal enough anyway to satisfy the distributional requirements of the *t* distribution. Data from 500 babies in the Born in Bradford study

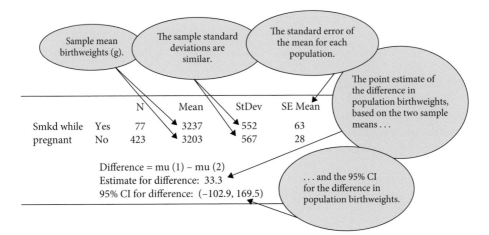

Figure 14.2 Output (edited slightly) from Minitab, showing the 95 per cent confidence interval for the difference in population mean birthweights between the babies of mothers who smoked while pregnant and those who did not. Minitab uses 'mu' to represent the population mean (usually denoted by μ)

follow that the population means are also not the same. This is because a sample is inevitably an imperfect representation of the population it was drawn from. The two population means could be the same and any difference in the sample means could just be due to chance. This is why we need to calculate a confidence interval to rule out this possibility.

Minitab calculates the 95 per cent confidence interval for the difference in population mean birthweights to be (-102.9 to 169.5) g. SPSS produces the results as shown in Figure 14.3. Notice the slight difference in the values given for the confidence interval. This difference arises from the slightly different computational methods used by the two programs.

> **Exercise 14.1.**   Can you think of one reason why the standard error of the smokers (in Figure 14.2) is considerably greater than that of the non-smokers.

Now, we come to a very important rule. If two population means are identical and if we are to subtract one from the other, the result would be 0. If the two means are not the same, the result would not be 0. We can use this idea to give us a rule for interpreting a confidence interval for the difference between two population parameters, thus:

> If the 95 per cent confidence interval for the difference between two population parameters includes zero, then you can be 95 per cent confident that there is *no* difference in the two parameter values. If the interval *doesn't* contain zero, then you can be 95 per cent confident that there *is* a statistically significant difference in the parameters.

In other words, if you want to know if there is a statistically significant difference between two population means, calculate the 95 per cent confidence interval for the difference and see if

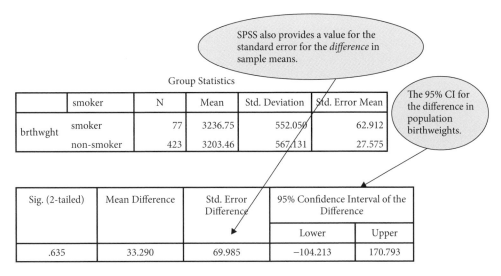

Figure 14.3 Output (edited slightly) from SPSS, showing the 95 per cent confidence interval for the difference in population mean birthweights between the babies of mothers who smoked while pregnant and those who did not. Source: McCreadie *et al.* (1998). Reproduced by permission of BMJ Publishing Group Ltd

it contains zero. If it does, the means are most probably the same. But bear in mind that there is a five per cent chance that the means are not the same. In our birthweights example, and using Minitab's results, the confidence interval from (−102.9 to 169.5) g includes 0, so we can be 95 per cent confident that the population mean birthweight of the babies whose mothers smoked while pregnant is the same as that of the babies whose mothers did not smoke.

Assessing the evidence using the confidence interval (and was the sample size large enough?)

There are two other important points that I must mention. First, even though this confidence interval includes 0, the most likely value for the difference in population means is still the *point estimate* of the difference in sample birthweights, that is, 33 g. Or to interpret the confidence interval in a slightly different way, there probably is a difference in birthweights, and it is likely to be closer to 33 g than it is to either −102.9 g or 169.5 g.

The second point relates to the way we assess the evidence contained in the confidence interval about the likely difference in the population means (and what it tells us about the adequacy of the sample size). I can best illustrate this idea with Figure 14.4. This shows four 95 per cent confidence intervals, each represented by a Normal curve. The height of the Normal curve anywhere in its range corresponds to the probability that the true difference in population means is likely to be found. So most likely under the middle bit of the curve, less likely as we move into the tails of the curve. The confidence intervals are for the percentage *decrease* in systolic blood pressure (SBP) from each of the four hypothetical trials of a new drug to reduce hypertension (compared to an established drug). The horizontal axes show the change in SBP (decreases

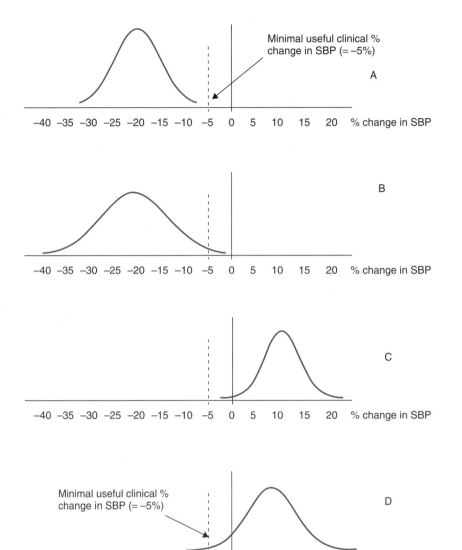

Figure 14.4   Four 95 percent confidence intervals (shown as Normal curves) for four hypothetical trials of a new drug to treat hypertension. The horizontal axes show the change in systolic blood pressure for each trial. Also shown is the percentage minimal useful clinical change (of −5 percent)

to the right). Let us assume that to make the introduction of the new drug worthwhile, the minimal clinical useful percentage decrease has to be 5 per cent.

In trial A, the *point estimate* of the decrease in SBP is −20 mmHg (under the peak of the confidence interval curve), and this represents the most likely true value for the decrease in percentage SBP. As we move away, both to left and to right from this value, there is less and less likelihood that values reflect the true decrease in SBP, as is reflected in the declining height (i.e. the probability) of the Normal curve. The confidence interval, (−28 to −12)%, does *not* include 0, and the top end exceeds the minimal useful clinical percentage decrease. As these two conditions are satisfied, we can say that trial A is both *positive* (statistically significant) and *definitive* (conclusive).

In trial B, with a smaller sample size than trial A, and thus a wider confidence interval of (−30 to −10)%, the point estimate of the decrease in SBP is again 20 per cent, and the confidence interval (as in trial A) does *not* include 0, so the trial is significant (*positive*). But the upper limit of the confidence interval is less than the clinically useful decrease in SBP of 5 per cent, so this result is positive but *not conclusive (not definitive)*. This implies that the sample size was possibly too small. If the sample had been larger, it would have produced a narrower confidence interval, and the top end of the confidence interval might shift enough to the left, to exceed the minimal clinically useful decrease of 5 per cent.

In trial C (with a small sample size), the point estimate of the decrease in SBP was +10 mmHg, so this is the most likely value for the difference in SBPs. The confidence interval of (−2 to 22)%, includes 0, so the trial is not significant (i.e. is deemed *negative)*. And because the lower value is less than the clinically useful decrease in SBP of 5 per cent, the trial is both negative and *definitive* – there is no point in an increased sample size as this would produce a narrower confidence interval, which would shift both ends of the curve inwards, and the left-hand end would be even further away from the mimimal clinically useful decrease.

The sample size in trial D is smaller than in trial C. The point estimate of the decrease in SBP was +10 mmHg as in trial C. The confidence interval includes 0 so the trial is *negative*. But because the lower limit of the confidence interval exceeds the clinically useful decrease in SBP of 5 per cent, the trial does not completely exclude a patient–benefit effect and therefore cannot be considered definitive. So trial D is negative but not definitive (or not significant and also inconclusive). A trial with a larger sample is required to provide a more definite conclusion.

In general, when you are interpreting the result from a study giving a negative, non- significant, result (as in C), you should look at the lower value of the confidence interval. Would a larger trial improve things? This is unlikely because with a 95 per cent confidence interval, a larger trial can only decrease the lower value by 2.5 per cent (the other 2.5 per cent lies above the upper limit of the confidence interval), so there is only a 1 in 40 chance that the true difference will be as much as the upper value or more. Would this extra bit be enough to make the upper value of the confidence interval exceed the minimal clinically useful value?

The point I am (perhaps) labouring to make is that we should view confidence intervals as a continuum rather than as a definite Yes/No result (as a hypothesis test does – we will see how in Chapter 16). We should interpret them as offering various *levels of evidence* as to whether two population parameters are equal or not. Ultimately, to reach a more reliable conclusion, we really need to turn to meta-analysis, which amalgamates a large number of studies. We will discuss this approach in Chapter 24.

I should acknowledge my debt for the above treatment of confidence interval interpretation to Guyatt *et al.* (1995) and Greenhalgh (1997).

Exercise 14.2. Figure 14.5 is from a randomised placebo controlled trial to assess the effect of continuous positive airway pressure (CPAP) on 24 hour ambulatory blood pressure monitoring in patients (with untreated systemic hypertension) with new onset and obstructive sleep apnea. It shows 95 per cent confidence intervals for the difference in various blood pressure measurements between the treatment group ($n = 169$) receiving continuous positive airway pressure (CPAP), and the placebo (sham) group ($n = 171$). Ignore the 'p value' column for now. (a) Which confidence intervals indicate strong evidence for a true difference in blood pressures between the CPAP and the sham groups? (b) What is the best guess for the true difference between the CPAP and sham groups in diurnal systolic and diurnal diastolic blood pressures? (c) If the minimal clinical worthwhile difference in blood pressure is plus 2 mmHg, which confidence intervals indicate a potentially patient-useful difference between the CPAP and the sham groups?

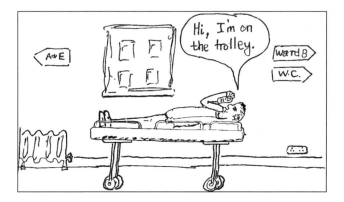

	Difference* (95% CI)	p value[†]
Diurnal systolic blood pressure	1.6 (−0.2 to 3.3)	0.07
Diurnal diastolic blood pressure	1.1 (−0.1 to 2.3)	0.07
Diurnal mean blood pressure	1.3 (−0.1 to 2.5)	0.06
Nocturnal systolic blood pressure	3.1 (0.9 to 5.2)	0.005
Nocturnal diastolic blood pressure	1.5 (0.1 to 3.0)	0.03
Nocturnal mean blood pressure	2.1 (0.5 to 3.6)	0.01
Mean systolic blood pressure	2.1 (0.4 to 3.7)	0.01
Mean diastolic blood pressure	1.3 (0.2 to 2.3)	0.02
Mean blood pressure	1.5 (0.4 to 2.7)	0.01

*Differences in blood pressure (mm Hg) between continuous positive airway pressure (CPAP) and sham groups.
[†]Calculated by t test; compares treatment effects.

Figure 14.5 95 per cent confidence intervals for the difference at 12 weeks in various blood pressure measures between the treatment group receiving continuous positive airway pressure (CPAP) and the placebo (or sham) group, for the treatment of patients with new onset untreated systemic hypertension and obstructive sleep apnea. Data from Durán-Cantolla *et al.* (2010)

Exercise 14.3. Figure 14.6 is from a randomised placebo controlled trial to determine the efficacy of intraoperative treatment with low-dose tranexamic acid in reducing the rate of perioperative transfusions in patients undergoing radical prostatectomy. (a) What are the single best guesses for the difference in blood loss for each of the three outcomes? (b) For each of the three confidence intervals draw a figure like that in Figure 14.4. If the minimum clinically worthwhile blood loss reduction is 50 ml, which confidence intervals are indicative of both a positive *and* a definitive outcome (significant and conclusive, if you prefer)?

Volume (ml)	Placebo group ($n = 100$)	Tranexamic acid group ($n = 100$)	p	Difference (95% CI)
Suctioned blood	1012 (608.1)	810 (390.2)	0.009	202 (59 to 345)
Blood absorbed in gauzes	322 (151.8)	293 (188.6)	0.053	29 (−19 to 78)
Total intraoperative blood loss	1335 (686.5)	1103 (500.8)	0.01	232 (30 to 371)

Data are mean values (standard deviation) unless stated otherwise.

Figure 14.6 Confidence intervals for intraoperative blood loss (ml). Data from Crescenti *et al.* (2011)

Comparing two *paired* population means

When we are dealing with paired data, we again use a confidence interval based on the *t* distribution but adapted for the paired samples situation. Before we look at an example, we need to examine the idea of *within-subject* and *between-subject* variations.

Within-subject and between-subject variations

Cast an eye on the values for heart rate (beats per minute) in four groups of individuals shown in Figure 14.7. Taking Groups A and B first. The spread (or variation) in the values for individuals

	Heart rate (beats/min)			
	Group			
	A	B	C	D
The spread or variation in the values for the individuals in each of these groups is called the *between-subjects* variation.	45	45	53	46
	47	49	56	49
	44	42	55	49
	56	52	54	47
	59	50	54	48
	57	51	54	48
	60	40	55	48
	49	48	53	47
	62	48	53	48
	65	55	56	49

Figure 14.7 Heart rate (beats per minute) in four groups of individuals

in both groups is quite wide, although the variation in Group A is wider than it is for Group B. In fact the standard deviations are 7.55 beats per minute (Group A) and 4.57 beats per minute (Group B). We call the variation in each group, the *between-subject variation*.

The mean heart rates for the two groups are 54.40 beats per minute and 48.00 beats per minute, and these are significantly different – the 95 per cent confidence interval is (0.4167 to 12.3832) beats per minute, which does not include 0. However, it is not easy to spot this by looking at the heart rate data because it is quite widely spread in both groups. Because of this wide spread nature, we need a bigger sample size than we would if these variations were smaller. Which is not good news.

If the variation was smaller, as it is for Groups C and D in Figure 14.7, (standard deviations are 1.160 and 0.994, respectively) it is much easier to spot that the means are significantly different (the 95 per cent confidence interval is (5.38086 to 7.41914) beats per minute). Other things being equal, smaller sample sizes would be sufficient to discover that the means are different. Which is better news.

Now see Figure 14.8. Suppose that the heart rates in the 'Before' column were those of 10 individuals who were experiencing anxiety, and we had given them some appropriate treatment to deal with this. After 30 minutes, their heart rate values were as shown in the 'After' column. So we are taking two measurements on each individual: a 'before' measurement and an 'after' measurement. These observations are essentially *paired* or *matched*. The variation in this measurement for the 10 individuals is called the *within-subject* variation.

Heart rate (b/m)			
Before	After	Difference	
56	49	7	
56	49	7	
55	49	6	The spread or variation in
55	48	7	the values for the same
54	48	6	person, each measured
54	48	6	before and after, is called
54	48	6	the *within-subject*
53	47	6	*variation.*
53	47	6	
53	46	7	

Figure 14.8 Heart rates for 10 individuals before and after the administration of an appropriate treatment for anxiety. The spread in the values in the Difference column are known as *within-subject variation*

The between-subject variation is usually larger than the within-subject variation. In this example, the between-subject variations (as measured by the standard deviation) for the before and after values are 1.160 beats per minute and 0.994 beats per minute, respectively, while that for the within-subject variation is 0.516 beats per minute. We are usually more interested in the within-subject variation than we are in the between-subject variation, which as we saw earlier can hamper our investigations.

The advantage of the paired sample approach (which we are discussing in this section) is that by looking only at the within-subject differences, we can get rid of the between-subjects variability. This means that we end up with a simpler analysis of a single sample. Importantly, because the two measurements are on the same person, we eliminate the individual differences that inevitably arise between people. This means that the anaysis becomes more powerful, and we are likely to need fewer participants to achieve the same power as the two-sample t analysis. As a consequence, you can achieve better precision (narrower confidence intervals) without having to increase sample size. This is an attractive feature as finding appropriate participants can sometimes be difficult.

Why, you may be asking yourself, with these advantages, paired analyses do not appear more often in the literature? Well, the main reason is that not as many situations are suitable for the paired design as those for which we can use the two-sample t approach.

Exercise 14.4.   Explain the difference between within-subject and between-subject variations. What advantage(s) does the within-subject design have over the between-subject design?

As an example of the paired design, Figure 14.9 is taken from a cohort study to investigate the effectiveness of combining statin treatment and fitness on all-cause mortality in a cohort of US veterans. The figure shows the 95 per cent confidence intervals for a number of lipid concentrations in participants before and after treatment with statins (ignore the 'p value' column). In other words, this is paired data.

Exercise 14.5.   Interpret the 95 per cent confidence intervals in Figure 14.9.

	Patients treated with statins		Mean difference (95% CI)	p value
	Before statin treatment ($n = 2959$)	After statin treatment ($n = 2959$)		
Total cholesterol (mmol/l)	6.1 (0.8)	4.4 (1.2)	1.7 (1.6–1.7)	<0.0001
Triglycerides (mmol/l)	1.6 (0.9)	1.5 (1.0)	0.2 (0.1–0.2)	<0.0001
HDL cholesterol (mmol/l)	1.2 (0.3)	1.2 (0.3)	0.1 (0.0–0.1)	<0.0001
LDL cholesterol (mmol/l)	4.2 (0.7)	2.6 (1.0)	1.6 (1.5–1.6)	<0.0001

Data are mean (SD) unless stated otherwise. p values calculated by paired t test.

Figure 14.9 An example of the paired design. Lipid and lipoprotein concentrations in patients before and after treatment with statins. Data from Kokkinos *et al.* (2013)

You can also calculate a confidence interval for the difference in two population *percentages* provided they derive from two metric variables, such as percentage mortality or percentage change in cholesterol. However, if the variable in question is nominal, for example, the proportion or percentage of females or the proportion of schoolchildren who have asthma, then a different approach is needed. This is an extension of the single proportion case discussed in Chapter 13, as you will now see.

Comparing two independent population proportions

When we want to calculate the 95 per cent confidence interval for the difference in two population proportions, then provided neither proportion is close to 0 or 1, and the sample size is not too small, we can use the *Normal approximation* to the binomial distribution (as we did for the single proportion in Chapter 13). Under these assumptions, the formula for the confidence interval for the difference in two proportions is:

$$[(p_1 - p_2) - 2 \times \text{s.e.}(p_1 - p_2)] \text{ to } [(p_1 - p_2) + 2 \times \text{s.e.}(p_1 - p_2)]$$

where p_1 and p_2 are the sample proportions and s.e $(p_1 - p_2)$ is the standard error of the sampling distribution of the difference in two sample proportions. Once again, I am using the value 2 for convenience in place of the proper value, which in any case will be close to 2, and anyway you will not, in practice, be calculating this expression by hand. I am not including the formula for s.e.$(p_1 - p_2)$ as it is rather cumbersome (although not difficult).

As an example, suppose that you want to calculate a 95 per cent confidence interval for the difference between the population proportion of white women who smoked during pregnancy and the population proportion of non-white women who smoked, among the Born in Bradford sample. The smoking data is in Figure 1.3 (the study also contains eithnicity information on the 500 mothers). Minitab produces the following results.

	White	Percent	Non-white	Percent
Smoking	68	31.78	9	3.15
Not smoking	146	68.22	277	96.85

As you can see, the proportion smoking among white mothers was 0.3178, and among non-white mothers, the proportion was only 0.0315, the difference being 0.2863, which is the point estimate (the single best guess) of the difference in the two proportions. Although common sense tells us that these proportions are significantly different, we still need a formal test to confirm this. Minitab produces the following result for the confidence interval:

Difference $= p\,(1) - p\,(2)$
Estimate for difference: -0.286288
95% CI for difference: $(-0.351870, -0.220707)$

The confidence interval does not include 0 so this confirms what we thought. The fact that the confidence interval goes from a negative to a negative is simply because of the way I had arranged the columns of data in Minitab's worksheet. The confidence interval could equally be expressed as (0.2207 to 0.3519).

An example from practice

Figure 14.10 is from a randomised controlled trial to test the hypothesis that individuals would be motivated to change their smoking habits, if they knew that the risk of developing Crohn's disease among smokers at familial risk can be reduced by stopping smoking. One

Outcomes	DNA arm ($n = 251$)	Non-DNA arm ($n = 246$)	% difference in proportion (95% CI)
Primary outcome			
$\geq$One 24 hour quit attempts, measured at six months	35 (73/209)	36 (78/217)	−1 (−10 to 8)
Secondary outcomes			
7 day abstinence:			
Measured at one week (self report)	11 (27/251)	8 (20/246)	3 (−3 to 8)
Measured at six months: (self report)	17 (42/251)	20 (48/246)	−3 (−10 to 4)
Biochemical validation	4 (9/251)	5 (12/246)	−1 (−5 to 2)

Figure 14.10   Confidence intervals for difference in proportions of individuals at familial risk of Crohn's disease quitting smoking between two groups. One group was advised that quitting smoking would reduce the risk of developing Crohn's disease, along with information on predictive genetic testing (the DNA arm) and the other group was informed only of the smoking cessation information (the non-DNA arm). Data from Hollands *et al.* (2012)

group was given this smoking cessation information along with additional predictive genetic testing (the DNA arm) and the other group was given the smoking cessation information only (the non-DNA arm).

All the confidence intervals include 0 so there is no difference in the proportions between the two groups changing their smoking habits. Giving those at familial risk the extra DNA evidence seemed to make no difference to their smoking habits.

> **Exercise 14.6.**   Interpret the point estimates in Figure 14.10, for the differences in the proportion for each outcome.

Comparing two *independent* population medians – the Mann–Whitney rank sums method

It will be useful to start with an explanation of the difference between *parametric* and *non-parametric* methods. A parametric method requires not only that the data are metric but also that it has some particular distribution, most commonly the Normal distribution. A non-parametric method does not make these distributional requirements (and in consequence, they are sometimes referred to as *distribution-free* methods) and are mostly rank based, that is, they involve ranking the data.

So if you are analysing data that are metric and Normally distributed, you can use parametric methods based on the *t* distribution, as we did at the beginning of this chapter to compare two population means. You would want to use a parametric method if possible beccause they are more powerful than non-parametric methods. That is, for samples of the same size, they are more likely to detect an effect or a difference if there is one. But if your data are metric but not Normal, or are ordinal, then it' is appropriate to use a non-parametric approach and compare medians rather than means. How?

Well, in place of a method which uses the t distribution, you can use the *Mann–Whitney* test,[3] which is the non-parametric equivalent of the two-sample t approach discussed earlier. I know that we are not discussing tests until we get to Chapter 16, but some statistics computer programs will produce a confidence interval for the difference in the medians of the two groups concerned.

Here is a quote from a recent paper:

> To compare the distributions of data between the two study groups, we used the t test for continuous variables if the data were normally distributed, and the Mann–Whitney U test for data that were not normally distributed.
>
> *Kobayashi* et al. *(2012)*

However, there is a bit of a problem, because the Mann–Whitney test is not in fact a method for seeing if the population medians of two groups are equal but whether the two groups come from the same population (two groups can have the same mean or median but not necessarily the same distribution). The Mann–Whitney test does not produce a confidence interval for the difference in two population medians directly, but many computer programs (including Minitab, Stata and so on) will produce an associated confidence interval using what are known as *bootstrapping methods*.[4] In practice, the Mann–Whitney test is commonly used to compare two population medians.

I will give a brief expalnation of how the Mann–Whitney test works in Chapter 16, when we come to discuss hypothesis tests, but suffice to say here that it is a method based on the *ranks* of the sample data.

An example from practice

Figure 14.11 is from a randomised controlled trial in an emergency department to compare the cost effectiveness of two treatments (ketorolac versus morphine) in relieving pain after a blunt instrument injury. The figure shows the median times spent by two groups of patients in various clinical situations. The last column contains the 95 per cent confidence intervals for the difference in these median treatment times (minutes), between the groups, derived from a Mann–Whitney procedure.

The confidence interval for the difference in median 'Interval between receiving analgesia and leaving emergency department' is (4 to 39) mins, and this is the only confidence interval which does not include 0, so it offers strong evidence that there is a difference in the population median times for the ketorolac and morphine groups, for this outcome.

---

[3] Also known as the Mann–Whitney U test. The procedure produces a statistic called the U statistic. In the old days (before computers) tables of the values of U were available which could be used to decide if there was a significant result.

[4] Briefly, bootstrapping means taking repeated (different) sub-samples each of the same size from the original sample. So if you take 1000 samples, then order them, then the 95 percent confidence interval would be the 25th value to the 975th value.

	Ketorolac group (n = 75)	Morphine group (n = 73)	Median difference (95% confidence interval)
Interval between arrival in emergency department and doctor prescribing analgesia	38.0 (30.0 to 54.0)	39.0 (29.0 to 53.0)	1.0 (−5.0 to 7.0)
Preparation for analgesia	5.0 (5.0 to 10.0)	10.0 (5.5 to 12.5)	2.0 (0 to 5.0)
Undergoing radiography	5.0 (5.0 to 10.0)	5.0 (4.0 to 10.0)	0 (−1.0 to 0)
Total time spent in emergency department	155.0 (112.0 to 198.0)	171.0 (126.0 to 208.5)	15.0 (−4.0 to 33.0)
Interval between receiving analgesia and leaving emergency department	115.0 (75.0 to 149.0)	130.0 (95.0 to 170.0)	20.0 (4.0 to 39.0)

Figure 14.11 95 per cent confidence intervals for the median time spent by two groups of patients (one group received ketorolac, the other morphine) in various clinical situations, and the differences in these median times. Results from a Mann–Whitney test. From a randomised controlled trial in an emergency department to compare the cost effectiveness, of two treatments in relieving pain after blunt instrument injury. Data from Rainer *et al.* (2000)

Comparing two *matched* population medians – the Wilcoxon signed-ranks method

Once again, we will not discuss tests until we get to Chapter 16, but if you have two groups of paired or matched data, and the data are either ordinal or metric, and if the metric is noticeably skewed, you can obtain a confidence interval for the difference in population medians using the non-parametric *Wilcoxon signed-ranks test*. Like the Mann–Whitney test, this is a rank-based procedure and comes with a similar warning. Strictly speaking, the null hypothesis is that there is no tendency for the outcome under one set of conditions (say a treatment group) to be higher or lower than under a comparitive set of conditions (say a placebo group) but if you choose this method in Minitab, for example, you will be provided with a confidence interval for the difference in medians. This confidence interval does not stem directly from the Wilcoxon procedure but it is produced by the computer program using various assumptions about large sample aproximations to the binomial and/or Normal distributions.

The Wilcoxon approach is the non-parametric equivalent of the parametric matched-pairs *t* method described earlier. The matching will reduce the variation within groups, so narrower (and therefore more precise) confidence intervals are available for a given sample size.

Briefly, the Wilcoxon method starts by calculating the difference between each pair of values (these differences should be symmetrically distributed), and these differences are then ranked (ignoring any minus signs). Any minus signs are then restored to the rank values, and the negative and positive ranks are separately summed. If the medians in the two groups are the same, then these two rank sums should be similar. If different, the Wilcoxon method provides a way of determining whether this is due to chance or it represents a statistically significant difference in the population medians.

Intake/day	Patients (cases) (n = 30)	Controls (n = 30)	Median difference (95% CI)*	p
Energy (MJ)	9.71 (5.07–17.94)	11.98 (5.25–23.22)	2.06 (0.26–4.23)	0.04
Protein (g)	84.5 (38.4–157.4)	96.0 (40.5–633.0)	15.9 (−1.1–32.8)	0.07
Total fibre (g)	12.6 (7.3–20.8)	18.9 (8.7–86.2)	7.0 (3.6–10.6)	0.0001
Retinol (µg)	590 (288–7556)	817 (134–12 341)	310 (93–1269)	0.02
Carotene (µg)	1443 (219–4657)	2798 (523–11 313)	1376 (549–2452)	0.004
Vitamin C (mg)	40.5 (3.0–204)	80.5 (14.0–219)	33.5 (2.0–64.0)	0.03
Vitamin E (mg)	4.7 (2.3–18.0)	7.8 (2.2–32.0)	2.9 (1.45–5.35)	0.0002
Alcohol (g)	0 (0–19.4)	5.7 (0–80)	5.4 (1.2–9.9)	0.009

*Wilcoxon signed ranks test

Figure 14.12   95 per cent confidence intervals from the Wilcoxon signed-ranks method for the difference in population food intakes per day, for a number of substances, from a study of the dietary habits of schizophrenics. Values are median (range). Reproduced from *BMJ*, 317, 784–5, courtesy of BMJ Publishing Group. McCreadie *et al.* (1998). Reproduced by permission of BMJ Publishing Group Ltd

An example from practice

Figure 14.12 contains the results of a case–control study into the dietary intake of schizophrenic patients residing in the community in Scotland. It shows the daily energy intake of eight dietary substances for the cases (17 men and 13 women diagnosed with schizophrenia) and the controls, each individually matched on sex, age, smoking status and employment status (ignore the last column). If you focus on the penultimate column, you can see that only the confidence interval for daily protein intake, (−1.1 to 32.8) g, contains zero, which implies that there is no difference in population median protein intake between schizophrenics and normal individuals. For all other substances, the difference is statistically significant.

Exercise 14.7.   Explain the meaning of the 95 per cent confidence interval for difference between the two groups in (a) median protein intake, and (b) median alcohol intake, for the two groups in Figure 14.12.

15

Confidence intervals for the *ratio* of two population parameters

Medical Statistics from Scratch: An Introduction for Health Professionals, Third Edition. David Bowers.
© 2014 John Wiley & Sons, Ltd. Published 2014 by John Wiley & Sons, Ltd.

Using confidence intervals for ratios

Getting a confidence interval for the *ratio* of two independent population means

When you compare two population means, you usually would want to know if they are the same or not, and if not, get some idea on how big the difference between them is. Sometimes though, you might want to know *how many times bigger* one population mean is than another. The *ratio* of the two means will tell you that. The ratio of the sample means might be 1 or close to 1, suggesting that one population mean is no bigger (or smaller) than the other population mean. If the ratio differs from 1, this suggests that one population mean might be bigger than the other. The bigger the ratio of sample means is (the further away from 1), the more likely it is that one population mean is bigger than the other, but you need to eliminate the possibility that the result is just due to chance.

You can do this if you look at a 95 per cent confidence interval for the *ratio of population means*. This will help you decide whether one population mean is bigger than the other. And here is the rule:

> If the confidence interval for the *ratio* of two population parameters contain the value 1, then you can be 95 per cent confident that one population mean is no bigger (or smaller) than the other population mean.

Compare this with the rule for the *difference* between two population parameters, where the rule is that if the confidence interval contains 0, then we can be 95 per cent confident that the two population means are the same.

Clinical outcome	Integrated care (n ≥ 296)	Conventional care (n ≥ 277)	Ratio of means
No. of bronchodilators prescribed	10.1 (9.2 to 11.1)	10.6 (9.7 to 11.7)	0.95 (0.83 to 1.09)
No. of inhaled steroids prescribed	6.4 (5.9 to 6.9)	6.5 (6.1 to 7.1)	0.98 (0.88 to 1.09)
No. of courses of oral steroids used	1.6 (1.4 to 1.8)	1.6 (1.4 to 1.9)	0.97 (0.79 to 1.20)
No. of general practice asthma consultations	2.7 (2.4 to 3.1)	2.5 (2.2 to 2.8)	1.11 (0.95 to 1.31)
No. of hospital admissions for asthma	0.15 (0.11 to 0.19)	0.11 (0.08 to 0.15)	1.31 (0.87 to 1.96)

Means and 95% confidence interval are estimated from Poisson regression models after controlling for initial peak flow, forced expiratory volume (as % of predicted), and duration af asthma.

Figure 15.1   95 per cent confidence intervals for the ratio of integrated care to conventional care, for a number of clinical outcomes over 12 months for asthma patients. The treatment group patients received integrated care and the control group received conventional GP care. Data from Grampian Asthma Study of Integrated Care (1994)

An example from practice

See the last column in Figure 15.1 (this is Figure 13.2 reproduced for convenience), which shows a number of outcomes from a randomised trial to compare integrated versus conventional care for asthma patients. The last column contains the 95 per cent confidence intervals for the ratio of population means for the treatment and control groups. You will see that *all* of the confidence intervals contain 1, indicating that the population mean number of bronchodilators used, the number of inhaled steroids prescribed, and so on was no larger (or smaller) in one population than in the other.

The *sample* ratio furthest away from 1 is 1.31 (this is the point estimate of the ratio – the best guess as to its value), for the ratio of mean number of hospital admissions, that is, the *sample* of integrated care group patients had 31 per cent more admissions than the conventionally treated control group patients. However, the 95 per cent confidence interval of (0.87 to 1.96) includes 1, which implies that this is generally *not* the case in the populations.

Exercise 15.1.   Figure 15.2 is from a randomised controlled trial to study the effect of screening for mosquito control. One group of houses (the controls) had no screening, the second group had total screening and the third group had screened ceilings only. The table shows the ratio of the mean number of mosquitos trapped for the total screening group compared to the controls, and for the screened ceilings group compared to the controls. Interpret the 95 per cent confidence interval for the ratio of mean number of mosqquitos trapped in each case.

---

	n^*	Anopheles gambiae sensu lato mosquitos		
		Mean number of mosquitoes	Ratio of means (95% CI)	*p* value
Control	731	37.5	..	..
Full screening	1463	15.2	0.41 (0.31–0.54)	<0.0001
Screened ceilings	1376	19.1	0.53 (0.40–0.70)	<0.0001

*Total number of house visits for analysis of mosquitoes caught per trap per night and number of houses for analysis of mosquitoes caught per house.

Figure 15.2 Comparison of mosquito densities between intervention and control groups. Ratios of means are for intervention versus control. Intention to treat analysis. (Table abbreviated by current author). Source: Adapted from Kirby *et al.* (2009). Reproduced by permission of Elsevier

Confidence interval for a population risk ratio

Look again at Figure 8.2, which is a contingency table from a cohort study showing the risk of coronary heart disease (CHD) as an adult, among men who weighed 18 lbs or less at 12 months old (the risk factor). The risk ratio of CHD among the sample of men who weighed ≤18 lbs at 1 year compared to men who weighed more than this is (using the formula above Figure 12.3):

$$\text{risk ratio} = \frac{4/15}{38/275} = \frac{0.2667}{0.1382} = 1.9298$$

So the sample data indicates that men who weighed less than 18 lbs at one year have nearly twice the risk of CHD as adults as those weighing more than 18 lbs. But is this true in the *population* of such men, or no more than a *chance* departure from a population ratio of 1? You now know that you can answer this question by examining the 95 per cent confidence interval for this risk ratio.

As it happens, the 95 per cent confidence interval for the CHD risk ratio turns out to be (0.793 to 4.697).[1] As this interval contains 1, you can conclude, that despite a *sample* risk ratio of nearly 2, weighing 18 lbs or less at one year is *not* a significant risk factor for coronary heart disease in adult life in the *population*. Notice that, in general, the value of a sample risk (or odds) ratio, as in this example, does *not* lie in the centre of its confidence interval, but it is usually closer to the lower value.

An example from practice

Figure 15.3 is from a cohort study of 552 men surviving acute myocardial infarction, in which each participant was assessed for depression at the beginning of the study and after six months. The six-month levels of depression were 13.3 per cent severely depressed, 22.5 per cent moderately depressed and 64.2 per cent had low levels of depression. A number of participant outcomes were measured, including suffering angina, returning to work, emotional stability, and smoking. The researchers were interested in examining the role of moderate and severe depression (compared to low depression), as risk factors for each of these outcomes.

The results show the crude and adjusted relative risks (risk ratios) for each outcome. The crude relative risks are *not* adjusted for any confounding factors, whereas the adjusted relative risks *are* adjusted for those factors listed in the table footnote, namely, age, social class, recurrent infarction, rehabilitation, cardiac events and helplessness. (see Chapter 7 for a reminder of confounding and adjustment).

Let's interpret the 95 per cent risk ratios for 'Return to work'. The *crude* risk ratios for return to work indicate lower rates of return to work for men both moderately depressed (relative risk = 0.41) and severely depressed (relative risk = 0.39) compared to men with low levels of depression. In other words, compared to those participants with low depression, moderately depressed men had only 41 per cent chance of returning to work and severley depressed men only a 39 per cent chance of returning to work. Neither of the confidence intervals, (0.22 to 0.77) and (0.18 to 0.88), include 1, indicating statistical significance. However, after adjusting for possible confounding variables, the *adjusted* relative risks are 0.58 and 0.54, respectively and are no longer statistically significant because both confidence intervals now include 1 – for moderate depression (0.28 to 1.17), and severe depression (0.22 to 1.31).

---

[1] The calculation of confidence intervals for risk ratios and odds ratios is a step too far for this book. Those interested in doing the calculation by hand can consult Altman (1991) who gives the necessary formulae.

Depression level	Relative risk (95% CI)	
	Crude	Adjusted*
Angina pectoris		
Moderate	1.36 (0.83 to 2.23)	0.97 (0.55 to 1.70)
Severe	3.12 (1.58 to 6.16)	2.31 (1.11 to 4.80)
Return to work		
Moderate	0.41 (0.22 to 0.77)	0.58 (0.28 to 1.17)
Severe	0.39 (0.18 to 0.88)	0.54 (0.22 to 1.31)
Emotional Instability		
Moderate	2.21 (1.33 to 3.69)	1.87 (1.07 to 3.27)
Severe	5.55 (2.87 to 10.71)	4.61 (2.32 to 9.18)
Smoking		
Moderate	1.39 (0.71 to 2.73)	1.19 (0.56 to 2.51)
Severe	2.63 (1.23 to 5.60)	2.84 (1.22 to 6.63)
Late potentials		
Moderate	1.30 (0.76 to 2.22)	1.54 (0.86 to 2.74)
Severe	0.70 (0.33 to 1.47)	0.75 (0.35 to 2.17)

*Adjusted for age, social class, recurrent infarction, rehabilitation, cardiac events, and helplessness

Figure 15.3 The crude and adjusted relative risks (risk ratios) for a number of outcomes related to the risk factors: experiencing moderate and severe levels of depression compared to low depression. Data from Ladwig *et al.* (1994)

Exercise 15.2. Intepret the confidence intervals in Figure 15.3 for the relative risks associated with angina pectoris.

An example from practice

Figure 15.4 is from a cohort study to investigate frequency and risk factors for prevalent, incident and persistent carcinogenic human papillomavirus (HPV) in young women before the introduction of immunisation against HPV types 16 and 18 for schoolgirls. The table gives crude and adjusted relative risks (risk ratios) and their 95 per cent confidence intervals for participants with the characteristics listed (the risk factors) compared to those without the characteristic. As you can see, although a number of the crude (unadjusted) relative risks appear to be significant (the confidence interval does not include 1), having had only 2 or more sexual partners in the previous 12 months remains significant after adjustment.[2] In this case, having two or more sexual partners means that the individual is nearly twice as likely to contract HPV compared to a participant who has had less than two sexual partners.

---

[2] And co-infection with *C trachomatis* or concurrent bacterial vaginosis was also independent predictors of carcinogenic HPV infection.

Characteristic	No (%) of women with characteristic	Relative risk (95% CI) of HPV infection	
		Crude	Adjusted[*]
Age < 20 years[†]	292/821 (36)	1.51 (1.13 to 2.03)	1.20 (0.89 to 1.63)
Black ethnicity	148/820 (18)	1.44 (1.03 to 2.02)	1.37 (0.96 to 1.94)
Smoker[†]	216/819 (26)	1.18 (0.85 to 1.62)	0.98 (0.70 to 1.37)
≥2 sexual partners in previous year[‡]	297/819 (36)	2.10 (1.57 to 2.82)	1.99 (1.46 to 2.72)
Age <16 years at first sex	228/812 (28)	1.24 (0.91 to 1.70)	1.20 (0.86 to 1.65)
Use of oral contraception[‡]	448/819 (55)	1.10 (0.81 to 1.48)	–
Use of condoms[‡]	439/800 (55)	1.56 (1.34 to 2.14)	1.25 (0.91 to 1.72)

[*]Controlled for all significant variables from the unadjusted analysis and for age <20 and age <16 at first sex.
[†]Reported at baseline.
[‡]Reported at follow-up. No data on frequency of condom use.

Figure 15.4   Crude and adjusted relative risks (risk ratios) for risk factors for incident carcinogenic HPV infection ($n = 145$) in 821 women who provided follow-up samples after a median of 16 months. Data from Oakeshott *et al.* (2012)

Exercise 15.3.   Figure 15.5 is from the study referred to in Figure 12.1, a randomised placebo controlled trial whose objective was to test the hypothesis that a relative deficiency in L-arginine may be associated with the development of pre-eclampsia in a population at high risk.

The participants were pregnant women with a history of pre-eclampsia. A total of 222 women were allocated to the placebo group; 228 received L-arginine plus antioxidant vitamins and 222 recieved antioxidant vitamins only. The upper table shows the relative risks (and 95 per cent confidence intervals) of treatment comparisons and the lower table the absolute risk reductions (and their 95 per cent confidence intervals). Ignore the (χ^2 and p) row. Interpret and compare the relative risk and the absolute risk reduction results (you may want to refer to Chapter 12 to refresh your understanding of absolute risk reduction).

Confidence intervals for a population odds ratio

Figure 8.7 shows the data for the case–control study into exercise between the ages of 15 and 25, and stroke later in life. The risk factor was 'not exercising', and in Chapter 12 (see Figure 12.8 and Exercise 12.9), you calculated the *sample* crude odds ratio of 0.411 for a stroke in those

	Relative risk (95% CI)		
	L-arginine + vitamins vs placebo	Vitamins alone vs placebo	L-arginine + vitamins vs vitamins alone
Pre-eclampsia or eclampsia	0.42 (0.28 to 0.62) (χ^2: $p < 0.001$)	0.74 (0.54 to 1.02) (χ^2: $p = 0.052$)	0.56 (0.37 to 0.85) (χ^2: $p = 0.004$)

	Absolute risk reduction (95% CI)		
	L-arginine + vitamins vs placebo	Vitamins alone vs placebo	L-arginine + vitamins vs vitamins alone
Pre-eclampsia or eclampsia	0.17 (0.12 to 0.21)	0.07 (0.005 to 0.15)	0.09 (0.05 to 0.14)

Figure 15.5 Relative risks (top table) and absolute risk reduction (bottom table), for three groups of women participating in a randomized placebo controlled trial of L-arginine and antioxidant treatment for the reduction of pre-eclampsia or eclampsia. One group of women ($n = 222$) were given a placebo, the second group ($n = 228$) were given L-arginine plus antioxidant vitamins and the third group ($n = 222$) antioxidant vitamins only. Data from Vadillo-Ortega *et al.* (2011)

who had exercised compared to those who had not. So the exercising group appear to have only about 40 per cent of the odds for a stroke as the non-exercising group. However, you need to examine the confidence interval for this odds ratio to see if it contains 1 or not, before you can come to a conclusion about the statistical significance of the *population* odds ratio.

The 95 per cent confidence interval is (0.2597 to 0.6536). This does not contain 1, so you can be 95 per cent confident that the odds ratio for a stroke in the *population* of those who did exercise compared to the population of those who did not exercise is somewhere between 0.2597 and 0.6536. It seems that early-life exercise does appear to reduce the odds for a stroke later on in life. Of course, this is a crude, unadjusted odds ratio, which takes no account of the contribution, positive or negative, of any other relevant variables.

An example from practice

Figure 15.6 shows the results from this same exercise/stroke study, where the authors provide both crude odds ratios and ratios *adjusted* for age and sex, stratified by age when exercising.

We have been looking at exercise between the ages of 15 and 25, the first row of the table. Compared to the *crude* odds ratio calculated above of 0.411, the authors report an odds ratio for stroke, *adjusted* for age and sex, among those who exercised compared to those who did not exercise, as 0.33, with a 95 per cent confidence interval of (0.20 to 0.60). So even after the effects of any differences in age and sex between the two groups have been adjusted for, there is good evidence that exercising between the ages of 15 and 25 reduces the odds for a stroke in later life.

	Exercise not undertaken		Exercise undertaken	
	Odds ratio	No of cases: no of controls	Odds ratio (95% CI)	No of cases: no of controls
Age when exercise undertaken (years):				
15–25	1.0	70:68	0.33 (0.2 to 0.6)	55:130
25–40	1.0	103:136	0.43 (0.2 to 0.8)	21:57
40–55	1.0	101:139	0.63 (0.3 to 1.5)	10:22

Figure 15.6   Odds ratios (and 95% CIs) for stroke, according to whether, and at what age, exercise was undertaken, by cases (those with stroke), compared to controls (without stroke). Data from Shinton and Sagar (1993)

Adjustment for possible confounders is crucial if your results are to be of any use, and we discussed this topic in Chapter 8, but I will return to adjustment in Chapters 21 and 22.

Exercise 15.4. (a) Explain briefly why age and sex differences between the groups are usually adjusted for. (b) What do the results in Figure 15.6 indicate about not exercising as a risk factor for stroke among the three age groups?

Exercise 15.5. Returning to the randomised controlled trial on the use of a cervical pessary in women with a short cervix to prevent pre-term births (see Exercise 5.1), Figure 15.7 contains odds ratios and their 95 per cent confidence intervals for a number of outcomes for women in the treatment group (cervical pessary) and in the expectant management group (ignore the p value column). For each outcome, do you think the evidence supports the use of a cervical pessary to reduce pre-term births? What about the last two outcomes?

Confidence intervals for hazard ratios

Odds ratios and risk ratios (relative risks) are the ratios that you will often see in the literature, but the *hazard ratio* (HR) is also important, mainly in the context of survival analysis, which I will discuss in detail in Chapter 23. Put simply, the hazard ratio is the probability of death (or some other end point) in one group compared to that in another group, measured over some period of time (the study period). More in Chapter 23!

But as an example of the interpretation of the confidence intervals for hazard ratios, the table in Figure 15.8 is from a chort study to examine all cause and disease-specific mortality in patients with osteoarthritis of the knee or hip and shows the hazard ratios for a number of demographic and clinical characteristic of the patients in the study, along with the 95 per cent confidence intervals.

Pregnancy outcome	Cervical pessary group	Expectant management group	Odds ratio (95% CI)	p value
Spontaneous delivery before 28 weeks	4 (2%)	16 (8%)	0.23(0.06 to 0.74)	0.0058
Spontaneous delivery before 34 weeks	12 (6%)	51 (27%)	0.18(0.08 to 0.37)	< 0.0001
Any delivery before 34 weeks	14 (7%)	53 (28%)	0.21(0.10 to 0.40)	< 0.0001
Spontaneous delivery before 37 weeks	41 (22%)	113 (59%)	0.19(0.12 to 0.30)	< 0.0001
Chorioamnionitis*	5 (3%)	6 (3%)	0.82 (0.20 to 3.32)	0.76
Pregnancy bleeding	7 (4%)	9 (5%)	0.77(0.24 to 2.38)	0.61

*Chorioamnionitis is the inflammation of the foetal membranes due to a bacterial infection. It typically results from bacteria ascending into the uterus from the vagina.

Figure 15.7   Odds ratios (and 95% CIs) for pregnancy outcomes. From a randomised controlled trial on the use of a cervical pessary in women with a short cervix to prevent pre-term births. Data from Goya *et al.* (2012)

Characteristic at baseline	Patients died		Crude hazard ratio*(95% CI)
	Yes (*n* = 438)	No (*n* = 725)	
Age (years) at baseline:			
35–54	6 (1)	169 (23)	1.00 (reference)
55–74	273 (62)	503 (69)	12.4 (5.53 to 27.9)
≥ 75	159 (36)	53 (7)	40.7 (18.0 to 92.0)
Male sex	204 (47)	299 (41)	1.21 (1.00 to 1.46)
Lower social class (IIIM to V)	228 (52)	342 (47)	1.21 (1.00 to 1.46)
Smoking	70 (16)	115 (16)	0.94 (0.74 to 1.19)
Previous joint replacement	42 (10)	38 (5)	1.61 (1.17 to 2.22)
Type of osteoarthritis:			
Knee only	130 (30)	233 (32)	1.00 (reference)
Hip only	120 (27)	222 (31)	0.98 (0.77 to 1.26)
Knee and hip	188 (43)	270 (37)	1.20 (0.96 to 1.50)
Knee or hip pain	289 (66)	477 (66)	1.00 (0.82 to 1.22)
Walking disability	152 (35)	136 (19)	1.93 (1.59 to 2.36)

Values are numbers (percentages) unless stated otherwise.
*Univariable hazard ratios, 95% confidence intervals, and p values were derived from Cox regression models after multiple imputation of missing covariate data; hazard ratios >1 indicate lower mortality in the reference category.

Figure 15.8   Crude (unadjusted) hazard ratios and 95 per cent confidence intervals, for a number of demographic and clinical characteristic of the patients, from a cohort study to examine all cause, and disease-specific, mortality in patients with osteoarthritis of the knee or hip (abbreviated by author). Source: Adapted from Nüesch *et al.* (2011). Reproduced by permission of BMJ Publishing Group Ltd

Exercise 15.6.   Which characteristics of the patients in Figure 15.8, represent a significant hazard of death?

You may be wondering where all these odds ratios and risk ratios come from (and you will see more of both in Chapter 18), in other words how are they calculated? With two-by-two contingency tables, the calculations are easy enough (although calculation of the confidence intervals is not so easy), but when the problem becomes one of adjusting for confounders, and there may be many of these, we have to use regression models to get odds ratios and risk ratios – we will deal with these models in Chapters 21, 22 and 23.

VII

Putting it to the Test

16

Testing hypotheses about the *difference* between two population parameters

Learning objectives

When you have finished this chapter, you should be able to:

- Explain how a research question can be expressed in the form of a testable hypothesis.

- Explain what a null hypothesis is.

- Summarise the hypothesis test procedure.

- Explain what a *p*-value is.

- Explain what the significance level of a test is.

- Use the *p*-value to appropriately reject or not reject a null hypothesis.

- Summarise the principal tests described in this chapter, along with their most appropriate application, and any distributional and other requirements.

Medical Statistics from Scratch: An Introduction for Health Professionals, Third Edition. David Bowers.
© 2014 John Wiley & Sons, Ltd. Published 2014 by John Wiley & Sons, Ltd.

- Explain types of error.

- Describe what is meant by the power of a test and how it relates to a particular type of error.

- Be able to calculate an appropriate sample size for testing the difference between two means or two proportions.

Answering the question

As we have seen, almost all clinical investigations begin with a question. For example, is malathion a more effective drug for treating head lice than *d*-phenothrin? Is there a difference in the mean birthweight of babies born to mothers who smoked while pregnant and those who did not? Does a cervical pessary reduce pre-term births in women with a short cervix? And so on. In the preceding three chapters, we answered questions of this sort by calculating a confidence interval and seeing if it contains 0 (in the case of a difference) or 1 (in the case of a ratio).

We could then make statements like, 'We are 95 per cent confident that the range of values defined by the confidence interval will include the value of the population parameter,' or 'The confidence interval represents a plausible range of values for the population parameter.'

The hypothesis

But there is an alternative approach, which I want to discuss in this chapter, which is to transform the *research question* into a *testable, working,* or *research hypothesis* (also called the *null hypothesis*).

Hypothesis testing, which uses exactly the same sample data as the confidence interval approach, focuses not on using a confidence interval to answer the research question but on *testing* whether a value (e.g. a difference or a ratio) is the same as a previously *hypothesised* value. In recent years, the confidence interval approach has become more generally favoured, primarily because the results from a confidence interval provide *more information* than the results of a hypothesis test (as you see later in this chapter).

However, hypothesis testing is still common in research publications as confidence intervals are not always appropriate (as we saw with the difference between two medians in Chapter 14), and therefore later in this chapter I describe a few of the more common tests.

Here are three examples from the literature where authors declare their interest in testing hypotheses (my italics and bolding):

> We **hypothesised** that long term intake of low or high calcium increases the risk of cardiovascular mortality.
>
> *Michaëlsson* et al. *(2013)*

To test the **hypothesis** that a relative deficiency in L-arginine, the substitue for synthesis of the vasidilatory gas nitric oxide, may be associated with the development of pre-eclampsia in a population at high risk.

Vadillo-Ortega et al. *(2011)*

There have been claims that statins might be more beneficial in people with raised C-reactive protein (CRP) concentrations and might even be ineffective in people with low concentrations of CRP and LDL cholesterol. This study aimed to test this **hypothesis**.

Heart Protection Study Collaborative Group (2011)

Before we go any further, bear in mind that not all investigations lend themselves to being expressed as a hypothesis, typically those to do with determining a prevalence or a rate. For example, 'what is the prevalence and incidence of genital carcinogenic human papillomavirus infection in sexually active women?' 'What is the hospital mortality rate following an infarction?' And so on.

The null hypothesis

The hypothesis is often expressed as a *null* hypothesis, denoted as H_0, which we (usually) hope to disprove. For example:

Null hypothesis, H_0: Long-term intake of low or high calcium has *no* effect on the risk of cardiovascular mortality.

Null hypothesis, H_0: A relative deficiency in L-arginine is *not* associated with the development of pre-eclampsia in a population at high risk.

Notice that both of these null hypotheses reflect the conservative position of *no* difference, *no* effect, *no* association, and so on; hence the '*null*'. Notice also that these null hypotheses contradict the research hypotheses as stated by the authors above. There is a good reason why we express our hypothesis in this null form because it is impossible to *prove* a hypothesis. Suppose our hypothesis is that all men aged 70 or more have grey hair. We could see 1000 or 100 000 or a million men, or more, and find that they all had grey hair, but this hasn't proved our hypothesis. However, if we come across just *one* 70+ man with *black* hair, we have disproved the hypothesis.

To *test* a null hypothesis, researchers take samples and measure outcomes and decide whether the sample data provides strong enough evidence to be able to refute or *reject* the hypothesis or not. If the evidence against the null hypothesis is strong enough for us to be able to reject it, then we implicitly accept that some specified alternative hypothesis, usually labelled as H_1, is probably true. We'll see in a moment how we can judge whether the evidence from the sample supports or refutes the null hypothesis, but first let me summarise the hypothesis testing procedure.

The hypothesis testing process

The hypothesis testing process can be summarised thus:

- Select a suitable outcome variable.

- Use your research question to define a testable null hypothesis involving this outcome variable.

- Collect the appropriate sample data and determine the relevant sample statistic. For example, the difference in sample means, or in sample proportions, or in a risk ratio or an odds ratio.

- Use a decision rule that will enable you to judge whether the sample evidence supports or does not support your null hypothesis.

- Thus, on the strength of this evidence, either reject or do not reject your null hypothesis.

Let's illustrate this process with a simple example. Imagine that you are approached by a shady character on a train. He suggests playing a simple coin tossing game. For every tail, he will give you a euro; for every head, you give him a euro. Being sceptical by nature (you are a statistician after all), you want to test whether the coin is fair, that is, not weighted to produce more heads than it should, before you agree to play. Your null hypothesis is that the coin is fair, that is, it will produce as many heads as tails, so that the population proportion, which is denoted as π, is 50 per cent, that is, the probability is 0.5. That is:

$$H_0 : \pi = 0.5 \,(\text{coin is fair})$$

Your outcome variable is the sample proportion of heads, p. You toss the coin 100 times and get 42 heads, so $p = 0.42$. Is this outcome compatible with your hypothesised value of 0.5? Does the difference between 0.5 and 0.42 reflect a real difference or could it be due to chance, that is, is it just sampling error? If you had to bet on it, you would probably think that this value of 0.42 is reasonably compatible with your null hypothesis H_0: $\pi = 0.5$, so it appears that the coin is fair.

But suppose that you get 30 heads from 100 tosses of the coin, so that now $p = 0.30$. Is *this* value compatible with your null hypothesis of a fair coin? More difficult to judge now. You probably would not want to bet a large amount of money on it.

You can see the problem. How do we decide on how far the sample proportion p has to be from 0.5 before we begin to doubt that our null hypothesis is true? What is the critical value of p? Our line in the sand, as it were. As it happens, there is a generally accepted rule, which involves something known as the *p-value*.

The *p*-value and the decision rule

The hypothesis test decision rule is:

Supposing the null hypothesis is true. If you now get a certain number of heads when you toss the coin, and if the probability of getting this number of heads (or even fewer) is less than 0.05,[1] then this is strong enough evidence against the null hypothesis, and it can be rejected.

Again supposing that the null hypothesis is true, then the probability of getting the outcome observed (e.g. some particular number of heads or fewer), is called the p-value.

In other words, if the p-value is less than 0.05, then the evidence against the null hypothesis is strong enough for you to be able to reject it.

You will get your *p*-value from a computer. The beauty of this rule is that you can apply it in any situation where the probability of an outcome can be calculated and not just to coin tossing.

As a matter of interest, the probability of getting say 42 *or fewer* heads if the coin is fair, is 0.0666, which is *not* less than 0.05. This is *not* strong enough evidence against the null hypothesis.

However, if you had got 41 heads or fewer, the probability of which is 0.0443, this *is* less than 0.05, and so now the evidence against H_0 *is* strong enough and it can be rejected. The coin is not fair. This crucial threshold outcome probability, the *p*-value, is 0.0443 in this example.

So, in the end, the decision rule is simple:

- Determine the *p-value* for the output you have obtained (using a computer).

- Compare it with the *critical value*, usually 0.05.

- If the *p*-value is *less* than 0.05, reject the null hypothesis; otherwise, do not reject it.

Note that the critical value, usually 0.05 or 0.01, is called the *significance level* of the hypothesis test and is denoted as α (alpha). We will return to α again shortly. It is important to note that if the *p*-value is ≥ 0.05, you can neither reject the null hypothesis nor can you say that it is true; it is only that there is insufficient evidence to reject it. Maybe, H_0 is not true but your sample size was not big enough to find the evidence!

When you reject a null hypothesis, it's worth remembering that although there is a probability of 0.95 that you are making the correct decision, there is a corresponding probability of 0.05 that your decision is incorrect. In fact, you *never* know whether your decision is correct or not,[2] but there are 95 chances in 100 that it is. Compare this with the conclusion drawn from a confidence interval where you can be 95 per cent confident that a confidence interval will include the population parameter, but there is still a 5 per cent chance that it will not.

It is important to stress that the *p*-value is *not* the probability that the null hypothesis is true (or not true). It is a measure of the *strength of the evidence against* the null hypothesis. The smaller the *p*-value, the stronger the evidence (the less likely it is that the outcome you got occurred by chance, that is, it was due to sampling error).

---

[1] Or 0.01. There is nothing magical about these values, they are quite arbitrary, but 0.05 is most often used and is compatible with the 95 per cent confidence interval.
[2] Because you will never know what the actual value of any population parameter is.

Exercise 16.1.   Suppose you want to check your belief that as many males as females use your genito-urinary clinic. (a) Frame your belief as a research question. (b) Write down an appropriate null hypothesis. (c) You take a sample of 100 patients on Monday and find that 40 are males. The *p*-value for 40 or fewer males from a sample of 100 individuals is 0.028. Do you reject the null hypothesis? (d) Your colleague takes a sample of 100 patients on the following Friday and gets 43 males, the *p*-value for which is 0.097. Does your colleague come to the same decision as you did? Explain your answer.

A brief summary of a few of the commonest tests

Some hypothesis tests are suitable only for metric data, some for metric and ordinal data and some for ordinal and nominal data. Some require data to have a particular distribution (often Normal); these are *parametric* tests. Some have no (or less strict) distributional requirements; the *non-parametric* tests. Before I discuss a few tests in any detail, I have listed in Figure 16.1 a brief summary of the more commonly used tests, along with their data and distributional requirements if any (I am ignoring tests of single population parameters as these are not required often enough to justify any discussion).

In this chapter, I want to talk about the first five tests listed in Figure 16.1 (so I will!). In Chapter 17, I will provide some insights into the chi-squared test – what it is and how it is calculated. In Chapter 18, I will give a few examples from the literature to illustrate the various applications of the chi-squared test. Let's kick off with a look at the use of *p*-values in comparing independent population means.

Using the *p*-value to compare the means of two independent populations

When we are using the two-sample *t* test to compare two independent population means, we can write the null hypothesis as:

$$H_0 : \mu_A = \mu_B$$

The alternative hypothesis is:

$$H_1 : \mu_A \neq \mu_B$$

where, μ_A = the mean of one population and μ_B = the mean of the second population. We then calculate the appropriate *p*-value to see if the sample evidence is, or is not, strong enough for us to reject H_0 in favour of H_1.

As an example, look at Figure 16.2 (if it looks vaguely familiar it's because it's Figure 14.5 again). The table is from a randomised placebo controlled trial to assess the effect of continuous positive airway pressure (CPAP) on 24 hour ambulatory blood pressure monitoring values in patients with new onset untreated systemic hypertension and obstructive sleep apnea. The table shows the difference in mean blood pressures between the groups for a number of blood

Two-sample *t* test. Used to test whether or not the difference between the means of two *independent* populations is zero (i.e. the two means are equal). The null hypothesis is that it is. Both variables must be metric and Normally distributed (this is a parametric test). In addition, the two population standard deviations should be similar (but for larger sample sizes, this becomes less important).

Matched-pairs *t* test. Used to test whether the difference between the means of two *paired* populations is zero. The null assumption is that it is, that is, the two means are equal. Both variables must be metric and the *differences* between the two must be Normally distributed (this is a parametric test).

Mann–Whitney rank sums test. Often used to test whether the difference between the medians of two *independent* populations is zero. The null assumption is that the two medians are equal. Variables can be either metric or ordinal. More accurately this is a test of whether the two groups come from the same population. This is the non-parametric equivalent of the two-sample *t* test.

Kruskal–Wallis test. Used to test whether the medians of three or more *independent* groups are the same. Variables can be either ordinal or metric. Distributions can be of any shape but all need to be similar. This non-parametric test is an extension of the Mann–Whitney test.

Wilcoxon signed ranks test. Often used to test whether the difference between the medians of two *paired* populations is zero. The null assumption is that it is, that is, the two medians are equal. Strictly speaking, the null hypothesis is that there is no tendency for the outcome under one set of conditions (say a treatment group) to be higher or lower than under a comparative set of conditions (say a placebo group). Variables can be either metric or ordinal. Distributions can be of any shape, but the *differences* should be distributed symmetrically. This is the non-parametric equivalent of the matched-pairs *t* test.

Chi-squared test. (χ^2). Used to test whether the proportions across a number of categories of two or more *independent* groups are the same. The null hypothesis is that they are. Variables must be categorical.* The chi-squared test is also a test of the independence of the two variables (and has a number of other applications). We will deal with the chi-squared test in Chapter 17.

Chi-squared test (χ^2) for trend. Used as a test for a *trend* in the proportions or percentages across categories, when the categories can be *ordered*. The ordinary chi-squared test is much less powerful than the chi-squared test for trend. Note that establishing a linear trend across categories implies a relationship between the two variables in question. Variables must be categorical. The null hypothesis is that there is no trend, that is, no relationship.

Chi-squared test with odds ratios, **relative risk**, **etc**. Used as a measure of the statistical significance of odds and risk ratios, and the like. The null hypothesis is that the ratio is not significant.

Fisher's exact test. Used to test whether the proportions in two categories of two *independent* groups are the same. The null hypothesis is that they are. Variables must be categorical. This test is an alternative to the 2 × 2 chi-squared test, when cell sizes are too small (I will explain this later).

McNemar's test. Used to test whether the proportions in two categories of two *matched* groups are the same. The null hypothesis is that they are. Variables must be categorical.

---

*Categorical will normally be nominal or ordinal, but metric discrete or grouped metric continuous might be used provided the number of values or groups is small. For example: aged less than 50, or 50 or more; an Apgar score of less than 7, or 7 or more.

Figure 16.1   Some of the more common hypothesis tests

	Difference* (95% CI)	p value[†]
Diurnal systolic blood pressure	1.6 (−0.2 to 3.3)	0.07
Diurnal diastolic blood pressure	1.1 (−0.1 to 2.3)	0.07
Diurnal mean blood pressure	1.3 (−0.1 to 2.5)	0.06
Nocturnal systolic blood pressure	3.1 (0.9 to 5.2)	0.005
Nocturnal diastolic blood pressure	1.5 (0.1 to 3.0)	0.03
Nocturnal mean blood pressure	2.1 (0.5 to 3.6)	0.01
Mean systolic blood pressure	2.1 (0.4 to 3.7)	0.01
Mean diastolic blood pressure	1.3 (0.2 to 2.3)	0.02
Mean blood pressure	1.5 (0.4 to 2.7)	0.01

*Differences in blood pressure (mmHg) between continuous positive airway pressure (CPAP) and sham groups.
[†]Calculated by t test; compares treatment effects.

Figure 16.2 p-values and 95 per cent confidence intervals for the difference at 12 weeks, in various mean blood pressure outcomes, between the treatment group receiving continuous positive airway pressure (CPAP) and the placebo (sham) group. Taken from a randomised controlled trial of the effectiveness of continuous positive airway pressure for the treatment of patients with new onset and obstructive sleep apnea, who have untreated systemic hypertension. Durán-Cantolla *et al.* (2010)

pressure outcomes. The last column shows the p-values derived using the two-sample t test (see the table footnote).

As you can see, the first three p-values are >0.05 (and the 95 per cent confidence intervals include 0), so there is not enough evidence to reject the null hypothesis of no difference between the two groups in these three outcomes. The remaining p-values are all <0.05, so the evidence against the null hypothesis is strong enough for us to reject it.

Exercise 16.2.   Figure 16.3 (Figure 14.6 again) is from a randomised placebo controlled trial to determine the efficacy of intraoperative treatment with low-dose tranexamic acid in reducing the rate of perioperative transfusions in patients undergoing radical prostatectomy. For which outcomes do the p-values indicate sufficient evidence for us to reject the null hypothesis (of no difference in the blood loss between the placebo and tranexamic groups)?

Interpreting computer hypothesis test results for the difference in two independent population means – the two-sample t test

As the two-sample t test is one of the more commonly used hypothesis tests, it will be helpful to have a look at the computer output. As an example, we can test the hypothesis that the mean birthweight of babies (in a random sample of 500 from the Born in Bradford cohort) born to

Volume (ml)	Placebo group ($n = 100$)	Tranexamic acid group ($n = 100$)	p
Suctioned blood	1012 (608.1)	810 (390.2)	0.009
Blood absorbed in gauzes	322 (151.8)	293 (188.6)	0.053
Total intraoperative blood loss	1335 (686.5)	1103 (500.8)	0.01

Data are mean values (standard deviation) unless stated otherwise.

Figure 16.3 *p*-values for differences in mean blood loss between placebo and tranexamic groups. From a randomised controlled trial into the effectiveness of intraoperative treatment with low-dose tranexamic acid in reducing the rate of perioperative transfusions in patients undergoing radical prostatectomy. Crescenti *et al.* (2011)

White mothers (μ_{White}) is the same as babies born to non-White mothers ($\mu_{\text{non-White}}$). Notice that if $\mu_{\text{White}} = \mu_{\text{non-White}}$, then $\mu_{\text{White}} - \mu_{\text{non-White}} = 0$.

Output from Minitab – two-sample *t* test of difference in mean birthweights of babies born to White mothers and to non-White mothers

The output from Minitab for the two-sample *t* test of the null hypothsis that the population mean birthweights are the same as is shown in Figure 16.4. This is a test that $\mu_{\text{White}} - \mu_{\text{non-White}} = 0$.

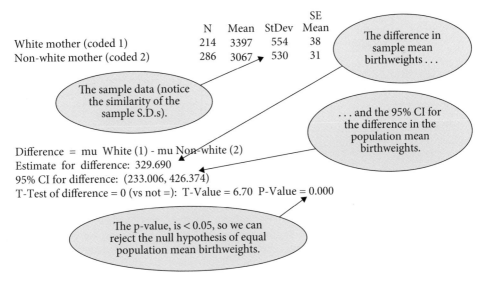

Figure 16.4 Minitab output for the hypothesis test that the population mean birthweights of babies born to White mothers is the same as babies born to non-White mothers. In fact the null hypothesis that $\mu_{\text{White}} - \mu_{\text{non-White}} = 0$

You will see that the p-value, given as 0.000 is <0.05, so there is enough evidence for us to reject the null hypothesis of equal population mean birthweights of babies born to White and non-White mothers. Note that the p-value is not 0, it is just that Minitab (and SPSS – see below) only gives three decimal values in the p-value result. We can only say that the p-value is <0.000. It might be 0.0009 or 0.00001, we have no way of knowing.

Output from SPSS: two-sample t test of difference in mean birthweights of babies born to White mothers and to non-White mothers

Figure 16.5 shows the output from SPPS for the two-sample t test of the null hypothesis that the mean birthweight of babies of White mothers is the same as the mean birthweight of

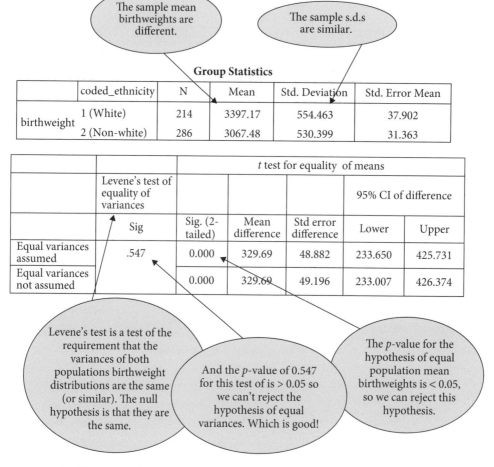

Figure 16.5   SPSS output for the hypothesis test that the population mean birthweights of babies born to white mothers is the same as that of babies born to non-white mothers (slightly abbreviated by present author)

babies born to non-White mothers. The SPPS output is slightly more complicated than that of Minitab for the same problem.

As you will recall, one of the requirements for the t test is that the variances (which are the squares of the standard deviations) are approximately the same.[3] SPSS gives two complete sets of results: one where equality of variances is assumed and the other where it is not assumed. Levene's test is a test of this equality, the null hypothesis being that the variances are equal. As you can see, the p-value for Levene's test is 0.547, which is >0.05, so we can't reject the hypothesis of equal variances. Thus, this requirement for using the two-sample t test appears to be satisfied.

The p-values (shown in the Sig. (two-tailed column)) are both <0.05, so the hypothesis of equal birthweights can be rejected.

Exercise 16.3.   Refer back to Figure 1.7, showing the basic characteristics of women in the breast cancer and stressful life events case–control study. Comment on what the p-values tell you about the equality or otherwise, between cases and controls, of the means of the seven metric variables (shown with an* – see the table footnote).

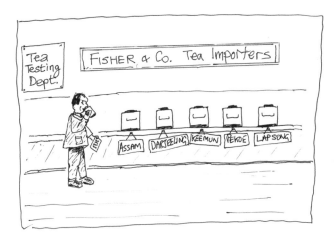

Comparing the means of two paired populations – the matched-pairs t test

You will remember that for pairs to be treated as being properly matched or paired, each individual in one group had to be matched with an individual in the second group. Frequency matching, where percentages in each group are about the same, for example, same percentage of individuals over 60, or similar percentages of males, and so on does not achieve this. Often, this matching can take the form of before and after designs, where the same individual is involved, thus being the perfect match. When matching exists, we can use the matched-pairs

---

[3] Just a reminder that the other two requirements are, first that the data are metric and second that both population distributions are Normal.

t test to test the hypotheses of equal population means. We will illustrate this situation with an exercise.

Exercise 16.4. In Figure 14.9, we looked at the 95 per cent confidence intervals (derived from the paired t test) for the difference in the mean lipid and lipoprotein concentrations for a number of outcomes, before and after patients were treated with statins. The data were from a cohort study of the interactive effects of fitness and statin treatment on mortality risk in veterans with dyslipidaemia. If you look back at that figure, you will see that the differences between the mean values in the before and after groups were all significant for all of the lipid outcomes. That is, we were able to reject the null hypothesis of no difference between the before and after mean lipid values – none of the confidence intervals included 1.

Figure 16.6 is from the same study and shows the initial and follow-up lipid levels for the same outcomes. What do the p-values, derived from the paired t test, tell you about the strength of the evidence against the null hypothesis of no difference between the lipid values intially and at follow-up?

Using p-values to compare the medians of two independent populations: the Mann–Whitney rank-sums test

As you saw in Chapter 14, if your data is ordinal or skewed metric, the Mann–Whitney approach, which compares population medians and not means, is appropriate. The null hypothesis is that the two medians are the same.[4] As we noted briefly in Chapter 14, the

	Patients not treated with statins			
	Initial ($n = 1433$)	At follow-up ($n = 1433$)	Mean difference (95% CI)	p value
Total cholesterol (mmol/l)	6.0 (0.8)	5.1 (1.1)	0.9 (0.8 to 0.9)	<0.0001
Triglycerides (mmol/l)	1.5 (0.9)	1.5 (0.8)	0.1 (0.0 to 0.2)	0.03
HDL cholesterol (mmol/l)	1.2 (0.4)	1.2 (0.4)	0.0 (0.0 to 0.0)	0.22
LDL cholesterol (mmol/l)	4.0 (0.8)	3.6 (0.9)	0.4 (0.4 to 0.5)	<0.0001

Data are mean (SD) unless stated otherwise. p values calculated by paired t test.

Figure 16.6 p-values for the initial and follow-up values for a number of lipid and lipoprotein concentration outcomes for a group of patients not treated with statins. You need to compare this table with Figure 14. 9 taken from the same study for before and after values for patients *treated with statins*. Data is from a cohort study of the interactive effects of fitness and statin treatment on mortality risk in veterans with dyslipidaemia (Kokkinos *et al.*, 2013).

---

[4] As you saw in Chapter 14, the Mann–Whitney approach is not strictly speaking, a test of the equality of two population medians, but of whether the two groups come from the same population. However, it is popularly used to compare medians.

Mann–Whitney test is a rank-based method. You need to know whether any observed difference in the rank sums is because there really is a significant difference in the two population medians or is it simply due to chance (sampling error). The *p*-value from the Mann–Whitney test will help you decide between these alternatives.

How the Mann–Whitney test works

The Mann–Whitney test is a rank-based method. As the test will often be used with ordinal data (as well as non-Normal metric data), and we know that ordinal numbers are not real numbers (see Chapter 1) which thus prevents us from applying the common numeric operators (+, −, × and ÷) to the data, we have to rank the data first.

As a very simple illustration of the rank method underlying the Mann–Whitney test, suppose that we have sample Injury Severity Scores (ISS),[5] for two groups of individuals and we want to know if their population ISS median scores are the same. ISS being a scale produces ordinal values. The data and working are shown in Figure 16.7.

The procedure is relatively simple:

Step 1. Amalgamate the two sets of scores, making sure you can identify which group each score came from.

Step 2. Rank these amalgamated scores from the smallest to the largest.

Step 3. Separate the ranks into their respective groups and sum each set of ranks.

Step 4. Compare the rank sums. Are they same (or similar) or different?

Group A ISS score	Group B ISS score	Joined Values	Ranks	A	B
60	50	50 (B)	1		1
55	65	55 (A)	2	2	
71	68	58 (A)	3	3	
58	75	60 (A)	4	4	
62	70	62 (A)	5	5	
		65 (B)	6		6
		68 (B)	7		7
		70 (B)	8		8
		71 (A)	9	9	
		75 (B)	10		10
			Rank sums	23	32

Figure 16.7 The ranking procedure of the Mann–Whitney rank-sums test for comparing the population median Injury Severity Scores (ISS) of two independent groups

---

[5] The Injury Severity Score is a measure of anatomical injury. It ranges from 1 to 75; higher scores indicate more severe injury.

As you can see, the rank sums are 23 and 32 for groups A and B, respectively. Even if the population medians were the same, we would not expect these rank sums to be identical because of sampling error. But how far apart do they have to be before we can feel that the evidence is strong enough for us to reject the null hypothesis of equal population medians? This is a decision that the *p*-value will help us make. If it is <0.05, we can reject the null hypothesis, otherwise we cannot.

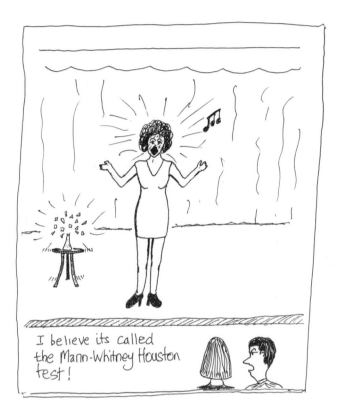

I believe its called the Mann-Whitney Houston test!

Interpreting computer output for the Mann–Whitney test

With Minitab

Suppose that we want to compare the median booking weight (kg) of White and non-White mothers from the Born in Bradford data. Although weight is a metric variable, it is not Normally distributed in either population, as you can see from Figure 16.8, so the Mann–Whitney test seems appropriate.

The output from Minitab for the Mann–Whitney test is shown in Figure 16.9. As you can see, the sample median weights are different, 70 kg and 61 kg for the White and non-White mothers, respectively. The Mann–Whitney test results indicate that the evidence against the null hypothesis of equal median population booking weights of White and non-White mothers

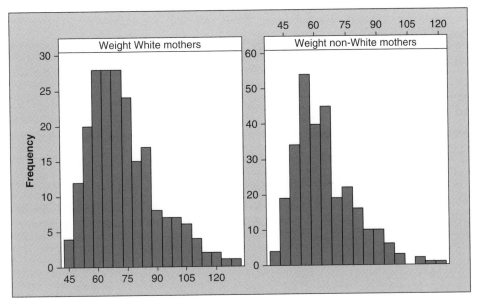

Figure 16.8 Distribution of booking weight (kg) of white and non-white mothers, for a random sample from the Born in Bradford cohort. As you can see, neither distribution is Normal (both positively skewed)

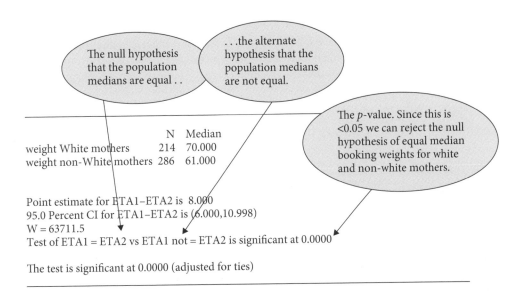

Figure 16.9 Output from Minitab for the Mann–Whitney test of the null hypothesis that the population medians of booking weight for white mothers and non-white mothers are equal. Data from a random sample drawn from the Born in Bradford cohort

is strong enough for us to reject it, the *p*-value is <0.05. (Note that Minitab uses ETA to denote the population median).

With SPSS

The output for the Mann–Whitney test of equal population booking weights is shown in Figure 16.10. As you can see, the result is the same as for Minitab – we can reject the null hypothesis of equal population median booking weights in White and non-White mothers.

> **Exercise 16.5.**   Interpret the *p*-values in Figure 16.11 for the differences in the medians of six procedure characteristics between two groups of patients, one group receiving a biodegradable stent and the other group a durable stent. (We first encountered this study in Figure 3.19).

Two matched medians – the Wilcoxon signed-ranks test

In the same circumstances as that for the Mann–Whitney test described earlier, but with *matched* populations, the non-parametric Wilcoxon signed-ranks test is appropriate. (see Chapter 14 for a brief explanation of the procedure). Look back at Figure 14.12, which is from a matched case–control study into the dietary intake of schizophrenic patients living in the community in Scotland. Here, the authors have used the Wilcoxon matched-pairs to test the null hypothesis that there is no difference in population median daily intakes of a number of substances between 'All Patients' and 'All Controls'. The *p*-values are in the column headed 'P'.

As you can see, the only *p*-value *not* less than 0.05 is that for protein (*p*-value = 0.07), so this is the only substance whose median daily intake for which the evidence is not strong enough for us to reject the null hypothesis that median intakes are the same (which is confirmed by the confidence intervals).

Confidence intervals versus hypothesis testing

I said at the beginning of this chapter that confidence intervals are preferred to hypothesis tests. Why is this? Because the confidence intervals are more informative. To illustrate this, look

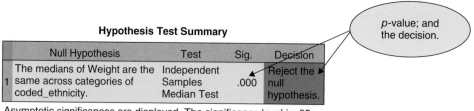

Figure 16.10   Output from SPSS for Mann–Whitney test of equal population median booking weights of White and non-White mothers from a sample drawn from the Born in Bradford cohort

	Biolimus-eluting stent ($n = 1229$)	Sirolimus-eluting stent ($n = 1239$)	p value
More than one stent			
Per patient	448 (36.5%)	450 (36.3%)	0.56
Per lesion	279 (18.3%)	300 (19.2%)	0.79
Total stent length (mm)			
Per patient	22.0 (14.0 to 32.0)	23.0 (13.0 to 33.0)	0.22
Per lesion	15.0 (10.0 to 20.0)	15.0 (10.0 to 20.0)	0.51
Direct stenting	329 (21.6%)	345 (22.4%)	0.60
Stent delivery failure	26 (1.7%)	31 (2.0%)	0.54
Maximum pressure (atm)	16.0 (14.0 to 20.0)	18.0 (15.0 to 20.0)	<0.0001
Length of procedure (min)	24.0 (16.0 to 38.0)	24.0 (15.0 to 38.0)	0.94
Fluoroscopy time (min)	6.5 (4.0 to 12.0)	6.9 (4.0 to 12.2)	0.27
Contrast (ml)	100.0 (60.0 to 130.0)	100.0 (60.0 to 140.0)	0.64
Use of glycoprotein IIb/IIIa inhibitors	195 (15.9%)	209 (16.9%)	0.50

Data are number (%) or median (IQR).

Figure 16.11 Use of the Mann–Whitney test to determine if there is a difference in the medians of six procedure characteristics. From a study to investigate the effects of a biodegradable polymer biolimus-eluting stent compared with a durable polymer-coated sirolimus-eluting stent. Data from Christiansen *et al.* (2013)

again at the Minitab output for the Mann–Whitney test of the difference in population median booking weights of White and non-White mothers Figure 16.9. The 95 per cent confidence interval for the difference in median weights is (6.000 to 10.998) kg and the *p*-value = 0.0000.

What do these two pieces of information tell us? The *p*-value (being <0.05) tells us that the evidence is plenty strong enough to reject the null hypothesis of equal population median weights. And that is all. But the confidence interval not only tells us that the median weights are different because the confidence interval does not include 0, but in addition, it also tells us that the difference in median weights is probably somewhere between 6.000 kg and 10.998 kg. This useful extra information comes completely free of charge!

So the confidence interval does everything that the hypothesis test does – it tells us if the medians are equal or not, but it *also* gives us extra information – on the likely range of values for this difference. Moreover, unlike a *p*-value, the confidence interval is in *clinically meaningful* units (in this case kg), which helps with the interpretation. So whenever possible, it is a good practice to use confidence intervals in preference to *p*-values. Although, of course, you can present both and many authors do.

There is one final and important point to make before we leave this discussion on *p*-values. It is very important not to be blinded by the <0.05 decision rule. A *p*-value just above 0.05 (e.g. for the difference in mean diurnal mean blood pressure in Figure 14.5) does not mean that there is no effect, that is, say no difference in the two means. It might be that a bigger sample would have given a *p*-value <0.05. When you come to interpret a *p*-value (in conjunction with a confidence interval), do not feel too restricted by the 0.05 threshhold. Don't forget that the point estimate of a difference is the single best guess of its value (1.3 mmHg in the diurnal blood pressure example). You should re-read the discussion on the interpretation of confidence intervals in

Chapter 14. And a useful discussion on the interpretation of p-values can be found in the study by Hackshaw and Kirkwood (2011).

Exercise 16.6.   Explain why it is better to present a confidence interval rather than a p-value.

What could possibly go wrong?

Again see Figure 16.2, from a randomised placebo controlled trial of the effectiveness of CPAP for the treatment of patients with new onset and obstructive sleep apnea, who also have untreated systemic hypertension. Your null hypothesis is that there is no difference in various blood pressure outcomes between the CPAP group and the sham (placebo) group.

If you consider the results for the difference in Diurnal mean blood pressure, the 95 per cent confidence interval is (-0.1 to 2.5) mmHg and the p-value $= 0.06$. Both of these measures indicate that the evidence against the null hypothesis is *not* strong enough for it to be rejected. So you don't reject it. But what if you have made the wrong decision and there is in fact a significant effect but you do not detect it.

How can this be? Well, your sample size might not be large enough, and the consequence is that your two-sample t test is not powerful enough to detect the differences between the CPAP and the sham groups, which smaller than 2 mmHg.

Now consider the results in Figure 16.2 for Nocturnal diastolic blood pressure. The 95 per cent confidence interval is (0.1 to 0.3) mmHg and the p-value $= 0.03$. Both of these measures indicate that the evidence against the null hypothesis is strong enough for it to be rejected. But suppose that this is also the wrong decision! It is possible that sampling error has given us a sample which is not representative of the populations (don't forget that we are only 95 per cent confident not 100 per cent), and there is actually *no* difference in Nocturnal blood pressure between the two groups in the population.

These two different types of failure to make the correct decision about the null hypothesis raises three interesting questions. First, what exactly is the power of a test and how can we measure it? Second, how can we increase the power of the test we are using? Third, is there a more powerful test that we can use instead? Before I address these questions, a few words on *types of error*.

Types of error

Whenever you decide either to reject or not reject a null hypothesis, you could be making a mistake. After all, you are basing your decision on *sample* evidence. Even if you have done everything right, your sample could still, by chance, not be very representative of the population, or it might be too small, and as a consequence your test might not be powerful enough to detect an effect if there is one. There are two possible errors:

- *Type I error*: Rejecting a null hypothesis when it is true. Also known as a *false positive*. In other words, concluding there *is* an effect when there isn't. The *probability* of committing a type I error is denoted as α (alpha), and it is the *same* α as that of the significance level of a test (see above).

- *Type II error*: Not rejecting a null hypothesis when it is false. Also known as a *false negative*. That is, concluding there is *no* effect when there is. The probability of committing a type II error is denoted as β (beta).

Ideally, you would like a test procedure which minimises the probability of a type I error because in many clinical situations such an error is potentially serious – judging some procedure to be effective when it is not. When you set the significance level of a test at $\alpha = 0.05$, it is because you want the probability of a type I error to be no more than 0.05.

Nonetheless, if there *is* a real effect you would certainly like to detect it, so you also want to minimise the probability of β, a type II error, or put another way, you want to make $(1 - \beta)$ as large as possible.

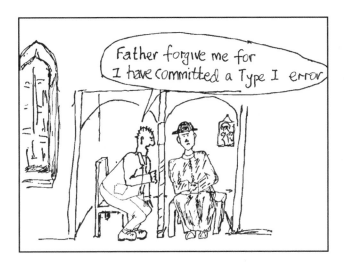

Exercise 16.7.   Explain, with examples, what is meant in hypothesis testing by: (a) a false positive, (b) a false negative. (c) How do we denote the probability of committing each type of error?

The power of a test

We can now come back to the three questions above.

What is meant by the *power* of a test? To answer the first question – the *power* of a test is a measure of the capacity of the test to reject the null hypothesis when it is false. In other words, the power to detect what is called the *smallest effect of clinical interest* if one is present in the population. This the smallest beneficial effect that clinicians would consider worthwhile in any intervention. Power is defined as $(1 -$ probability of a type II error), that is, $(1 - \beta)$.

In practice, β is typically set at 0.2 (or sometimes 0.1). This provides a power value of 0.80 (or 80 per cent). So if there *is* an effect, then the probability of the test detecting it is 0.80.

To answer the second question. How can you increase the power of the test you are using? Although you would like to minimise both α and β, unfortunately, they are, for a given sample size, interconnected. You can't make β smaller without making α larger and vice versa. Therefore, when you decide a value for α, you are also inevitably fixing the value for β. The only way to reduce both values simultaneously (and increase the power of a test) is to increase the sample size.

To answer the third question. Is there a more powerful test? Briefly, parametric tests are more powerful than non-parametric tests (see Figure 16.1 on the meaning of these terms). For example, a Mann–Whitney test has 95 per cent of the power of the two-sample t test.[6] The Wilcoxon matched-pairs test similarly has 95 per cent of the power of the matched-pairs t test. As for the chi-squared test, there is usually no obvious alternative when used for categorical data, so comparisons of power are less relevant, but it is known to be a powerful test. Generally, you should of course use the most powerful test that the type of data, and its distributional shape, will allow.

An example from practice

The following is an extract from the randomised controlled trial of epidural analgesic in the prevention of stump and phantom pain after amputation. The authors of the study outline their thinking on power thus:

> The natural history of phantom pain after amputation shows rates of about 70%, and in most patients the pain is not severe. Since epidural treatment is an invasive procedure, we decided that a clinically relevant treatment should reduce the incidence of phantom pain to less than 30% at week 1 and then at 3, 6, and 12 months after amputation. Before the start of the study, we estimated that a sample size of 27 patients per group would be required to detect a between-group difference of 40% in the rate of phantom pain (type I error rate 0.05; type II error rate 0.2; power $= 0.8$).

Exercise 16.8. (a) Explain, with the help of a few clinical examples, why you would normally want to minimise α while testing a hypothesis. (b) α is conventionally set at 0.05 or 0.01. Why, if you want to minimise it, do you not set it at 0.001 or 0.000001, or even 0?

Maximising power – calculating sample size

Before I say anything about calculating how big a sample you will need to answer your research question, the strongest possible advice I can give you is to consult a medical statistician for

---

[6]In view of the restrictions associated with the 2-sample t test, the Mann–Whitney test seems an excellent alternative!

help with this question. It is disastrous to embark on a piece of research, collect the data, then discover – too late – that your sample is not big enough to answer your research question!!! What follows is no more than a fairly superficial coverage of the topic – really to give you some idea of the numbers involved. If you are embarking on some clinical research project, I would strongly advise you to consult a statistician who will offer you reliable advice on sample size.

Generally, the bigger the sample, the more powerful the test.[7] The minimum size of a sample for a given power is determined both by the chosen level of α and the smallest effect of clinical interest. The sample size calculation can be summarised thus:

- Decide on the smallest effect of clinical interest.

- Decide the significance level of α, usually 0.05.

- Decide the power required, usually 80 per cent.

- Do the sample size calculation, using some appropriate software, or the rule of thumb described below.

Minitab has an easy-to-use sample size calculator for the most commonly used tests. Machin *et al.* (1987) is a comprehensive collection of sample size calculations for a large number of different test situations.

Rule of thumb 1. Comparing the means of two independent populations (metric data)

Assuming a significance level of 0.05 and a power of 0.8, the required sample size n is given by the following expression:

$$n = \frac{16 \times \text{s.d.}^2}{E^2}$$

where s.d. is the population standard deviation (assumed equal in both populations) in the outcome variable concerned. This can be estimated using the sample standard deviations, if they are available from a pilot study say. Otherwise the s.d. will have to be guessed using whatever information is available. E is the minimum difference in the means that would be clinically useful or otherwise interesting.

For example, suppose that you propose to use a case–control study to examine the efficacy of a program of regular exercise as an alternative to your current drug of choice in treating moderately hypertensive patients. The smallest effect of clinical interest is a difference of 10 mmHg in mean systolic blood pressures between the cases (given the exercise program) and the controls (given the existing drug). You will have to make an intelligent guess as to the standard deviation of systolic blood pressure (assumed the same in both groups – see above). Let's assume that the

---

[7] These sample-size calculations also apply if you are calculating confidence intervals. Samples that are too small produce wide confidence intervals, sometimes too wide to enable a real effect to be identified.

systolic blood pressure standard deviation is 15 mmHg (information on this, and many other measures, can be found in reference sources, from the research literature, from colleagues, etc.)

If power required is 80 per cent, with a significance level of 0.05, then the sample size required per group is:

$$n = \frac{16 \times 15^2}{10^2} = 36$$

So you will need at least 36 subjects in each of the two groups (always round up to next highest integer) to detect a difference of 10 mmHg between the means. In addition, you should add more participants to this sample size to allow for drop-outs from the study (you will have to make some sort of sensible asssessment of this number). Note that these sample sizes will also be large enough for two matched populations since these require smaller sample sizes for the same power.

Rule of thumb 2. Comparing the proportions of two independent populations (binary data)

The required sample size, n, for a significance level of 0.05, is given by:

$$\frac{[P_a(1 - P_a)] + [P_b \times (1 - P_b)]}{(P_a - P_b)^2} \times 8$$

where P_a is the proportion with treatment a, P_b is proportion with treatment b, so $(P_a - P_b)$ is the smallest effect of clinical interest.

For example, suppose that the percentage of elderly patients in a large district hospital with pressure sores is currently around 40 per cent or 0.40. So $P_a = 0.40$ and $(1 - P_a) = 0.60$. You want to test a new pressure-sore-reducing mattress, and you would like the percentage with pressure sores to decrease to at least 20 per cent or 0.20, so $P_b = 0.20$, and $(1 - P_b) = 0.80$. Therefore, $(P_a - P_b) = (0.40 - 0.20) = 0.20$. If power required is 80 per cent and significance level $\alpha = 0.05$, then required sample size per group is:

$$\frac{(0.40 \times 0.60) + (0.20 \times 0.80) \times 8}{(0.4 - 0.2)^2} = 80$$

Thus, you would need at least 80 subjects *in each group*, which would also be big enough for the matched samples case.

An interesting view on sample size calculation is found in a paper by Norman *et al.* (2012). To finish, here are two extracts from recent papers on the calculation of sample size.

Sample size
The original sample size was revised because fewer patients meeting the eligibility criteria were available for recruitment within practices than had been anticipated. For 80% power at 5% significance level (two sided test), 464 eligible patients (average of eight per practice) from 58 general practices were required to detect an absolute 0.5% reduction in mean HbA$_{1c}$ between the intervention and control groups at 18 months.

Sample size was based on a two sample *t* test, a standard deviation of 1.44. This value was then inflated by 1.3 to allow for the correlation of outcomes of patients within the same practice, assuming an intracluster correlation of 0.05 and variation in sample cluster size, and a further 20% for attrition over 18 months.

Blackberry et al. *(2013)*

The sample size calculation was based on our primary outcome (disability). On the basis of a power of 80% and an α of 0.05 (two tailed testing), and an expected treatment difference of at least 2.0 points on the Groningen Activity Restriction Scale, the required sample size was 80 per group (160 in total). Accounting for a dropout rate of 30% and a cluster effect of 1.73 (intraclass correlation coefficient 0.05), assuming equal cluster sizes, the final sample size had to be 180 per group (360 in total).

Metzelthin et al. *(2013)*

17

The chi-squared (χ^2) test – what, why, and how?

Medical Statistics from Scratch: An Introduction for Health Professionals, Third Edition. David Bowers.
© 2014 John Wiley & Sons, Ltd. Published 2014 by John Wiley & Sons, Ltd.

- Interpret SPSS and Minitab chi-squared test results.

- Interpret the published results of chi-squared tests.

- Outline the procedure for a chi-squared test for trend.

Of all the tests in all the world – you had to walk into my hypothesis testing procedure

As we discuss the use of the chi-squared (χ^2) test, quite a lot in the next chapter, it seems like a good idea to say something about the chi-squared test itself; what it is and how it works?

As we noted in Chapter 16, three hypothesis tests are quite common in clinical research. The first is the two-sample t test (see Chapter 14) which, as you have seen, is used with metric data to compare the means of two independent populations. The second is the Mann-Whitney test, which is used with ordinal or non-Normal metric data to compare the medians of two independent populations (Chapter 14). The third is the *chi-squared test*[1] (χ^2, pronounced as the first syllable in *Kylie* Minogue). The chi-squared test is probably the most common of the three.

The chi-squared test has three common applications: first, as a test of whether the proportions of a categorical variable are the same across two or more groups; second, to test whether two variables are related (i.e. dependent) or not (as you will see these tests are in fact equivalent), and third, to test the significance of relative risks (risk ratios), odds ratios, and other ratios (hazard ratios and incidence ratios immediately spring to mind).

Using chi-squared to test for related-ness or the equality of proportions

The chi-squared test is used with frequency data[2] in the form of a contingency table (i.e. a table of cross-tabulations), with the rows representing groups or categories of one variable and the columns representing the groups or categories of the second variable. The groups must be *independent* – this is an essential requirement of the chi-squared test.[3] The null hypothesis is that the two variables are unrelated.

Let me illustrate the idea of a chi-squared test with an example from the literature. Figure 17.1 is from a cohort study to assess whether mild iodine deficiency during early pregnancy was

---

[1] So called because it uses what is called the chi-squared distribution. If a variable X is Normally distributed, then X^2 has a chi-squared distribution. The chi-squared distribution is very skewed for small samples but becomes more and more like the Normal distribution as the sample size increases.

[2] The method works only with counts (i.e. numbers of persons or things); it does not work with proportions or percentage values.

[3] If the groups are matched then McNemar's test is appropriate.

		Outcome		
		Sub-optimum reading speed?		
		No	Yes	Total
Urinary iodine-to-creatinine ratio	<150 μ/mg	441	170	611
	≥150 μ/mg	231	62	293
	Total	672	232	904

Figure 17.1 The numbers of children aged nine years (out of the total sample of 904 children) with a sub-optimum reading speed, by maternal iodine status (urinary iodine-to-creatinine ratio). From a cohort study to assess whether mild iodine deficiency during early pregnancy is associated with an adverse effect on child cognitive development. Data from Bath *et al.* (2013)

associated with an adverse effect on child cognitive development. The table shows the numbers of children with a sub-optimum reading speed at nine years (out of the total sample of 904 children) by maternal iodine status: urinary iodine-to-creatinine ratio of <150 μ/mg and ≥150 μ/mg.

The rows of this table represent the two groups of the variable: urinary iodine-to-creatinine ratio, that is, <150 μ/mg and ≥150 μ/mg. The columns of the table represent two groups of the variable sub-optimum reading speed (no and yes). These groups are clearly independent. Notice that both variables are categorical.[4]

The question is: is there a relationship between mild iodine deficiency during early pregnancy and child cognitive development in the population? In other words, are the two variables related? The null hypothesis is that there is no relationship, that is, the two variables are independent of each other. That is:

H_0: Urinary iodine-to-creatinine ratio and sub-optimum reading speed at nine years are not related in the population (i.e. are independent).

We can use the chi-squared test and its associated *p*-value to provide us with a measure of the evidence against the null hypothesis.

Here is the important bit. If the two variables are unrelated, then there is no reason why the proportion of children with sub-optimum reading speed should be any different among mothers with a urinary iodine-to-creatinine ratio of <150 μ/mg compared to the proportion among children of mothers with a ratio of ≥150 μ/mg.

However, if the two variables were related, that is, if mild iodine deficiency during early pregnancy did adversely affect child cognitive development, then we would expect to find that the proportion of children with a sub-optimum reading speed would be different in the two categories of iodine levels.

In this example, the sample proportions of nine-year-old children with sub-optimum reading speeds are $170/611 = 0.2782$ in the < 150 μ/mg group and $62/293 = 0.2116$ in the ≥150 μ/mg group, respectively. These proportions are different, but (the usual question) are they different

---

[4]Urinary iodine-to-creatinine ratio is a metric variable but has been ordinalised by dividing it into these two groups.

		Outcome		
		Sub-optimum reading speed?		
		No	Yes	Total
Urinary iodine-to-creatinine ratio	<150 µ/mg	*454*	*157*	611
	≥150 µ/mg	*218*	*75*	293
	Total	672	232	904

Figure 17.2 Expected values (in italics for emphasis) assuming the null hypothesis between the urinary iodine-to-creatinine ratio and sub-optimum reading speed is true, that is, there is no relationship between these two variables

enough for us to think that the null hypothesis should be rejected? Is this difference due to a true difference in the proportions in the population or is it due to sampling error, and the population proportions are in fact the same? We need a way of answering this question, which we'll come to it shortly.

As it happens, we have already discussed a method for deciding whether two proportions are the same – by calculating a confidence interval for the difference in two population proportions (see Chapter 14). In fact, the two methods – asking if two variables are independent or if two proportions are the same, are equivalent whenever one of the variables *has only two* categories. However, although we can calculate the confidence interval in the two proportions approach, as we saw in Chapter 14, we can't with a chi-squared approach.

The crucial question is this, 'what proportions would we *expect* to find if the null hypothesis of unrelated variables was true?' The answer is that as we have got a total of 232 children with sub-optimum reading speed in the total sample of 904, that is, a proportion of 232/904 = 0.2566, we would expect to find 0.2566 or 25.66 per cent of the total in each category. That is, 25.66 per cent of the 611 in the <150 µ/mg category and 25.66 per cent of the 293 in the ≥150 µ/mg. This gives us 0.2566 × 611 = 157 and 0.2566 × 293 = 75 respectively. So you would expect about 157 nine-year-old children with a sub-optimum reading speed in the <150 µ/mg category and 75 in the ≥150 µ/mg category, rather than the observed values of 170 and 62.

The table in Figure 17.2 is what we would *expect* to find if the null hypothesis of no relation between the variables was true (rounded to the nearest whole number).

So the table in Figure 17.1 contains the values we actually *observe* in the sample, and the values in the table in Figure 17.2 are the values we would *expect* to find if the null hypothesis was true. We are back to the crucial question. How close are the observed and expected values? Are they close enough for us to put the difference down to sampling error and accept the null hypothesis of no relationship between the two variables, or is the difference between them too great to put down to mere sampling error and thus cause us to reject the null hypothesis. I will deal with this question in a moment.

Incidentally, if you do this calculation by hand (particularly as the number of rows and columns gets larger) an easier way to calculate *expected* frequencies is to use the expression:

$$\text{Expected cell frequency} = \frac{\text{total of row that cell is in} \times \text{total column that cell is in}}{\text{overall total frequency}}$$

So, for example, for the top left-hand cell, expected value $= (611 \times 232)/904 = 157$, which is correct!

Exercise 17.1.   From the same study as that of the data in Figure 17.1, the IQ of the children at eight years old was measured. The results were in the $<150\,\mu/mg$ group, 177 of 646 children had sub-optimum IQ; in the $\geq 150\,\mu/mg$ group, 65 of 312 children had sub-optimum IQ. Set this data out in the form of a contingency table as in Figure 17.1. Assuming a null hypothesis of no relationship between the two variables, calculate a table of expected values.

The chi-squared test can be used with more than two categories in each variable but with small sample sizes, the maximum number of either is limited by the proviso that none of the *expected* values should be less than 1 and that 80 per cent of expected values should be greater than 5. There are two ways round the problem of low expected values. First, increase the sample size – usually impractical. Second, amalgamate two or more rows or columns, if this can be done and still make sense.

Applying the chi-squared test

As you know, even if the null hypothesis is true and if there is no relationship between the variables, you would not expect the difference between each observed (O) value and each expected (E) value to be *exactly* zero, because of sampling error. But how far away does this difference have to be from zero before you accept that the sample results *are* indicative of a true difference in the proportions in the population rather than being due to sampling error?

You can use the *chi-squared test* to answer this question: if the p-value associated with the chi-squared test is less than 0.05 (or 0.01), you can reject the null hypothesis and conclude that the two variables are not independent or, put another way, there is a statistically significant difference in the proportions.

But anyway we can't use the value of $\sum (O - E)^2$ because it is always zero, so we have to do some cunning arithmetical manipulation to overcome this problem, as you will now see. The procedure (perhaps tedious but not difficult to do by hand if the number of categories is small) is as follows:

- Calculate the expected value, E, for each cell in the table.

- For each cell, calculate the value of $(O - E)$, where O is the observed value.

- Square each $(O - E)$ value, to get a set of $(O - E)^2$ values.

---

[5] Using the Greek letter $\sum$, which means the sum of the values.

- Divide each $(O - E)^2$ value by the E value for that cell, to get a set of $(O - E)^2/E$ values.

- Add all of the $(O - E)^2/E$ values. This gives the value of $\sum \left\{ \dfrac{(O - E)^2}{E} \right\}$

This final result is called the *chi-squared statistic*.

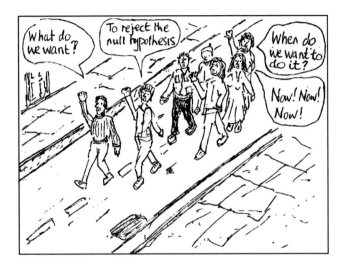

When all the observed values (the Os) are equal to their respective expected values (the Es), the chi-squared statistic will be equal to 0, so, for significance, we are looking for the value of chi-squared to be large. This chi-squared statistic has a chi-squared distribution when the null hypothesis is true: a property that we can use in our decision as to whether to reject or not the null hypothesis. Essentially, if the chi-squared statistic exceeds a critical value, we can take this as showing sufficient evidence against the null hypothesis of no relationship between the variables, and reject it.

For this purpose, we use critical values, the values of the chi-squared statistic at a 0.05 level of significance as shown in the table of Figure 17.3. The first column of this table is the number of degrees of freedom (d.f.) that the table has,[6] which is equal to the (number of rows - 1) × (the number of columns - 1). So, for example, a 2×2 table has $(2 - 1) \times (2 - 1) = 1$ d.f. For any given table size (numbers of rows and columns), the value of the chi-squared statistic must exceed the value in the table for us to reject the null hypothesis.

For example, the chi-squared statistic must *exceed* 3.84 for a 2×2 table for us to reject the null hypothesis that the two variables are independent, that is, the proportions are equal across categories. In practice, you will, no doubt, use a computer program to supply the p-value for the chi-squared test and thus to reject or not reject the null hypothesis.

---

[6] You do not need to know what degrees of freedom (d.f.) means for the purposes of reading this book. But I am sure that if you wish, you can find good explanations using a search engine.

Degrees of freedom (No. rows - 1) × (No. cols - 1)	Critical values, when $\alpha = 0.05$. The value to be exceeded if the null hypothesis of unrelated variables, (or equal proportions) is to be rejected
1	3.84
2	5.99
4	9.49
6	12.59
9	16.92

Figure 17.3 Table of critical p-values for the χ^2 test with statistical significance of 0.05. To reject the null hypothesis of unrelated, that is, independent variables (or equal proportions) the value of the test statistic must exceed the value in column two for the given table sizes in column one

Let's apply the chi-squared test to the data in Figure 17.1 to see if there is a relationship in the population between maternal iodine status and the sub-optimum reading speed of nine-year-old children.

Step 1. The $(O - E)$ terms from Figures 17.1 and 17.2, are:

$$(441 - 454), (170 - 157), (231 - 218) \text{ and } (62 - 75), \text{ i.e. } -13, 13, 13, -13^7$$

Step 2. Squaring each of these values gives: 169, 169, 169 and 169

Step 3. Dividing each of these by its E value, gives:

$$\frac{169}{454} = 0.372, \frac{169}{157} = 1.076, \frac{169}{218} = 0.7752 \text{ and } \frac{169}{75} = 2.253.$$

Step 4. Sum all of the values in the previous step. This gives:

$$(0.372 + 1.076 + 0.7752 + 2.253) = 4.476$$

So the chi-squared statistic $= 4.476$.

A 2×2 table has $(2 - 1) \times (2 - 1) = 1 \times 1 = 1$ d.f. So from Figure 17.3, the critical value is 3.84. As our chi-squared statistic of 4.476 comfortably exceeds this critical value, we can reject the null hypothesis. Therefore, there does appear to be a relationship between maternal mild iodine deficiency during early pregnancy and a sub-optimum reading speed in the children of these mothers at nine years.

---

[7]The differences in the $(O - E)$s are all the same, apart from the sign, in all four cells. This is true for all 2×2 tables.

Yate's correction (continuity correction)

The way the chi-squared test works is by approximating the *discrete* count (frequency) data in the contingency table with the *continuous* chi-squared distribution. If your sample size is small, however, even if more than 20 per cent of the expected values are greater than 5, or if any of the expected values is less than 1, this approximation is not satisfactory. The effect is to inflate the value of the chi-squared statistic. With a 2×2 table, we can use a continuity correction to improve the fit, by correcting this upwards bias. This sort of correction is called a continuity correction and in the 2×2 case, it is known as Yate's correction. This involves subtracting a value of 1/2 from each of the $(O - E)$ terms, *ignoring* its sign, thereby bringing the values closer to zero. You will not need to do this by hand.

Fisher's exact test

The chi-squared test is basically a test used with large samples, but when all the expected values are less than 5 (usually when the sample size is small) and we have a 2×2 table, we can turn to an alternative test called the Fisher's exact test. Most computer statistics programs perform this test, some by default if they find that the expected values are too small for the chi-squared test.

As an example of both Yate's correction and Fisher's exact test, Figure 17.4 shows the early (before hospital admission) and late deaths (after hospital admission) of children who

	Early death group (n = 19)	Late death group (n = 51)	p value
Median age (years; IQR)	6 (2–14)	7 (2.5–12)	0.9761*
Ethnic origin			
White British	12 (63%)	25 (49%)	0.7547[†]
Asian or Asian British (any)	6 (32%)	21 (41%)	
Black or Black British (any)	1 (5%)	3 (6%)	
Healthy or mild pre-existing disorders	9 (47%)	8 (16%)	0.0109[‡]
Presumed or confirmed bacterial sepsis	9 (47%)	19 (37%)	0.5842[‡]
Pre-hospital antivirals	2 (10%)	1 (2%)	0.1770[‡]
Duration from symptom onset to death (days; median, IQR)	2 (1–2.5)	10 (5.5–16.5)	<0.0001*
Duration from symptom onset to first medical consult (days; median, IQR)	1 (0.25–2)	2 (0–3.75)	0.4533*

Data are number of patients (%) unless otherwise stated.
*Mann–Whitney U test.
[†] χ^2 with Yates correction.
[‡] Fisher's test.

Figure 17.4 Examples of the use of the chi-squared test with Yate's correction and Fisher's exact test (as well the Mann–Whitney test of equal population medians – see Chapter 16). The table shows the characteristics of children presenting with rapid deterioration leading to death before, or at the point of, hospital admission (early death) and of those who died after hospital admission (late death). Data from Sachedina and Donaldson (2011)

died from AH1N1 influenza between June 2009 and March 2010, with a number of basic demographic and clinical characteristics. The table shows *p*-values for both tests (as well as for the Mann–Whitney test – see Chapter 16) and is taken from a study to analyse paediatric mortality to inform clinical and public health policies for future influenza seasons and pandemics.

> **Exercise 17.2.**   (a) Why do you think the authors of the study in Figure 17.4 used both the chi-squared test with Yate's correction and Fisher's exact test? (b) Assess the evidence for the rejection (or not) of the null hypothesis that there is no relationship between being White British (or not) and early or late death.

The chi-squared test with Minitab

Suppose that we want to know, using the Born in Bradford data ($n = 500$), if there is a relationship between ethnicity (two categories – White, and Non-White) and smoking while pregnant (Yes or No). The null hypothesis is that there is no relationship. Minitab produces the output shown in Figure 17.5. Both Minitab and SPSS (see below) produce more than one version of the chi-squared test. We are only interested in Pearson's chi-squared test.

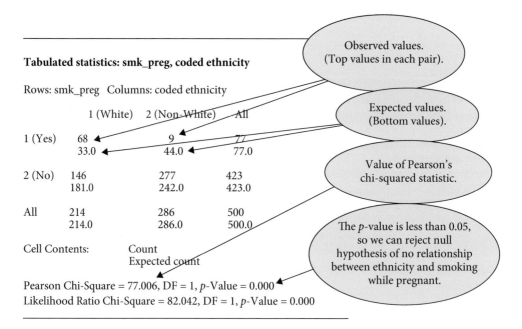

Figure 17.5 Output from Minitab for chi-squared test of relationship betwen ethnicity (White and Non-White mothers) and smoking while pregnant (Yes or No). Data is a random sample ($n = 500$) from the Born in Bradford cohort

As you can see, the value for the chi-squared statistic is large (77.006) and the p-value is <0.05, so we can reject the null hypothesis. Smoking while pregnant and ethnicity (White versus Non-White) appear to be related.

The chi-squared test with SPSS

SPSS produces the output as shown in Figure 17.6. The null hypothesis is the same as that shown for Minitab as described earlier, that is, there is no relationship between ethnicity of the mothers (White and Non-White) and smoking while pregnant. You will see that SPSS also provides a value for the chi-squared statistic with a continuity correction and the results for the Fisher's exact test. Notice also that at the foot of the results table, SPSS gives information on the number (and percentage) of expected value cells with a value less than 5.

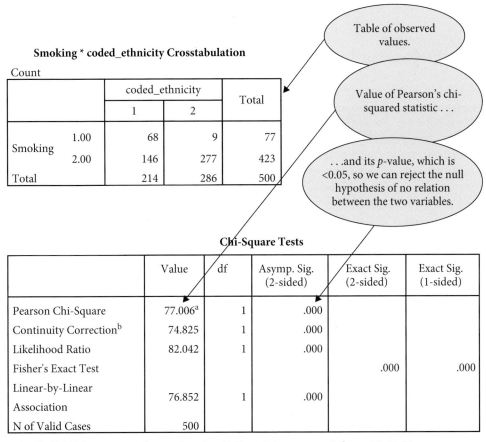

Smoking * coded_ethnicity Crosstabulation

Count

		coded_ethnicity		Total
		1	2	
Smoking	1.00	68	9	77
	2.00	146	277	423
Total		214	286	500

Table of observed values.

Value of Pearson's chi-squared statistic . . .

. . .and its p-value, which is <0.05, so we can reject the null hypothesis of no relation between the two variables.

Chi-Square Tests

	Value	df	Asymp. Sig. (2-sided)	Exact Sig. (2-sided)	Exact Sig. (1-sided)
Pearson Chi-Square	77.006[a]	1	.000		
Continuity Correction[b]	74.825	1	.000		
Likelihood Ratio	82.042	1	.000		
Fisher's Exact Test				.000	.000
Linear-by-Linear Association	76.852	1	.000		
N of Valid Cases	500				

a. 0 cells (0.0%) have expected count less than 5. The minimum expected count is 32.96.
b. Computed only for a 2×2 table

Figure 17.6 SPSS output for the null hypothesis that there is no relationship between the ethnicity of the mothers (White and Non-White) and smoking while pregnant

Exercise 17.3.   Following your calculation of expected values in Exercise 17.1, calculate the value of the corresponding chi-squared statistic and use the table of critical values (Figure 17.3) to reject or not reject the null hypothesis of no relationship between maternal mild iodine deficiency during early pregnancy and a sub-optimum IQ in children aged nine years.

Exercise 17.4.   Figure 17.7 is from a study to examine the associations between hospital volume and outcomes following cholecystectomy. Low volume is <173 cholecystectomies per year; medium volume is 173–244 cholecystectomies per year, and high volume is >244 cholecystectomies per year. The null hypothesis is that there is no relationship between each of the outcomes shown and hospital volume. Do you think that there is enough evidence to support the hypothesis of no relationship between each of the outcomes and hospital volume?

The chi-squared test for trend

An important extension of the chi-squared test is the *chi-squared test for trend*. This is a test of whether there is a systematic increase (or decrease) in proportions across categories when the categories in one of the variables can be *ordered*. For example, the categories might be hospital volume as in Figure 17.7 (low, medium or high), which are obviously ordered, against for example, the outcome mortality (died or not). The chi-squared test for trend can then be used to discover if there is a systematic trend in the proportion of deaths as volume increases. Note that this test is usually applied to 2 × 'something' contingency tables, for example, 2 × 3, 2 × 4 and 2 × 5. In the chi-squared test for trend, the null hypothesis is that there is *no* trend, and the *p*-value is used in the usual way.

The chi-squared test statistic for the trend test will always be less than that for the ordinary chi-squared test described earlier. However, because this is more powerful than the ordinary

	Hospital volume			p
	Low ($n = 20\ 959$)	Medium ($n = 20\ 534$)	High ($n = 18\ 425$)	
Mortality*	107 (0.51)	112 (0.55)	73 (0.40)	0.09[†]
Reoperation at 30 days	677 (3.23)	954 (4.65)	607 (3.29)	<0.001[†]
Readmission at 30 days	1583 (7.55)	1676 (8.16)	1403 (7.61)	0.024[†]

Data are number (%).
*Inpatient mortality and 30 day mortality combined.
[†] Pearson's χ^2 test.

Figure 17.7   Use of the chi-squared test to examine the equality of proportions across categories. Unadjusted outcomes after cholecystectomy. From a study to examine the associations between hospital volume and outcomes following cholecystectomy. (abbreviated by present author). Source: Adapted from Harrison *et al.* (2012). Reproduced by permission of BMJ Publishing Group Ltd

	Proportion of resistant isolates			Chi-squared and p-value	Chi-squared for trend and p-value
	Low prescribing	Medium prescribing	High prescribing		
Prescribing of erythromycin	7/164	24/441	19/223	3.60; 0.17	3.27; 0.07

Figure 17.8 Example of chi-squared for trend. From a study to quantify the relation between three levels of community-based antibacterial prescribing of erythromycin and antibacterial resistance in community acquired disease. Data from Priest *et al.* (2001)

chi-squared test, the trend test may produce a statistically significant result even when the ordinary chi-squared test does not (i.e. it is more likely to detect an effect if there is one). For this reason the chi-squared test for trend should always be used if categories can be ordered.

Note that establishing a linear trend across categories implies a relationship between the two variables in question.

As an example, of the use of the chi-squared test for trend, Figure 17.8 shows the results from a study to quantify the relation between three levels of community-based antibacterial prescribing of erythromycin and antibacterial resistance in community-acquired disease. The values of the chi-squared statistic and of the chi-squared test for trend, along with their respective *p*-values are shown. You can see that the *p*-value for the chi-squared test for trend is lower than that for the simple chi-squared statistic, and although neither is significant (both are >0.05), nontheless, the *p*-value of 0.07 for the trend test perhaps hints at a greater likelihood of the trend across the prescribing categories. As I noted in Chapter 16, you should not be too rigid in the interpretation of *p*-values.

SPSS output for chi-squared trend test

Minitab does not perform a chi-squared trend test but SPSS does, and does so automatically whenever the simple chi-squared test is requested. Figure 17.9 contains the output from SPSS for a chi-squared test of the education level of the mothers in the sample from the Born in Bradford cohort (1 is lowest) and whether they smoked during their pregnancy. SPSS refers to the trend test as the Linear-by-Linear Association, as you see in the figure. The null hypothesis for the trend test is that the proportion smoking decreases as education levels increase, that is, there is a consistent downward trend in the proportions smoking while pregnant.

You can see that the chi-squared statistic and the trend statistic are much the same, and they both have *p*-values less than 0.05, so we can reject the null hypotheses of no relationship between the variable and no trend across column categories. Note though, that in some circumstances, the trend test will pick up a significant result where the simple chi-squared test does not, since, as I mentioned earlier, the trend test is more powerful. In this case, the trend statistic will be larger than the chi-squared statistic.

The chi-squared test is a very versatile procedure and has other important applications, for example, in meta-analysis (see Chapter 24) and in logistic regression (see Chapter 22).

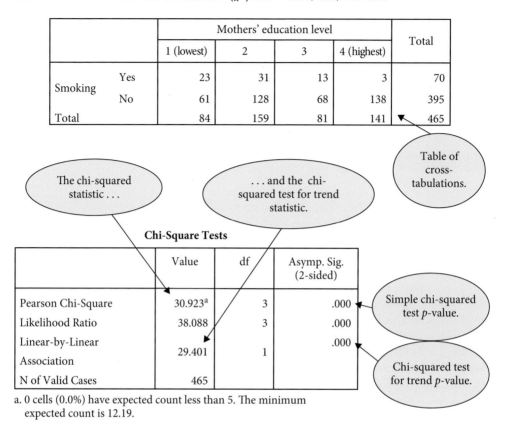

Figure 17.9   SPSS output for chi-squared test for trend of the educational levels of mothers and whether they smoked while pregnant. Data from the Born in Bradford cohort study

Exercise 17.5.   Refer back to Figure 1.7, the breast cancer and stress case – control study. The table footnote indicates four chi-squared trend tests. Comment on what each p-value reveals about the existence of a trend in the categories of each of the variables concerned.

18

Testing hypotheses about the *ratio* of two population parameters

Learning objectives

When you have read this chapter, you should be able to:

- Describe the usual form of the null hypothesis in the context of testing the ratio of two population parameters.

- Outline the differences between tests of ratios and tests of differences.

- Interpret published results on tests of risk, odds and hazard ratios.

Preamble

In the previous chapter, I introduced the basic idea of the chi-squared test. What it is? How it is calculated? How it is interpreted? I also discussed Yate's correction for the chi-squared test, the chi-squared test for trend and I briefly mentioned the Fisher's exact test for use in 2×2 tables when the sample size was small.

Another important use of the chi-squared test is to test for the significance of ratios, particularly the risk ratio and the odds ratio. In a later chapter, we will see how it has been used with the hazard ratio (Chapter 23).

The chi-squared test with the risk ratio

As an example of the use of the chi-squared test with risk ratios, see Figure 15.5, which I have very kindly reproduced here as Figure 18.1, taken from the investigation into whether a relative deficiency in L-arginine is associated with the development of pre-eclampsia in a population of high-risk women. The null hypothesis is that the risk ratio in the population is equal to 1. You can see that the supplementation with L-arginine plus vitamins reduces the risk of pre-eclampsia to 42 per cent compared to women receiving the placebo. This is significant because the confidence interval does not include 1, and this is confirmed by the p-value of <0.001, derived using the chi-squared test.

In other words, the probability of getting this result (a risk ratio of 0.42, referred to by the authors here as 'relative risk') by chance if the null hypothesis of no difference from the placebo group is true, is so small (much less than our critical value of 0.05) that we can be reasonably be confident in rejecting this null hypothesis. The same is true for the group receiving L-arginine plus vitamins versus vitamins alone. Here, the risk ratio is 0.56, and the p-value is again <0.001, that is, less than 0.05.

However, the result for the group receiving vitamins alone compared to the placebo group is not significant. The confidence interval includes 1, and the p-value of 0.052 exceeds 0.05, so the evidence is not strong enough for us to reject the null hypothesis of no difference between the

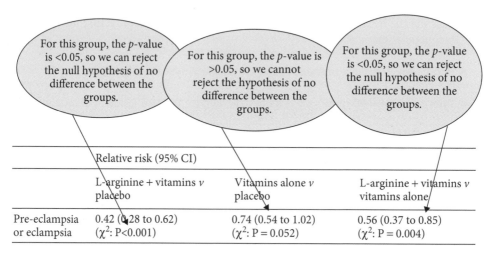

	Relative risk (95% CI)		
	L-arginine + vitamins v placebo	Vitamins alone v placebo	L-arginine + vitamins v vitamins alone
Pre-eclampsia or eclampsia	0.42 (0.28 to 0.62) (χ^2: P<0.001)	0.74 (0.54 to 1.02) (χ^2: P = 0.052)	0.56 (0.37 to 0.85) (χ^2: P = 0.004)

For this group, the p-value is <0.05, so we can reject the null hypothesis of no difference between the groups.

For this group, the p-value is >0.05, so we cannot reject the hypothesis of no difference between the groups.

For this group, the p-value is <0.05, so we can reject the null hypothesis of no difference between the groups.

Figure 18.1 Relative risks (risk ratios), 95 per cent confidence intervals and p-values for three groups of women participating in a randomised placebo controlled trial of L-arginine and antioxidant treatment for the reduction of pre-eclampsia or eclampsia. Data from Vadillo-Ortega *et al.* (2011)

groups in terms of getting pre-eclampsia. But we need to be careful not to be completely blinded by the p-value rule. The single best guess as to the risk ratio in this case is 0.74, which means that the group receiving vitamins were 26 per cent less likely to suffer from pre-eclampsia than those on a placebo. Besides, the confidence interval only just includes 1, and the p-value only just exceeds 0.05, implying, at least, that the effect of supplementation with vitamins versus placebo might be effective. A larger sample might confirm this.

Exercise 18.1.   From the results in Figure 18.1, by how much is the risk of pre-eclampsia reduced in the group receiving L-arginine + vitamins compared to those in the group receiving the placebo?

Exercise 18.2.   Figure 18.2 (from which I showed a small segment as Figure 8.3), is from a study to assess the main risk factors associated with stillbirth in a multi-ethnic English maternity population. Using the p-values, which characteristics appear to be significantly associated with stillbirth in the population?

Variables	Adjusted relative risk (95% CI)	p value
Parity:		
0	1.8 (1.3 to 2.5)	<0.01
≥3	1.6 (1.0 to 2.5)	0.05
Ethnic origin, place of birth:		
African*	2.4 (1.2 to 4.6)	0.01
African-Caribbean*	2.3 (1.3 to 4.1)	0.01
Indian*	2.1 (1.3 to 3.5)	<0.01
Pakistani, non-UK	3.0 (1.9 to 4.8)	<0.01
Body mass index:		
30–34.9	1.4 (1.0 to 2.0)	0.07
≥35	1.6 (1.1 to 2.4)	0.03
Mental health history	1.4 (1.0 to 1.9)	0.06
Pre-existing diabetes	3.9 (1.7 to 8.9)	<0.01
Antepartum haemorrhage	3.4 (2.6 to 4.5)	<0.01
Maternal smoking, no foetal growth restriction[†]		
Active smoker	2.5 (1.7 to 3.6)	<0.01
Passive smoker	1.3 (0.8 to 2.0)	0.28
Maternal smoking, foetal growth restriction[†]:		
Active smoker	5.7 (3.6 to 8.9)	<0.01
Passive smoker	10.0 (6.6 to 15.8)	<0.01
Foetal growth restriction[†], non-smoker	7.8 (5.6 to 10.9)	<0.01

Reference group: para 1, UK born, non-smoking, European mother; body mass index 18.5–24.9.
*UK and non-UK groups combined because of small numbers.
[†]Birth weight <10th gestation related optimal weight centile.

Figure 18.2   Adjusted relative risks (risk ratios), confidence intervals and p-values for risk factors for stillbirth. Source: Gardosi *et al.* (2013). Reproduced by permission of BMJ Publishing Group Ltd

The chi-squared test with odds ratios

As an example of the use of p-values with odds ratios, Figure 18.3 is from a cohort study to determine whether the use of paracetamol in early life is an independent risk factor for childhood allergic disease. The odds ratios reflect the increase in odds arising from an increase in the number of days of paracetamol use in early life (in fact a doubling). The null hypothesis is that the odds ratio is equal to 1, that is, there is no increase in of any of the allergic diseases shown in the table if days of paracetamol use increases (doubles).

As you can see, for the unadjusted odds ratios, only infantile wheeze and allergic rhinitis are significant (neither of the confidence interval contains 1 and both p-values are <0.05), and we can reject the null hypothesis for both outcomes. However, once the results are adjusted for possible confounders, allergic rhinitis becomes insignificant (we cannot reject the null hypothesis), but infantile wheeze remains significant, the evidence against the null hypothesis is still strong enough for us to reject it.

Exercise 18.3. Figure 18.4 is from a randomised controlled trial to examine whether the effect of tranexamic acid on the risk of death and thrombotic events in patients with traumatic bleeding varies according to baseline risk of death. It shows odds ratios, 95 per cent confidence intervals and p-values for a number of outcomes. Comment on what is revealed by the p-values for each event.

	Unadjusted		Adjusted*	
	Odds ratio (95% CI)	p value	Odds ratio (95% CI)	p value
Infantile wheeze	1.45 (1.23 to 1.71)	<0.01	1.44 (1.17 to 1.77)	<0.01
Infantile eczema	1.13 (0.99 to 1.30)	0.08	1.13 (0.97 to 1.31)	0.11
Positive skin prick test[†]	0.97 (0.82 to 1.14)	0.68	0.98 (0.82 to 1.18)	0.86
Asthma	1.18 (1.00 to 1.39)	0.05	1.08 (0.91 to 1.29)	0.39
Allergic rhinitis	1.21 (1.01 to 1.46)	0.04	1.17 (0.96 to 1.43)	0.12
Eczema	1.05 (0.90 to 1.22)	0.52	1.10 (0.93 to 1.29)	0.26

*Infant's sex, parental history of asthma, presence of older siblings at time of birth and frequency of infections (upper and lower respiratory tract infections, otitis media, and gastrointestinal infections) during first 2 years of life.
[†]≥3 mm to at least one of six allergens at 2 year test.

Figure 18.3 Unadjusted and adjusted odds ratios, 95 per cent confidence intervals and p-values for associations between total days of paracetamol use during early life and risk of allergic disease. The odds ratios reflect the risk when doubling the total number of days of paracetamol use. Table abbreviated by present author. Source: Adapted from Lowe *et al.* (2010). Reproduced by permission of BMJ Publishing Group Ltd

	Tranexamic acid (n = 6684)	Placebo (n = 6589)	Odds ratio (95% CI)	p value
Any event	98 (1.5)	140 (2.1)	0.69 (0.53 to 0.89)	0.005
Any arterial event	47 (0.7)	80 (1.2)	0.58 (0.40 to 0.83)	0.003
Myocardial infarction	23 (0.3)	46 (0.7)	0.49 (0.30 to 0.81)	0.005
Stroke	28 (0.4)	40 (0.6)	0.69 (0.43 to 1.11)	0.128
Any venous event	60 (0.9)	71 (1.1)	0.83 (0.59 to 1.17)	0.295
Pulmonary embolism	42 (0.6)	47 (0.7)	0.88 (0.58 to 1.33)	0.548
Deep vein thrombosis	25 (0.4)	28 (0.4)	0.88 (0.52 to 1.50)	0.641

Figure 18.4 Odd ratios, 95 per cent confidence intervals and p-values, for a number of events. From the study of the effect of tranexamic acid on fatal and non-fatal thrombotic events in patients with traumatic bleeding. Figures are numbers (percentages) of patients experiencing each event. Data from Roberts *et al.* (2012)

Exercise 18.4. Figure 18.5 is from an unmatched case–control study into the effect of passive smoking as a risk factor for coronary heart disease (CHD) in Chinese women who had never smoked. The cases were patients with CHD, the control women without CHD. The study considered both passive smoking at home from husbands who smoked and at work from smoking co-workers. The null hypotheses were that the population odds ratio was equal to 1, both at home and at work, that is, passive smoking had no effect on the odds for CHD. The table contains the adjusted odds ratios for CHD for a number of risk factors, with 95 per cent confidence intervals and p-values. Which factors do you think would increase the odds of coronary heart disease in the population of such women?

	Adjusted odds ratio (95% confidence interval)[*]	p value
Age (years)	1.13 (1.04 to 1.22)	0.003
History of hypertension	2.47 (1.14 to 5.36)	0.022
Type A personality	2.83 (1.31 to 6.37)	0.008
Total cholesterol (mg/dl)	1.02 (1.01 to 1.03)	<0.000
High density lipoprotein cholesterol (mg/dl)	0.94 (0.90 to 0.98)	0.0030
Passive smoking from husband	1.24 (0.56 to 2.72)	0.600
Passive smoking at work	1.85 (0.86 to 4.00)	0.120

[*]Adjusted for the other variables in the final model.

Figure 18.5 Odds ratios, 95 per cent confidence intervals and p-values, from an unmatched case-control study into the effect of passive smoking as a risk factor for coronary heart disease (CHD). The cases were patients with CHD, the control individuals without CHD. (Table is abridged by present author). Source: He *et al.* (1994). Reproduced by permission of BMJ Publishing Group Ltd

The chi-squared test with hazard ratios

Remember Figure 15.8? This contained a table of hazard ratios from a cohort study to examine all cause and disease-specific mortality in patients with osteoarthritis of the knee or hip. I have reproduced the figure below (see Figure 18.6) with p-values (which I suppressed in Figure 15.8). If I asked you to say which characteristics were significant hazards using the p-values, you would no doubt identify the same characteristics as you did in Exercise 15.6. I will have more to say on hazard ratios in Chapter 23 when I will discuss survival analysis.

Characteristic at baseline	Patients died		Crude hazard ratio* (95% CI)	p-value*
	Yes ($n=438$)	No ($n=725$)		
Age (years) at baseline:				
35–54	6 (1)	169 (23)	1.00 (reference)	<0.001
55–74	273 (62)	503 (69)	12.4 (5.53 to 27.9)	
≥75	159 (36)	53 (7)	40.7 (18.0 to 92.0)	
Male sex	204 (47)	299 (41)	1.21 (1.00 to 1.46)	0.048
Lower social class (IIIM to V)	228 (52)	342 (47)	1.21 (1.00 to 1.46)	0.050
Smoking	70 (16)	115 (16)	0.94 (0.74 to 1.19)	0.60
Previous joint replacement	42 (10)	38 (5)	1.61 (1.17 to 2.22)	0.003
Type of osteoarthritis:				
Knee only	130 (30)	233 (32)	1.00 (reference)	0.14
Hip only	120 (27)	222 (31)	0.98 (0.77 to 1.26)	
Knee and hip	188 (43)	270 (37)	1.20 (0.96 to 1.50)	
Knee or hip pain	289 (66)	477 (66)	1.00 (0.82 to 1.22)	0.97
Walking disability	152 (35)	136 (19)	1.93 (1.59 to 2.36)	<0.001

Values are numbers (percentages) unless stated otherwise.
*Univariable hazard ratios, 95% confidence intervals and p values were derived from Cox regression models after multiple imputation of missing covariate data; hazard ratios >1 indicate lower mortality in reference category.

Figure 18.6 Hazard ratios, 95 per cent confidence intervals and p-values, from a cohort study to examine all cause and disease-specific mortality in patients with osteoarthritis of the knee or hip (abbreviated by present author). Source: Adapted from Nüesch et al. (2011). Reproduced by permission of BMJ Publishing Group Ltd

VIII

Becoming Acquainted

19

Measuring the association between two variables

Medical Statistics from Scratch: An Introduction for Health Professionals, Third Edition. David Bowers.
© 2014 John Wiley & Sons, Ltd. Published 2014 by John Wiley & Sons, Ltd.

Preamble – plotting data

Suppose that you measure systolic blood pressure (SBP) in mmHg and waist circumference (waist) in cm in three patients. You get the following data:

	SBP	Waist
Patient A	120	75
Patient B	170	150
Patient C	150	100

Now, you plot the data, as in Figure 19.1, plotting values of SBP on the vertical axis and values of waist on the horizontal axis.[1] This plot is called a *scatterplot*. Note that it does not matter which axis you use for SBP and which for Waist. However, if you have a suspicion that changes in one of the variables causes changes in the other variable (in this example you might think that changes in Waist cause changes in SBP, that is, the larger your waist measurement, the higher will be your SBP *in consequence*) then you should put the *causing* variable on the horizontal axis, as I have here.

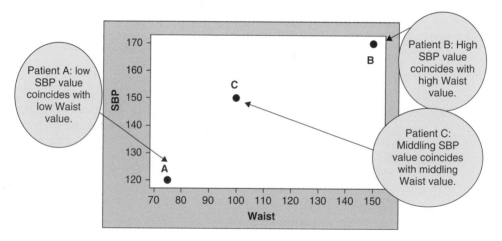

Figure 19.1   A scatterplot of systolic blood pressure (mmHg) against waist circumference (cm). Shows a *positive association* between the two variables

What do you see in the scatterplot? Well, for Patient A, a low SBP coincides with a low Waist measurement; for Patient B, a high SBP coincides with a high Waist measurement; for Patient C, a middling SBP coincides with a middling Waist measurement. In other words, the two variables seems to be *associated* in some way. Let's now discuss what we mean by association.

---

[1] For the three of you out there who may have forgotten how to draw a graph, the value for Patient A is drawn where the SBP of 120 on the vertical axis meets the value of 75 on the horizontal axis. And similarly for the other two points.

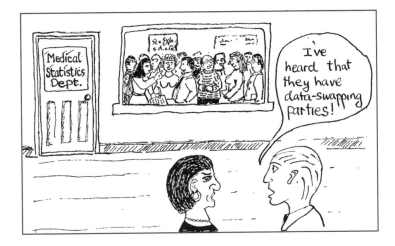

Association

When we say that two ordinal or metric variables are *associated*, we mean that they behave in a way that makes them appear 'interconnected' – changes in either variable seem to coincide with changes in the other variable. It is important to note (at this point anyway) that we are not suggesting that the change in either variable is *causing* the change in the other variable, simply that they exhibit this commonality. As you will see, association, if it exists, may take the form of:

- *Positive association* – low values of one variable tend to coincide with low values of the other variable, and high values with high values. If the value of one variable increases, we find that the value of the other variable also tends to increase. If the value of one variable decreases, we find that the value of the other variable also tends to decrease.

- *Negative association* – low values of one variable tend to coincide with high values of the other variable, and vice versa. If the value of one variable increases, we find that the value of the other variable also tends to decrease. If the value of one variable decreases, the value of the other variable tends to increase.

In this chapter, I want to discuss two alternative methods of finding out if an association exists between two variables. The first method relies on a plot of the sample data, the *scatterplot* (like that in Figure 19.1) in which the values of one variable are plotted on the vertical axis and the values of the other variable on the horizontal axis. The second approach is numeric, making both comparison and inference possible.

The scatterplot

A scatterplot will enable you to see if there is an association between the variables, and if there is, its strength and direction. It is always a good idea to draw a scatterplot before you move onto a numerical approach. This will often reveal interesting patterns, which may not be otherwise obvious. A weakness of the scatterplot is that it provides only a *qualitative* assessment, and thus has obvious limitations. First, it is not always easy to say which of the two sample scatterplots indicates a stronger association and second, it doesn't allow us to make *inferences* about possible associations in the population. Before I deal with the numeric approach to measuring association, let us have a look at a couple of scatterplots from the literature.

Figure 19.2 is from a cross-sectional study of the satisfaction by both patients and nurses with a particular hospital among a number of hospitals, in one of a number of countries. The measures captured by the researchers included what percentage of patients would recommend

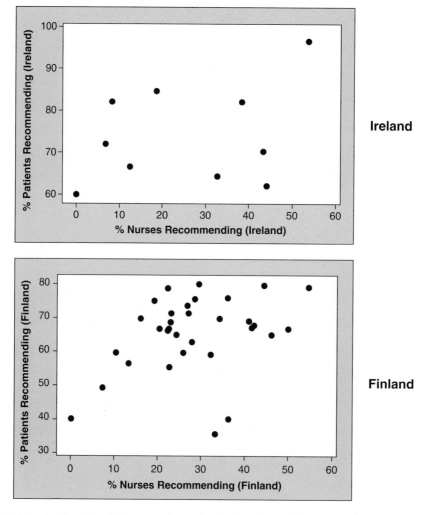

Figure 19.2 Scatterplots of the percentage of patients who would recommend a hospital and the percentage of nurses who would recommend the same hospital. Outcome for hospitals in Ireland (top chart), Finland (middle chart) and Spain (bottom chart – see overleaf). Source: Aiken *et al.* (2012). Reproduced by permission of BMJ Publishing Group Ltd

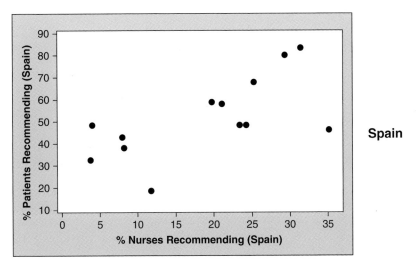

Figure 19.2 *(continued)*

each of the hospitals, and what corresponding percentage of nurses would recommend the same hospitals. The figure shows the results for hospitals in Ireland, Finland and Spain. What can we say about any possible associations indicated by the scatterplots?

If we look at the scatterplot for Ireland, we see no obvious association, apart from that corresponding to the lowest and highest patient percentages, which coincide with the lowest and highest percentages for nurses. Otherwise, the scatter seems completely random. The scatterplot for Finland shows a little more association. If it wasn't for the two values at the bottom middle of the plot, we would be able to say that higher and lower values for patients and nurses seem to coincide to some extent.

The scatterplot for Spain shows much clearer association. Lower values for patients coincide more or less with the lower values for nurses, and higher values with higher values. Later on, we will re-examine these conclusions when we look at numeric measures of association.

Exercise 19.1. The scatterplot in Figure 19.3 is from a cross-sectional study to describe variations in the incidence of ulcerative colitis (UC) and Crohn's disease (CD) in 52 postal areas in Manitoba. What does the scatterplot indicate about a possible association between the two illnesses?

I said earlier that when you set out to investigate a possible association between two variables, a scatterplot is almost always worthwhile, and will often produce an insight into the way the two variables co-behave. In particular, it may reveal whether an association between them is *linear*. Put simply, a linear association is one in which the points in the scatterplot seem to cluster around a straight line – the closer the clustering to the straight line, the more linear is the association. The Normality of the distributions can also be assessed visually – normally distributed variables produce a cigar-shaped or an elliptical scatter. When I talk about association in this chapter, I am talking about *linear association*. When you look at a scatterplot, you

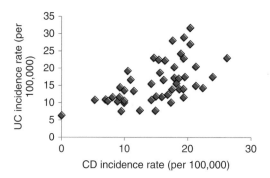

Figure 19.3   Scatterplot of incidence of ulcerative colitis (UC) and Crohn's disease (CD), in 52 postal areas in Manitoba. Source: Blanchard *et al.* (2001). Reproduced by permission of Oxford University Press

should ask yourself, do the points lie (even roughly) around an imaginary straight line? Is the scatter elliptical-ish?

Exercise 19.2.   Look at the two scatterplots in Figure 19.4. These plots are taken from a retrospective examination of hospital records, as part of a study into the relationship between hospital volume (number of cases dealt with per year) and hospital percentage mortality. Do you think these scatterplots show any association between the variables? If so, is it a linear association?

Exercise 19.3.   (a) Why is it always a good idea to draw a scatterplot when investigating a possible association between two variables? (b) What is the main shortcoming of a scatterplot?

The correlation coefficient

Despite being invaluable for looking at the shape of the scatter, a limitation of the scatterplot in assessing association is that it does not provide us with a *numeric* measure of the *strength* of the association. For this, we have to turn to the *correlation coefficient*. Loosely speaking, the correlation coefficient is a measure of the average distance of all of the points in the scatter from an imaginary straight line drawn through the scatter (analogous to the standard deviation measuring the average distance of each value from the mean). Two correlation coefficients are widely used: *Pearson's* and *Spearman's*. We will start with Pearson's.

Pearson's correlation coefficient

Pearson's correlation coefficient is denoted as ρ (Greek 'rho') in the population and r in the sample. It provides a measure of the strength of the *linear* association between the two variables.

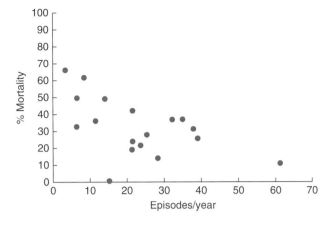

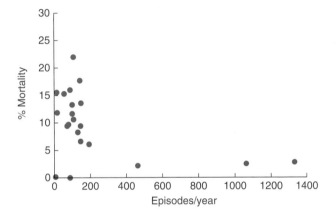

Figure 19.4 Scatterplots for the association between hospital volume (cases per year) and hospital percentage mortality. Top plot is for aortic aneurism and bottom plot is for carcinoma of the colon. Source: McKee and Hunter (1995). Reproduced by permission of BMJ Publishing Group Ltd

If you plan to use Pearson's correlation coefficient then both variables must be *metric continuous*, and at least one of the variables should be approximately Normally distributed. However, if a confidence interval is to be determined, both variables should be Normal. It is worth noting that, even with approximately Normal distributions, Pearson's correlation coefficient is sensitive to the presence of outliers. If you have outliers in either data set, you should interpret any results with suspicion, as these outliners can distort the results or you should consider using Spearman's correlation coefficient (see below).

The value of Pearson's correlation coefficient can vary as follows:

- From −1, indicating a perfect negative association. All the points lie exactly on a straight line sloping down from left to right.

- Through 0, indicating no association.

- To +1, indicating a perfect positive association. All the points lie exactly on a line sloping upwards from left to right.

In practice, with real sample data, you will never see values of −1, 0 or +1. The value of r can be found in a flash with a computer statistics program, such as SPSS or Minitab. These will usually provide the associated p-value as well.

Is the correlation coefficient statistically significant in the population?

Just because we get a non-zero *sample* correlation coefficient (as we invariably will) does not necessarily mean that the *population* correlation coefficient is also non-zero (this is the old familiar question). To discover whether the population correlation coefficient is non-zero or not, and hence decide whether there is a linear association between the two variables, means a hypothesis test of the hypotheses:

$$H_0 : \rho = 0$$

$$H_1 : \rho \neq 0$$

With the usual decision rule: if the p-value is <0.05, we can reject H_0, otherwise we can't. For example, for the data shown in the scatterplot in Figure 19.3, the authors report a sample $r = 0.577$, with a p-value less than 0.000. This indicates a significant positive[2] linear association in the population between incidence rate of Crohn's disease and ulcerative colitis.

In contrast, for the scatterplot in Figure 19.2, for the percentage of patients and nurses recommending their hospital in Ireland (which we have already noticed gave little indication of any association), $r = 0.304$ and the p-value $= 0.393$, much bigger than 0.05, so it is unlikely that there is any linear association in the population between these two variables. Calculation of a confidence interval for the population correlation coefficient is more complicated and many statistics programs do not provide one.

Finally, it is important to note that the statistical significance of r is related to the size of the sample. Very large samples can have a very small value for r, which is nonetheless significant, despite the linear association being possibly weak, whereas very small samples will require a large value for r before it is significant. That is why a close look of the scatterplot is critical in assessing the linearity of the association.

A useful rule of thumb, if you have a value for r but no confidence interval or p-value, for it to be statistically significant, r must be greater than $2/\sqrt{n}$, where n is the sample size. For example, if $n = 100$, then r has to be greater than $2/10 = 0.200$ to be statistically significant.

Exercise 19.4.   What conditions must the data satisfy for Pearson's correlation coefficient to be used?

---

[2] Positive because the value of r (0.577) is positive.

An example from practice

Figure 19.5 is from a study in which the authors investigated the role of the intrauterine environment in childhood adiposity (fatness), in 17 284 infants. Using Pearson's correlation coefficients, they calculated the maternal versus offspring body mass index (BMI) assciation and the paternal versus offspring BMI association, at birth and when the offsprings were one year and three years old, using the parental pre-pregnancy BMI. The null hypothesis was that there is no difference in the correlation of the maternal–offspring BMI association and the paternal–offspring BMI association.

	Offspring BMI (age of offspring)					
	At birth		At 1 year		At 3 years	
	r 95% CI	p-value	r 95% CI	p-value	r 95% CI	p-value
Maternal BMI	0.10 0.09, 0.12		0.11 0.09, 0.12		0.10 0.09, 0.12	
Paternal BMI	0.04 0.02, 0.05		0.08 0.07, 0.10		0.09 0.08, 0.11	
Statistical difference between maternal-offspring BMI r value, and paternal-offspring BMI r-value		<0.001		0.010		0.327

Figure 19.5 Pearson's correlations between parental pre-pregnancy body mass index (BMI) for both mother and father, and offspring BMI, among 17 284 Norwegian parent–offspring trios. (I have omitted the results of the two-year-old offsprings, which were not in any case significant). Data from Fleten *et al.* (2012)

In other words, is a mother's BMI related to her baby's BMI (is r significant), and is a father's BMI related to his baby's BMI (is r significant)? And is there a significant difference between the two correlation coefficients?

The table contains values for Pearson's correlation coefficient r, between maternal BMI and offspring BMI, and paternal BMI and offspring BMI, along with 95 per cent confidence intervals for each r, and in the last row, a p-value for the difference between the r values.

As you can see, maternal BMI and paternal BMI are associated with the baby's BMI at birth, at one year and at three years because none of the confidence intervals contains 0. However, the correlation coefficients beween maternal–offspring BMI and paternal–offspring BMI are only significantly different at birth (p-value <0.05).

Exercise 19.5. The table of correlation coefficients in Figure 19.6 is from a study whose objective was:

> To examine the geographical relation between mortality and deprivation in England and Wales at the start of the 20th and 21st centuries, and explore the evidence for a strengthening or weakening of this relation over the century, and test for relations between the mortality and deprivation patterns of a century ago and modern mortality and causes of death.

The table shows, for five common causes of death in 2001, the Pearson correlation coefficient between each cause of death and the standardised mortality rate (SMR) and deprivation, in 2001 and in the 1900s. Comment, for each cause of death, on what is revealed by the values in the table about the association between deprivation and the SMR between the start and end of the 20th century.

Cause of death	2001		1990s	
	SMR	Deprivation	SMR	Deprivation
Stomach cancer	0.474**	0.379**	0.299**	0.231**
Bowel cancer	0.378**	0.061	0.138**	0.076
Lung cancer	0.750**	0.584**	0.481**	0.407**
Breast cancer	0.273**	−0.013	−0.068	−0.019
Prostate cancer	0.284**	0.009	−0.014	−0.014

SMR, standardised mortality ratio

** $p < 0.01$.

Figure 19.6 Pearson's correlations (for five common causes of death) between deprivation and mortality (SMR) in 2001 and between deprivation and mortality in 2001 and in the 1900s. All data have been standardised on 1900s registration districts unless otherwise stated. (Abbreviated by present author). Source: Gregory (2009). Reproduced by permission of BMJ Publishing Group Ltd

Spearman's rank correlation coefficient

You have seen that to use Pearson's correlation coefficient as a measure of linear association, both variables must be metric and at least one should be approximately Normally distributed (or both should be Normal if you want a confidence interval). But if *either* (or both) of the variables is ordinal, or metric but not Normally distributed, then *Spearman's rank correlation coefficient* is appropriate. This is a *non-parametric* measure, which assesses a more general association rather than specifically a linear one.

As with Pearson's correlation coefficient, Spearman's correlation coefficient varies from −1, through 0, to +1, and its statistical significance can again be assessed with a *p*-value, or less

Descriptive variables	Measured temperatures			Spearman's rank correlation coefficient (p-value)
	<65°C	65–69°C	≥70°C	
Tea temperature:				
Warm or lukewarm	32 414	3749	467	
Hot	5385	4246	1757	0.46 (<0.001)
Very hot	37	48	421	
Interval between tea being poured and drunk (minutes)				
≥4	30 259	4678	675	
2–3	6836	2691	859	0.32 (<0.001)
<2	741	674	1111	

Table shows numbers of participants.

Figure 19.7 Spearman's correlation coefficients between tea temperature variables among 48 582 participants in Golestan Cohort Study, Golestan, northern Iran, 2004–2008. The first column shows the estimated temperatures and times. Data from Islami *et al.* (2009)

often, a confidence interval. It is usually denoted as ρ_s in the population and r_s in the sample. The null hypothesis is that the population correlation coefficient $\rho_s = 0$.

Note that if your data are metric for both variables but you are uncertain about how Normal the distributions are, you should use Spearman's correlation coefficient. If the data are Normal, then the values for Pearson's r and Spearman's r_s will be more or less the same. The more different the two values are, the less Normally distributed are the variables. In fact, if you calculate a Pearson's correlation coefficient for some ranked data, it will be the same as a Spearman's correlation coefficient on the same data.

Exercise 19.6. Explain the circumstances which would persuade you to use Spearman's correlation coefficient rather than Pearson's.

An example from practice

Figure 19.7 is from a study to investigate the association between tea drinking habits in Golestan province, northern Iran, and risk of oesophageal squamous cell carcinoma. The table shows the Spearman correlation coefficients between the actual temperature at which tea was drunk and its temperature as estimated by the participants, as well as the correlations between the interval between tea being poured and being drunk, among healthy participants in a cohort study.

As you can see, the correlation between actual tea temperature and estimated temperature was high and significant (*p*-value <0.05). So we can reject the null hypothesis of no linear association between the two variables in the population. The same is true of the tea temperature and the interval between it being poured and drunk.

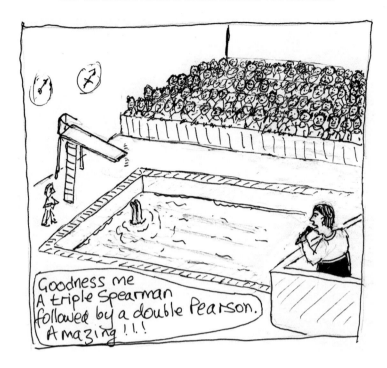

Exercise 19.7. The Spearman correlation coefficients in Figure 19.8 are from a cross-sectional study to investigate the relationship between community-based antibacterial prescribing and antibacterial resistance (to ampicillin or amoxicillan and to trimethoprim) in community-acquired disease. Data was collected for individual practices (from microbiological specimens sent to seven Public Health Laboratories) and from 10 primary care groups (each with 10–15 general practices). The correlations for these two groups are shown separately. Comment on what the correlation coefficients indicate.

Exercise 19.8. Figure 19.9 is from a time trend analysis study comparing the actual number of suicides in 2009 with the number that would be expected based on trends before the financial crisis (2000–2007). The object was to investigate the impact of the 2008 global economic crisis on international trends in suicide and to identify sex/age groups and countries most affected. The table shows Spearman's correlation coefficients, 95 per cent confidence intervals and p-values, between changes in unemployment rate and suicide rate between 2007 and 2009 in 50 countries, stratified by unemployment rate before the financial crisis in 2007. What do these results suggest about the association between changes in unemployment and suicide rates?

One other correlation coefficient can only be mentioned briefly. Kendall's rank-order correlation coefficient, denoted as τ (tau), is a non-parametric measure of association, appropriate in the same circumstances as that of Spearman's r_s, that is, with ranked categorical data. In most

Antibacterial resistance*	Antibacterial prescribing[†]	Primary care group			Practice		
		No	r_s[‡]	p value	No	r_s[‡]	p value
Ampicillin or amoxicillin	All β lactams	20	0.57	0.009	262	0.18	0.003
	Ampicillin and amoxicillin	20	0.44	0.05	262	0.20	0.001
Trimethoprim	Trimethoprim	32	0.31	0.09	371	0.24	0.0001

*Resistant isolates per 100 isolates.
[†]Prescriptions per 1000 patients a year.
[‡]Spearman's correlation coefficient.

Figure 19.8 Spearman correlations between antibacterial resistance and prescribing, at primary care group and practice level. Data from Priest *et al.* (2001)

	No of countries	Spearman's r_s (95% CI)	p value
All countries			
Men	50	0.25 (−0.03 to 0.50)	0.075
Women	50	0.10 (−0.18 to 0.37)	0.49
Countries with low unemployment level (<6.2%) before crisis			
Men	25	0.48 (0.10 to 0.73)	0.016
Women	25	0.13 (−0.28 to 0.50)	0.55
Countries with high unemployment level (≥6.2%) before crisis			
Men	25	0.31 (−0.10 to 0.63)	0.13
Women	25	0.20 (−0.21 to 0.55)	0.34

Figure 19.9 Spearman's correlation coefficients, 95 per cent confidence intervals and *p*-values between unemployment rate and suicide rate between 2007 and 2009, in 50 countries, stratified by unemployment rate before the financial crisis in 2007. Data from Chang *et al.* (2013)

cases, their values will be very similar, but when they differ, it is probably safer to use the value closest to 0. Kendall's tau and Spearman's rho have a different basis. Spearman's rho is the same as Pearson's *r* applied to the data when it has been ranked. However, Kendall's tau represents a probability, that is, the difference between the probability that the observed data are in the same order versus the probability that the observed data are not in the same order. Some statisticians consider Kendall's tau to be under-rated and under-represented in the general research literature. Tau is available in SPSS but not (as far as I know) in Minitab.

Finally, it must be emphasised that just because two variables are significantly associated does *not* mean that there is a cause–effect *relationship* between them. I will have more to say on this in Chapter 21.

20

Measuring agreement

Learning objectives

When you have finished this chapter, you should be able to:

- Explain the difference between association and agreement.

- Describe Cohen's kappa, calculate its value and assess the level of agreement.

- Interpret the published values for kappa.

- Describe the idea behind ordinal kappa.

- Outline the Bland–Altman approach to measuring agreement between metric variables.

To agree or not agree: that is the question

As you have seen in Chapter 19, association is a measure of the inter-connectedness of two variables: the degree to which they tend to change together, either positively or negatively. *Agreement*, in contrast, is the degree to which the values in two sets of data actually *agree*, that is, are the same. We commonly want to measure the degree of agreement in two situations:

- When two (or more) health practitioners, who, in this context, may also be referred to as *raters* (or *observers*) are assessing some clinical characteristic in a number of patients. In this context, the degree of agreement of the raters is known as *inter-rater* agreement.

Medical Statistics from Scratch: An Introduction for Health Professionals, Third Edition. David Bowers.
© 2014 John Wiley & Sons, Ltd. Published 2014 by John Wiley & Sons, Ltd.

- When a single health practitioner is making repeated assessments of some characteristics in a number of patients. The degree of agreement in this context is called *intra-rater* agreement.

We often need a measure of agreement in the context of diagnosis or in examining the properties of a new measurement scale. To illustrate this idea, see the hypothetical data in Figure 20.1, which shows the decision by a psychiatrist and by a psychiatric social worker (PSW) whether to section (Y) or not section (N), each of 10 individuals with mental ill-health. We would say that the two variables were in perfect *agreement* if every pair of values were the same. In practical situations, this will not happen, and in this case, you can see that only seven out of the 10 decisions are the same, so the observed level of *proportional agreement* is 0.70 (70 per cent).

Note however, that if you had asked each clinician simply to toss a coin to make the decision (heads = section, tails = don't section), some of their decisions would probably still have been in agreement – by *chance* alone. We need a method of measuring agreement which takes this random agreement into account. Cohen's kappa does this.

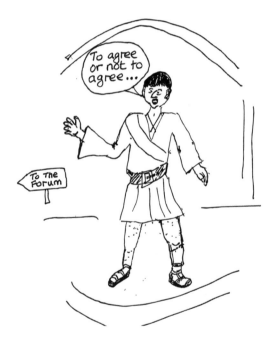

Patient	1	2	3	4	5	6	7	8	9	10
Psychiatrist	Y	Y	N	Y	N	N	N	Y	Y	Y
PSW	Y	N	N	Y	N	N	Y	Y	Y	N

Figure 20.1 Decision by a psychiatrist and a psychiatric social worker whether to section 10 individuals suffering from mental ill-health

> **Exercise 20.1.** What is the difference between association and agreement? Do variables that are associated also have high levels of agreement?

Cohen's kappa (κ)

We can adjust the observed level of agreement for the proportion you would have *expected* to occur by chance alone using a method due to Cohen and appropriate for categorical data. This adjustment gives us the *chance-corrected proportional agreement statistic*, known as Cohen's *kappa, κ*:

$$\kappa = \frac{(\text{proportion of observed agreement} - \text{proportion of expected agreement})}{(1 - \text{proportion of expected agreement})}$$

We can calculate the *expected* values for each cell in the contingency table in exactly the same way as we did for chi-squared (row total $\times$ column total/overall total – see Chapter 17). Figure 20.2 shows the data shown in Figure 20.1 expressed in the form of a contingency table, with the psychiatrist's scores in the rows, the PSW's scores in the columns and with the row and the column totals added. The expected values are shown in brackets in each cell.

We have seen that the *observed* agreement is 0.70, and we can expect the two clinicians to agree on 'Yes' three times and 'No' two times, making five agreements in total. So the expected agreement is five out of 10 or 0.50. Therefore:

$$\kappa = \frac{(0.70 - 0.50)}{(1 - 0.50)} = \frac{0.20}{0.50} = 0.40$$

So after allowing for chance agreement is reduced from 70 per cent to 40 per cent.

Kappa can vary between zero (agreement no better than chance) and 1 (perfect agreement), and you can use the table in Figure 20.3 to assess the quality of agreement (although this table has no theoretical basis). It is possible to calculate a confidence interval for kappa, but these intervals will usually be too narrow to add much insight to your result (except for quite small samples).

As an example of both inter-rated and intra-rated agreement, the following extract is from a paper which used video recording to investigate the causes of falls in elderly people in long-term care. The authors aimed to provide evidence of causes of falls by analysing real-life falls captured on video. They assessed inter-rater reliability of a questionnaire which probed the cause of

		Psychiatric social worker		
		Yes	No	Totals
Psychiatrist	Yes	4 (3)	2 (3)	6
	No	1 (2)	3 (2)	4
	Totals	5	5	10

Figure 20.2 Contingency table showing observed (and *expected*) decisions by a psychiatrist and a psychiatric social worker on whether to section 10 patients (data from Figure 20.1)

Kappa	Strength of agreement
≤ 0.20	Poor
0.21 – 0.40	Fair
0.41 – 0.60	Moderate
0.61 – 0.80	Good
0.81 – 1.00	Very good

Figure 20.3   How good is the agreement? Assessing kappa

imbalance and activity at the time of falling by comparing responses from two teams, each consisting of three members, who analysed 15 randomly selected videos.

> We assessed inter-rater reliability of the questionnaire by comparing responses from two teams, each consisting of three members, who analysed 15 randomly selected videos. For cause of fall, percentage agreement between teams was 87%. Corresponding Cohen's κ was 0.79 (95% CI 0.53 – 1.0), showing strong internal consistency. For activity at time of fall, the teams agreed in 93% of cases, with corresponding κ of 0.91 (0.73 – 1.0). We also examined intra-rater reliability by having one team reanalyse the same 15 videos 12 months after their first assessment. For cause of fall, percentage agreement was 93%, and κ was 0.90 (0.72 – 1.0). For activity at the time of the fall, percentage agreement was 93%, with a corresponding κ of 0.91 (0.74 – 1.0).
>
> *Robinovitch* et al. *(2013)*

As a further example from practice, Figure 20.4 is from a study into the development of a new quality-of-life scale for patients with advanced cancer and their families – the Palliative Care Outcome Scale (POS). It shows agreement between the patient and staff (who also completed the scale questionnaires) for a number of items on the POS scale. The table also contains values of Spearman's r_s and the proportion of agreements within one point on the POS scale. The level of agreement between staff and patient is either fair or moderate for all items and agreement within one point is either good or very good.

Exercise 20.2.   Do the highest and the lowest levels of agreement in Figure 20.4 coincide with the highest and lowest levels of correlation? Will this always be the case?

Exercise 20.3.   Figure 20.5 is from a study conducted in a major trauma unit into the variation between two experienced trauma clinicians in assessing the degree of injury of 16 patients from their case notes. The table shows the Injury Severity Score (ISS) awarded to each patient.[1] Categorise the scores into two groups: ISS scores of less than 16, and of 16 or more. Express the results in a contingency table and calculate (a) the observed and expected proportional agreement, and (b) kappa. Comment on the level of agreement.

---

[1] The ISS is used for the assessment of severity of injury, with a range from 0 to 75. ISS scores of 16 or above indicate potentially life threatening injury, and survival with ISS scores above 51 is considered unlikely.

Kappa	No of patients	Patient score (% severe)	Staff score (% severe)	κ	Spearman correlation	Proportion agreement within 1 score
At first assessment: 145 matched assessments						
Pain	140	24.3	20.0	0.56	0.67	0.87
Other symptoms	140	27.2	26.4	0.43	0.60	0.86
Patient anxiety	140	23.6	30.0	0.37	0.56	0.83
Family anxiety	137	49.6	46.0	0.28	0.37	0.72
Information	135	12.6	13.4	0.39	0.36	0.79
Support	135	10.4	14.1	0.22	0.32	0.79
Life worthwhile	133	13.6	16.5	0.43	0.54	0.82
Self worth	132	15.9	23.5	0.37	0.53	0.82
Wasted time	135	5.9	6.7	0.33	0.32	0.95
Personal affairs	129	7.8	13.2	0.42	0.49	0.96

Figure 20.4 Values of kappa from a Palliative Care Outcome Scale (POS) study showing levels of agreement between the patient and staff assessment for a number of items on the POS scale. Source: Hearn and Higinson (1999). Reproduced by permission of BMJ Publishing Group Ltd

								Case no.								
Observer	1	2	3	4	5	6	7	8	9	10	11	12	13	14	15	16
1	9	14	29	17	34	17	38	13	29	4	29	25	4	16	25	45
2	9	13	29	17	22	14	45	10	29	4	25	34	9	25	8	50

Figure 20.5 Injury Severity Score (ISS) values allocated to 16 patients by two experienced trauma clinicians in a major trauma unit from the evidence in case notes. Source: Zoltie and de Dombal (1993). Reproduced by permission of BMJ Publishing Group Ltd

Weighted kappa

The idea behind weighted kappa is best illustrated by referring back to the data in Figure 20.5. The two clinician's ISS scores agree for only five patients, so the proportional observed agreement is only $5/16 = 0.3125$ (31.25 per cent). However, in several cases, the scores have a 'near miss'; patient 2 for example, with scores of 14 and 13. Other pairs of scores are further apart, patient 15 is given scores of 25 and 8! Weighted kappa gives credit for near misses, but its calculation is too complex for this book.

A limitation of kappa is that it is sensitive to the proportion of subjects in each category (i.e. to prevalence), so caution is needed when comparing kappa values from different studies – these are only helpful if prevalences are similar. Bear in mind also the fairly arbitrary scale for judging the quality of any kappa value (Figure 20.3). Furthermore, kappa is not universally popular among clinicians and medical statisticians; see for example, the discussion in de Vet *et al.* (2013).

Measuring the agreement between two metric continuous variables

When it comes to measuring agreement between two metric continuous variables, the obvious problem is the large number of possible values – it is quite likely that *none* of them will be

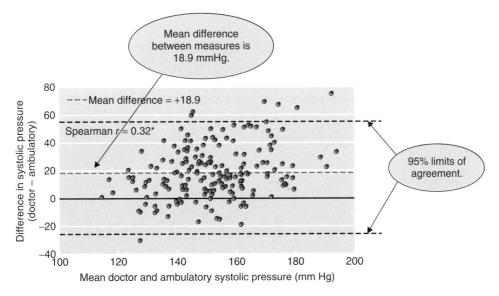

Figure 20.6 Bland–Altman plot of difference between doctor's measurement of systolic blood pressure and ambulatory systolic blood pressure. Source: Little *et al*. (3 August 2002). Reproduced by permission of BMJ Publishing Group Ltd

the same. One solution is to use a Bland–Altman chart (Bland and Altman 1986). This involves plotting, for each pair of measurements, the *differences* between the two scores on the vertical axis, against the *mean* of the two scores on the horizontal axis.

If the two methods of measurement are in exact agreement, all of the points will lie on a horizontal line drawn through the zero point on the difference (vertical) axis. If there is a difference in the results produced by the two methods, the horizontal difference line will be above or below the zero line (depending on which measure gives the higher values), and the points will form a cloud around this line.

A pair of tramlines, called the 95 per cent *limits of agreement*, are drawn at a distance of two standard deviations above and below the horizontal difference line. If all of the points on the graph fall between the tramlines, then this suggests that the agreement is 'acceptable', but the more points there are outside the tramlines, the less good the agreement. Moreover, the spread of the points should be reasonably horizontal, indicating that differences are not increasing (or decreasing) as the values of the mean of the two variables increase. A difference (bias) in the agreement between the two measures is shown by the plots having a tendency to be above or below the 0 line.

The idea is illustrated in Figure 20.6. This Bland–Altman plot is from a study to assess alternative ways of measuring systolic blood pressure in 200 hypertensive patients. The aim was to determine the level of agreement between the doctor-measured blood pressure and the ambulatory blood pressure; 24 hour ambulatory measurement – readings taken at half hourly intervals during the day (0700–2300) and hourly at night (2300–0700).

The horizontal line through 0 corresponds to no difference between the two methods, that is, doctor measurement minus ambulatory measurement equals zero. As you can see, most of the points were above this line, indicating that the measurement by the doctors was greater than the ambulatory measure. This upward bias (the mean of the difference in the two methods of measurement) was +18.9 mmHg, as shown on the graph by the horizontal dotted line drawn at 18.9. It is possible that the increased blood pressures when measured by the doctor might be due to the 'white coat effect'.

The standard deviation of the difference in measurements was 19 mmHg. This means that for 95 per cent of the patients, the difference in their systolic blood pressures is between plus and minus two standard deviations, that is, $2 \times 19 = 38.0$ from the mean of 18.9. That is, $18.9 - 38.0$ to $18.9 + 38.0$ or from -19.1 mmHg to 56.9 mmHg. These values, the limits of agreement, are shown on the graph; you can see that most of the points lie between the lines, so agreement seems acceptable. The larger discrepancies for high systolic blood pressures are worrying, however, and an indication of poor agreement in the higher ranges. The authors conclude:

> Readings made by doctors were much higher than ambulatory systolic pressure.

Notice that the authors provide a value for Spearman's correlation coefficient of $+0.39$, indicating that the difference between measures increases as the mean of the two measures increases.

Exercise 20.4.   What is the problem when trying to measure agreement between the values of two continuous variables?

Exercise 20.5.   The Bland–Altman plot in Figure 20.7 is taken from a study to investigate whether birthweight is associated with depression in young women. The horizontal axis shows the mean of recalled birthweight (by the woman or parents) and recorded birthweight from local hospital obstetric records The vertical axis shows the *difference* between the two measurements. What does the chart suggest about the level of agreement and possible bias?

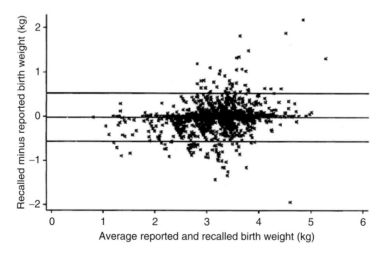

Figure 20.7   Bland–Altman plot of mean reported and recalled birthweight (on the horizontal axis) against the difference between the two measurements (vertical axis). From a study to investigate if birthweight is associated with depression among 1729 young women. Source: Inskip *et al.* (2008). Reproduced by permission of Oxford University Press

IX

Getting into a Relationship

21

Straight line models: linear regression

Learning objectives

When you have finished this chapter, you should be able to:

- Describe the difference between an association and a cause-and-effect relationship.

- Estimate the equation of a straight line from a graph and draw a straight line knowing its equation.

- Describe what is meant by a linear relationship and how the linear regression equation can be used to model it.

- Identify the constant and slope parameters, and the dependent and independent variables.

- Explain the role of the residual term.

- Summarise the model building process.

- Provide a brief explanation of the idea behind the method of ordinary least squares estimation.

Medical Statistics from Scratch: An Introduction for Health Professionals, Third Edition. David Bowers.
© 2014 John Wiley & Sons, Ltd. Published 2014 by John Wiley & Sons, Ltd.

- List the basic assumptions of the simple linear regression model.

- Interpret computer-generated linear regression results.

- Explain what goodness-of-fit is and how it is measured in the simple linear regression model.

- Explain the role of $\bar{R}^2$ in the context of multiple linear regression.

- Interpret published multiple linear regression results.

- Explain the adjustment properties of the regression model.

- Outline how the basic assumptions can be checked graphically.

Health warning!

Although the maths underlying the idea of linear regression is a little complicated, some explanation of the concept is necessary if you are to gain some understanding of the procedure and be able to interpret regression computer outputs sensibly. I have tried to keep the discussion as brief and as non-technical as possible. If you have an aversion to maths you might want to skim the material in the next few pages.

Relationship and association

In Chapter 19, I emphasised the fact that an *association* between two variables does *not* mean that there is a cause-and-effect *relationship* between them. For example, birthweight and systolic blood pressure (SBP) among a group of individuals may appear to be closely associated (i.e. those people with a high birthweight tend to have a high SBP), but this does not *necessarily* mean that an increase in birthweight will *cause* a corresponding increase in SBP (or indeed that an increase in SBP will cause an increase in birthweight). This association is illustrated as follows:

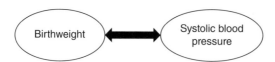

In this chapter and in the following chapter, I am going to deal with the idea of a *causal* relationship between variables. By causal relationship, I mean that a change in the value of one variable will bring about or *cause* a change in the value of some other variable. For example, variation in salt intake among a group of individuals *causes* variation in the blood pressure in those individuals – higher levels of salt intake lead to, that is, cause, higher levels of blood pressure (and vice versa). This causal action is illustrated as follows:

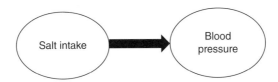

In the clinical world, demonstrating a cause–effect relationship is not easy and requires a number of conditions to be satisfied. Hill (1965), a British medical statistician, set out a number of criteria that should be satisfied if a relationship is to be defined as causal. These include:

Chronology (*temporality*). The effect has to occur *after* the cause. If factor Y is believed to cause disease Z, then factor Y must necessarily *always* precede the occurrence of the disease. This is the only absolutely essential criterion.

Dose–response relationship. An increasing amount of exposure increases the risk. If a dose–response relationship is present, it is a strong evidence for a causal relationship. However, the absence of a dose–response relationship does not rule out a causal relationship.

Consistency. The association is consistent when the results are replicated in studies in different settings using different methods and among different populations.

Plausibility. The association agrees with currently accepted understanding of pathological processes.

Coherence. The association should be compatible with existing theory and knowledge (although of course, existing theory and knowledge may be wrong).

I will assume from now on that a cause–effect relationship between the variables has been satisfactorily demonstrated, and that this relationship is *linear* (see Chapter 19, for an explanation of linearity).

A causal relationship – explaining variation

As a reminder, you may remember from your schooldays that the *equation of a straight line* can be written as:

$$y = mx + c$$

or

$$y = c + mx$$

where the y are the measurements on the vertical axis, the x are the measurements on the horizontal axis and m is the *slope* of the line. m will be positive if the line slopes up from left to right or negative if the line slopes down from left to right. c is called the *constant of intersection*; it is the point where the line crosses the y axis (c can be positive or negative).

Let us begin with a simple example. Suppose that the changes in systolic blood pressure (SBP), in mmHg, are caused by changes in body mass index (BMI) in kg/m^2, and the two variables are related by the following expression:

$$\text{SBP equals 110 plus } \tfrac{3}{4} \text{ of BMI}$$

As an equation this is:

$$\text{SBP} = 110 + 0.75 \times \text{BMI}$$

So, for example, when BMI $= 40$, SBP equals 110 plus 0.75 times 40, or 140 mmHg. This equation is a *linear* equation. If you plot it with pairs of values of BMI and SBP, you will see a straight line. For instance:

$$\text{when BMI} = 20, \text{SBP} = 125$$

$$\text{when BMI} = 28, \text{SBP} = 131.$$

We already know that when BMI $= 40$, SBP $= 140$, and if we plot these three pairs of values, and draw a line through them, we get Figure 21.1. This is clearly a straight line.

The equation mentioned earlier explains the *variation* in SBP from person to person, in terms of corresponding *variation* from person to person in body mass index (BMI). I have referred to this relationship as an equation, but I could also have described it as a *model*. We are *modelling* a relationship; that between the variation in SBP and the variation in BMI.

We can write this equation in a more general form in terms of two variables Y and X, thus:

$$Y = b_0 + b_1 \times X$$

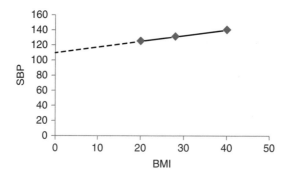

Figure 21.1   Linear relationship of systolic blood pressure (SBP) against body mass index (BMI). Note that when we are dealing with a causal relationship we talk about "a scatterplot of Y (in this case SBP) against X (in this case BMI)", and not the other way round.

The term b_0 is the usual coefficient of intersection, or *constant coefficient* – it's where the line cuts the Y axis (110 in Figure 20.1). The term b_1 is the *slope coefficient*, 0.75 in our equation, and will be positive if the line slopes upwards from left to right (as it does in Figure 20.1), and negative if the line slopes down from left to right (as in the top graph in Figure 19.4). Higher values of b_1 means more steeply sloped lines.

One important point: the value of b_1 (+0.75 in the example) is the amount by which SBP would increase if the value of BMI increased by 1 unit (BMI is measured in units of kg/m^2). I will come back to this later.

Refresher – finding the equation of a straight line from a graph

See Figure 21.2. Draw a right-angled triangle against the line with the line forming the hypoteneuse. The slope is equal to the length of the vertical side of this triangle divided by the length of the horizontal side. If the line slopes down from left to right, then the slope takes a negative sign. The constant of intersection c, is where the line cuts the vertical axis. Be careful if either or both axes are not shown going through the origin.

Exercise 21.1. Figure 21.3 is taken from a study of the effectiveness of health policies and shows the male smoking prevalence (per cent of males smoking) against level of tobacco control in a number of European countries. Tobacco control includes such measures as price increases, restriction on smoking in public places, advertising bans and so on. What is the equation of the regression line in Figure 21.3

Exercise 21.2. Plot the values in Figure 21.4 for the birthweight of baby (g) against weight of mother (kg) on a scatter plot. Draw a straight line through the points. What is the equation of this line?

The linear regression model

In Figure 21.1, all of the points lie *exactly* on the straight line. In practice, this will not happen of course, and the scatterplot in Figure 21.5 is more typical of what you might see. Here, we have birthweight (g) against mother's weight at booking, among a random sample of 500 babies

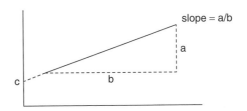

Figure 21.2 Calculating the slope of a straight line

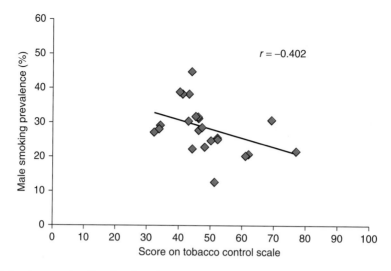

Figure 21.3 A regression line for the relationship between male smoking prevalence (per cent of males smoking) against the level of tobacco control in a number of European countries. Tobacco control includes such measures as price increases, restriction on smoking in public places, advertising bans, and so on Source: Mackenbach *et al.* (2013). Reproduced by permission of Elsevier

Birthweight (g)	2900	3120	3450	3780
Mother's weight (kg)	40.0	60.0	90.0	120.0

Figure 21.4 Birthweight (g) and mother's weight (kg) for four babies, based very roughly on values in the random sample of 500 babies from the Born in Bradford cohort study

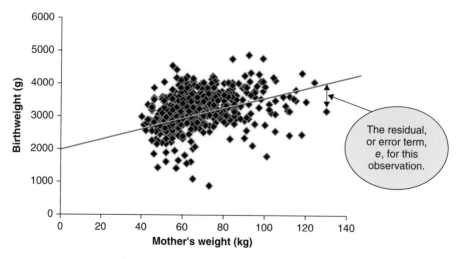

Figure 21.5 A scatterplot of birthweight against mother's weight at booking, among a random sample of 500 babies from the Born in Bradford cohort. The scatter of values appears to be distributed around a straight line. That is, the relationship between these two variables appears to be broadly *linear* (I will deal with the error term *e* shortly)

from the Born in Bradford cohort. Suppose that we believe that there is a causal relationship between mother's weight and baby's birthweight, that is, a variation in mother's weight causes variation in birthweight. If we want to investigate the nature of this relationship then we need to do three things:

- Make sure that the relationship is linear.[1]

- Find a way to determine the equation linking the variables, that is, get the values of b_0 and b_1.

- See if the relationship is statistically significant, that is, it is present in the population.

  I will deal with these issues one at a time.

First, is the relationship linear?

One way of investigating the linearity of the relationship is to examine the scatterplot, such as that in Figure 21.5.

The points in the scatterplot do seem to cluster (albeit loosely) along a straight line through the scatter. This suggests a *linear* relationship between birthweight and mother's weight. So far, so good. We can write the equation of this straight line as:

$$\text{birthweight} = b_0 + b_1 \times \text{mother's weight}$$

This equation is known as *the sample regression equation*. The variable on the left-hand side of the equation, birthweight, is known variously as the *outcome, response* or *dependent* variable. I am going to refer to this as the dependent variable in this chapter. It must be *metric continuous*. The value of this dependent variable is equal to the *mean* value of birthweight for any specified value of mother's weight. In other words, it would tell us (if we knew b_0 and b_1) what the mean birthweight would be for all those babies whose mothers had some particular booking weight.

The variable on the right-hand side of the equation, mother's weight, is known variously as the *predictor, explanatory* or *independent* variable, or the covariate. I will use the term *independent variable* here. This can be of any type: nominal, ordinal or metric. This is the variable that is doing the 'causing'. It is the changes in mother's weight that cause birthweight to change in response but not the other way round.

Incidentally, my 'by eye' line has the equation:

$$\text{birthweight} = 1950 + 17.1 \times \text{mother's weight}$$

This means that the *mean* birthweight of all those babies whose mothers weighed 70 kg is:

$$\text{birthweight} = 1950 + 17.1 \times 70 = 3147\,\text{g}$$

Clearly, drawing a line by eye through a scatter is not satisfactory – 10 people would get 10 different (although probably similar) lines. So the obvious question arises, 'What is the 'best'

---

[1] Because in this chapter, we are dealing only with linear relationships.

straight line that can be 'drawn' through a scatter of sample values, and how do I find out what it is?'

Exercise 21.3. (a) Draw by eye the best straight line you can through the scatterplot shown in Figure 19.3, and write down the regression equation. Assuming that there is a causal relationship between the two variables, that is, variation in the incidence of Crohn's disease (CD) brings about variation in ulerative colitis (UC), by how much would the mean incidence rate of ulcerative colitis change if the rate of Crohn's disease is changed by one unit? (b) Draw, by eye, the best straight line you can draw through the scatterplot shown in Figure 19.4 (top graph), and write down the regression equation. What change in mean percentage mortality would you expect if the mean number of episodes per year increased by 1?

Estimating b_0 and b_1 – the method of ordinary least squares (OLS)

The second problem is to find a method of getting the values of the sample coefficients b_0 and b_1, which will give us a line that fits the scatter of points better than any other line, and which will then enable us to write down the equation linking the variables. One of the most popular methods used for this calculation is called *ordinary least squares*, or OLS. This gives us the values of b_0 and b_1, and the straight line that *best* fits the sample data.

Roughly speaking, 'best' means the line that is, on average, closer to all of the points than any other line. How does OLS do this? See Figure 21.5. The distance of each point in the scatter from the regression line is known as the *residual*, or error, denoted as e. I have shown the e for just one of the observations. If all of these residuals are squared and then added together, to give the term $\sum e^2$,[2] then the 'best' straight line is the one for which the sum, $\sum e^2$, is smallest. Hence, the name ordinary 'least squares'.

The calculations involved with OLS are too tedious to do by hand, but you can use a suitable computer program to derive their values quite easily (both SPSS and Minitab will do this). It is important to note that the sample regression coefficients b_0 and b_1 are *estimates* of the population regression coefficients β_0 and β_1. In other words, we are using the sample regression equation:

$$Y = b_0 + b_1 X$$

to estimate the *population regression equation*:

$$Y = \beta_0 + \beta_1 X$$

We will need to see if this line is significant in the population – I will deal with this important issue shortly.

---

[2]Known as the sum of squares. $\sum$ is the Greek 'sigma', which means sum all the values.

Basic assumptions of the ordinary least squares procedure

The ordinary least squares procedure is only guaranteed to produce the line that best fits the data if the following assumptions are satisfied:

- The relationship between Y and X is linear.

- The dependent variable Y is metric continuous.

- The residual term, e, is Normally distributed, with a mean of zero – that is, it is centred on the regression line, for each value of the independent variable, X.

- The spread of the residual terms should be the same, whatever the value of X. In other words, e should not spread out more (or less) when X increases.

Let me explain the last two assumptions. These explanations are a bit technical and if you have difficulty understanding them, do not worry – you won't be alone! Besides which, an understanding is not essential to the basic idea of regression. Feel free to skip the next couple of paragraphs. Anyway, here goes.

Let us consider only those women in Figure 21.5 who weighed 80 kg. Suppose that there were 25 of them. As the scatterplot in Figure 21.5 indicates, most of these women will have a different birthweight baby. As you have seen, the difference between each observation and the regression line is the residual e. So we have 25 residual values (25 values of e). If you have arranged these 25 values into a frequency distribution, then the third assumption stipulates that this distribution should be Normal and centred on the regression line. And this should be true for the set of the residuals for *each value* of mothers weight. I have tried to illustrate this in Figure 21.6 (with a shaky hand – too much coffee!) for mothers who weighed 40, 60, 80 and 100 kg.

The fourth assumption demands that if you have repeated the exercise shown earlier for each separate value of mother's weight, then the spreads (the standard deviations) of each distribution of residual values should be the same for all mother's weights (as they

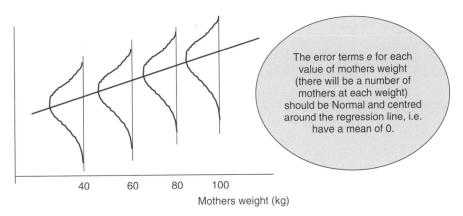

Figure 21.6 Showing how the error terms (the *es*) for the mothers weighing 40, 60, 80 and 100 kg, should be Normally distributed, and have a mean of 0, that is, should be centred on the regression line

are in Figure 21.6). If the residual terms have this latter property then they are said to be *homoskedastic*.

These assumptions may seem complicated, but the consequences for the accuracy of the ordinary least squares estimators may be serious if they are violated. Needless to say, these assumptions need to be checked. I will return to this later.

Exercise 21.4.   In linear regression, what is the relationship between b_0 and b_1 and β_0 and β_1?

Exercise 21.5.   What requirement does the dependent variable have to satisfy in a linear regression equation?

Back to the example – is the relationship statistically significant?

Having calculated b_1 and b_2, we now need to address the third question: is the relationship between birthweight and mother's weight statistically significant *in the population*? I want to say straight away that we are not much interested in whether β_0 is significant – it is only there to make up the numbers and basically we can ignore it.[3] The crucial parameter is β_1, and we can check whether this is significant by calculating a confidence interval for it and seeing if this confidence interval includes zero, and/or by performing a hypothesis test – the null hypothesis is that $\beta_1 = 0$ and seeing if the p-value is <0.05.

If the confidence interval for β_1 includes zero (or is its *p-value* > 0.05), then we *cannot* reject the null hypothesis that β_1 *is* equal to zero, which means that the relationship is not statistically significant. Whatever the value of mother's weight, once multiplied by a β_1 equal to zero, it disappears from the regression equation and can have no effect on birthweight.

Thus, the focus in linear regression analysis is to use b_1 to estimate β_1 and then examine its statistical significance. If β_1 *is* statistically significant, then the relationship is established (well, at least with a confidence level of 95 per cent).

Using SPSS to regress birthweight on mother's weight

The output from SPSS is shown in Figure 21.7. Ignore the top table for the moment. The bottom table gives us the sample regression equation:

$$\text{birthweight} = 2459.873 + 11.010 \times \text{mother's weight}$$

The 95 per cent confidence interval for β_1 is (8.084 to 13.935), which does not include 0 so the relationship between birthweight and mother's weight is significant in the population (confirmed by the p-value being < 0.05).

---

[3] Besides, in reality it has no sensible interpretation. For example, in the current example, β_0 would equal birthweight if a mother's weight was equal to zero!

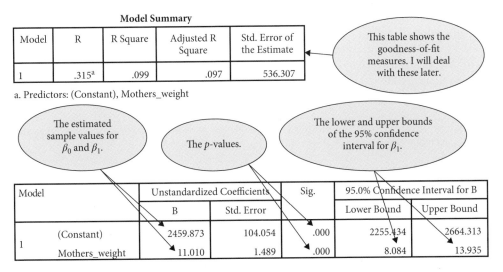

Model Summary

Model	R	R Square	Adjusted R Square	Std. Error of the Estimate
1	.315ᵃ	.099	.097	536.307

a. Predictors: (Constant), Mothers_weight

This table shows the goodness-of-fit measures. I will deal with these later.

The estimated sample values for β_0 and β_1.

The p-values.

The lower and upper bounds of the 95% confidence interval for β_1.

Model		Unstandardized Coefficients		Sig.	95.0% Confidence Interval for B	
		B	Std. Error		Lower Bound	Upper Bound
1	(Constant)	2459.873	104.054	.000	2255.434	2664.313
	Mothers_weight	11.010	1.489	.000	8.084	13.935

Figure 21.7 Output from SPSS for regression of birthweight on mother's booking weight for a random sample of 500 babies from the Born in Bradford cohort study

Using Minitab

With Minitab you get the output shown in Figure 21.8 (ignore the bottom line beginning S = for the moment). Minitab calculates only the *p-value*, otherwise the results are virtually the same as for SPSS (allowing for a bit of rounding). As you can see the p-value for β_1 is < 0.05, which means we can reject the hypothesis that $\beta_1 = 0$. Minitab actually supplies the sample regression equation – which is nice. Pity though about the lack of confidence intervals.

The value of +11.010 for b_1 means that for every unit (1 kg) increase in mother's weight, the mean birthweight will increase by 11.010 g. Knowing the equation, you can, if you wish, draw this best OLS estimated regression line onto the scatterplot. I hesitate to draw your attention to it, but my best straight line by eye (birthweight = 1950 + 17.1 × mother's weight), was not impressive!

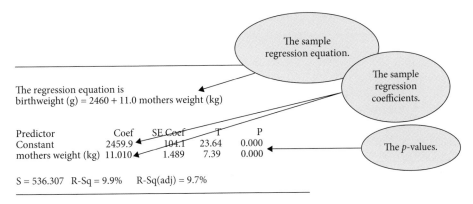

The sample regression equation.

The sample regression coefficients.

The regression equation is
birthweight (g) = 2460 + 11.0 mothers weight (kg)

Predictor	Coef	SE Coef	T	P
Constant	2459.9	104.1	23.64	0.000
mothers weight (kg)	11.010	1.489	7.39	0.000

The p-values.

S = 536.307 R-Sq = 9.9%   R-Sq(adj) = 9.7%

Figure 21.8 Output from Minitab for regression of birthweight on mother's booking weight for a random sample of 500 babies from the Born in Bradford cohort study

The regression equation also enables us to *predict* the value of the mean birthweight, for any value of mother's weight, *within the range* of the sample mother's weight values (30.0 kg – 140.0 kg). For example, for babies whose mothers weighed 70 kg at booking, their predicted mean birthweight is:

$$\text{birthweight} = 2460 + 11.010 \times 70 = 3230.7\,\text{g}$$

Prediction of birthweight for mother's weight values *outside* the original sample data range requires a more complex procedure, and will not be discussed here.

Exercise 21.6. What does the model described earlier predict for mean birthweight for the babies of women with a booking weight of 80 kg?

As an example from practice, Figure 21.9 is taken from a Norwegian study into the relationship between parent pre-pregnancy BMI and offspring BMI at three years of age.[4] The figure shows the results of a linear regression analysis of infant BMI against maternal BMI and separately against paternal BMI.

As you can see, neither confidence interval contains 0, so the relationship between both maternal and paternal BMI is significant in the population.

Exercise 21.7. Which do you think has a greater effect on the variation in offspring BMI, maternal BMI or paternal BMI?

Goodness-of-fit, R^2

Figures 21.6 and 21.7 contain values for something called R^2 and $\overline{R}^2$ (SPSS calls them R Square and Adjusted R Square; Minitab calls them R-Sq and R-Sq(adj)). What are these? Suppose

	Offspring BMI	
	β_1	95% CI
Maternal BMI	0.035	(0.031 – 0.039)
Paternal BMI	0.040	(0.040 – 0.051)

Figure 21.9   Results of a linear regression analysis of infant BMI against maternal BMI and separately against paternal BMI

---

[4] We first encountered this study in Figure 19.5 in the context of correlation.

that you think that mother's *height* might be causally related to birthweight, so you repeat the procedure mentioned above but use mother's height as your independent variable instead of mother's weight. Your results indicate that β_1 is again statistically significant. Now, you have two models, in both of which the independent variable has a statistically significant linear relationship with birthweight. But which model is best? The one with mother's weight or the one with mother's height?

In fact, the best model is the one whose independent variable 'explains' the greatest proportion of the observed variation in birthweight from subject to subject, that is, has the best *goodness-of-fit*. One such measure of this explanatory power is known as the *coefficient of determination* and is denoted as R^2.

As a matter of interest, when the mother's weight was used as the independent variable, $R^2 = 0.099$ (or 9.9 per cent). When mother's height was used, $R^2 = 0.075$ (or 7.5 per cent). So the variation in mother's weight explains almost 10 per cent of the observed variation in birthweight, while variation in mother's height explains only 7.5 per cent of the variation in birthweight. So using mother's weight as your independent variable gives you a better fitting model. However, the explanatory power of neither model is much to shout about. What about the other 90 per cent, or 75 per cent, of the variation in birthweight – what explains that?

One possibility is that the rest is due to chance – to random effects. A more likely possibility is that, as well as mother's weight, there are other variables that contribute something to the variation in birthweight from subject to subject. It would be naïve to believe that variation in birthweight, or any clinical variable, can be largely explained by only one variable. Which brings us neatly to the *multiple* linear regression model.

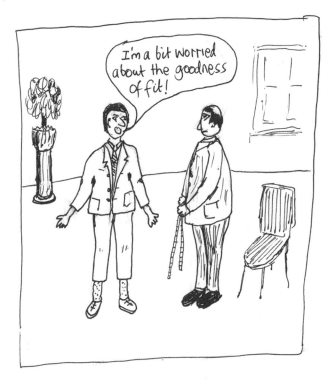

Multiple linear regression

A *simple* linear regression model is one with only one independent variable on the right-hand side. When you have *more* than one independent variable, the regression model is called a *multiple* linear regression model. For example, having noticed that both mother's weight and mother's height are each significantly related to birthweight, you might include them *both* as independent variables. Minitab gives the output shown in Figure 21.10.

So the estimated sample regression equation is:

$$\text{Birthweight (g)} = 147 + 15.3 \times \text{mothers height(cm)} + 8.61 \times \text{mothers weight(kg)}$$

This means that one unit (1 cm) increase in mother's weight will increase the mean birthweight by 15.3 g, and an increase of one unit (1 kg) in mother's weight will increase the birthweight by 8.61 g. Crucially, you can see that the goodness-of-fit has improved: $R^2 = 12.6$ per cent (compared to $R^2 = 9.9$ per cent for mother's weight alone or $R^2 = 7.5$ per cent when mother's height alone was used). Adding the extra variable seems to have improved the explanatory power of the model (although there is still a lot of variation in birthweight which is still unexplained).

SPSS produces a virtually identical output but includes 95 per cent confidence intervals (see Figure 21.11. I have omitted the table containing these values, but $R^2 = 12.6$ per cent and $\bar{R}^2 = 12.3$ per cent (I will come to $\bar{R}^2$ shortly). Note that in the multiple linear regression model, R^2 measures the explanatory power with *all* of the variables currently in the model *acting together*.

Note that when we move from the simple to the multiple linear regression model, we need to add a further basic assumption to the list in this chapter. That is, that there should be no perfect

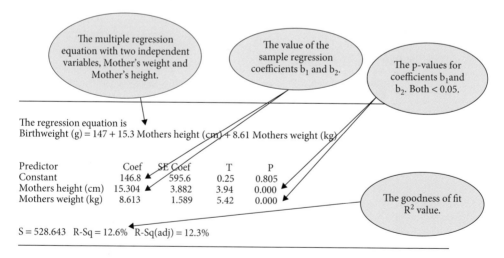

Figure 21.10 Output from Minitab for the regression of birthweight on mother's booking weight and mother's height. From a random sample of 500 babies from the Born in Bradford cohort study

Model	Unstandardized coefficients		Sig.	95.0% Confidence interval for B	
	B	Std. Error		Lower bound	Upper bound
1 (Constant)	146.794	595.582	.805	−1023.374	1316.962
Mothers_weight	8.613	1.589	.000	5.491	11.734
Height	15.304	3.882	.000	7.678	22.931

Figure 21.11 Output from SPSS for regression of birthweight on mother's booking weight and mother's height, for a random sample of 500 babies from the Born in Bradford cohort study

association or *collinearity* between any of the independent variables. When this assumption is not met (or only partially met), we refer to the model as having *multicollinearity*. The consequence of this condition is that the confidence intervals are wide and thus imprecise.

Exercise 21.8.   If we add mother's age (years) as a third independent variable to the birthweight model, then SPSS produces the results shown in Figure 21.12. (a) Comment on the statistical significance of the three independent variables. (b) How does an increase in mother's age affect mean birthweight values? (c) Has goodness-of-fit improved compared to the model with only mother's weight and mother's height included? (d) What is the mean birthweight of all of those babies in the sample with a mother's weight of 60 kg, height of 150 cm and age of 30?

As an example from practice, the following multiple regression equation is from a longitudinal ecological study to investigate whether the uneven rise in prosperity between 1999 and 2008 accounted for differential increases in life expectancy in English local authorities (we first encountered this study in connection with Figure 8.8). The authors measured trends in prosperity (the explanatory variables) in terms of changes in unemployment, in household income (GDHI), and in educational achievement (EDUC). A deprivation variable was also added to the model. The multiple linear regression model was[5]:

$$\Delta\text{Life expectancy} = \beta_0 + \beta_1 \times \Delta\text{Unemp} + \beta_2 \times \Delta\text{GDHI} + \beta_3 \times \Delta\text{EDUC} + \beta_4 \times \text{IMD} + +\epsilon$$

Model	R	R square	Adjusted R square
1	.359[a]	.129	.124

Figure 21.12 Output from SPSS with three independent variables: mother's weight, height and age

---

[5]I have amended this equation slightly, but not fundamentally, for pedagogic reasons.

where Δ is the 10 year *difference* in life expectancy, unemployment (Unemp), GDHI and EDUC, respectively. IMD is the level of deprivation in 1998. ϵ is the residual (or error) term.

The dependent variable is the 10 year change in life expectancy across a number of English local authorities. As you can see, there are four independent variables. The results of the linear regression analyses, for men and women separately, are shown in Figure 21.13. All variables are significant (none of the confidence intervals include zero nor are any of the p-values > 0.05).

Factor influencing life expectancy	Increase in life expectancy months (95% CI)	p value
Men ($R^2 = 0.27$)		
Additional increase in life expectancy with each 1% decline in unemployment rate	2.2 (0.5 to 3.8)	0.009
Additional increase in life expectancy with each £1000 increase in disposable household income per head	1.4 (0.3 to 2.5)	0.01
Additional increase in life expectancy for each point that LA's initial level of deprivation (IMD2000) is lower than average	0.2 (0.1 to 0.3)	<0.001
Women ($R^2 = 0.28$)		
Additional increase in life expectancy with each 1% decline in unemployment rate	1.7 (0.4 to 3.1)	0.013
Additional increase in life expectancy with each £1000 increase in disposable household income per head	1.1 (0.2 to 1.9)	0.016
Additional increase in life expectancy for each point that LA's initial level of deprivation (IMD2000) is lower than average	0.3 (0.2 to 0.4)	<0.001

Figure 21.13   Effect of baseline deprivation, decrease in unemployment and increase in average household income on increase in life expectancy. Data from Barr *et al.* (2012)

Exercise 21.9.   Using the results in Figure 2.12: (a) Do you think the model has a better fit (greater explanatory power) for men or for women? (b) Whose life expectancy changes the most when unemployment decreases – men or women? Does it increase or decrease? How can you tell?

Adjusted goodness-of-fit: $\bar{R}^2$

When you add an *extra* variable to an existing model and want to compare goodness-of-fit of the augmented model with the old model, you need to compare not R^2, but *adjusted R^2*, denoted as $\bar{R}^2$. The reasons do not need to concern us here, but R^2 will increase when an extra independent variable is added to the model, without there necessarily being any increase in explanatory power (its ability to explain more of the variation in the dependent variable).

However, if $\overline{R}^2$ increases, then you know that the explanatory power of the model *has* properly increased.

From Figures 21.7 or 21.8, $\overline{R}^2 = 0.097$ (9.7 per cent) in the *simple* regression model with only mother's weight as an independent variable. From Figures 21.9 or 21.12, with *both* mother's weight *and* height included, $\overline{R}^2$ increases to 0.123 (12.3 per cent), so this multiple regression model does show a small but real improvement in goodness-of-fit, and would be preferred to either of the simple regression models. Of course, you might decide to explore the possibility that other independent variables might also have a significant role to play in explaining variation in birthweight; age is one obvious contender, as is the sex of baby, and should be included in the model.

Exercise 21.10. If the sex of the baby is added to the model containing mother's weight and height, the output from Minitab is as shown in Figure 21.14. Comment on what the addition of sex to the model implies for the goodness-of-fit.

The regression equation is
Birthweight (g) = 190 + 15.2 Mothers height (cm) + 8.6 Mothers weight (kg)
      −20.7 sex

Predictor	Coef	SE Coef	T	P
Constant	190.2	604.4	0.31	0.753
Mothers height (cm)	15.228	3.889	3.92	0.000
Mothers weight (kg)	8.603	1.590	5.41	0.000
Sex	−20.68	47.48	−0.44	0.663

S = 529.075   R-Sq = 12.7%   R-Sq(adj) = 12.1%

Figure 21.14 Mintab output for model of birthweight against mother's weight, mother's height and sex of baby (1 = male, 2 = female)

Exercise 21.11. Researchers suggested that the value of the carbon isotope $\delta13C$ in human serum might reflect dietary consumption of corn-based and cane-based sweeteners. This might then offer a measure that objectively reflects intake of sweets and could thus replace unreliable self-reported dietary assessments. They investigated this possibility among a sample of 186 participants by using a linear regression model with the level of $\delta13C$ in serum as the dependent variable and the level of the consumption of sweetened drinks (estimated number of cans consumed per day) as the independent variable. They then successively added to the basic model: first, corn consumption then male gender and then consumption of animal fat (% total calories/day). For each model, they measured $\overline{R}^2$. The results are shown in Figure 21.15. Comment on what these successive $\overline{R}^2$ values suggest about goodness-of-fit for each addition to the simple model.

Model	β Coefficient for sweetened beverage consumption	95% CI	p-value	Adjusted r-squared value
1: Univariate (sweetened beverage alone)	0.21	0.09, 0.32	<0.001	0.06
2: +Corn consumption ($\geq$1/week)	0.20	0.08, 0.31	0.001	0.08
3: +Male gender	0.13	0.02, 0.25	0.02	0.13
4: +Animal fat (% total calories/day)	0.18	0.08, 0.29	0.001	0.29

Figure 21.15 Simple regression and multiple regressions of serum $\delta^{13}C$ values (dependent variable) against sweetened beverage alone (Model 1), plus corn consumption (Model 2), plus male gender (Model 3), plus animal fat consumption (Model 4). Data from Yeung *et al.* (2010)

Including nominal independent variables in the regression model: design variables and coding

In linear regression, many of the independent variables are likely to be metric, or at least ordinal. However, any independent variable that is *nominal* must be coded into a so-called *design* (or *dummy*) variable, before being entered into a model. There is only space for a brief description of the process here.

As an example, suppose that in a study of hypertension, you have SBP as your dependent variable and age (AGE) and smoking status (SMK), as your independent variables. Assume that SMK is a nominal variable, having the categories: non-smoker, ex-smoker and current smoker. This gives the model:

$$SBP = b_0 + b_1 AGE + b_2 SMK$$

To enter SMK into your computer, you would have to score the three smoking categories in some way – but how? As 1, 2, 3, or as 0, 1, 2 or what? As you can imagine, the scores you attribute to each category will affect your results. The answer is to *code* these *three* categories into *two* design variables. In this example, we set out the coding design as in Figure 21.16. Note that the number of design variables is always one *less* than the number of categories in the variable being coded.

Smoking status	Design variable values	
	D_1	D_2
Non-smoker	0	0
Ex-smoker	0	1
Current smoker	1	0

Figure 21.16 Coding design for a nominal variable with three categories

So you replace smoking status (with its dodgy numbering), with two new design variables, D_1 and D_2, which take the values in Figure 21.16, according to smoking status. The model now becomes:

$$SBP = b_0 + b_1 Age + b_2 D_1 + b_3 D_2.$$

For example, if the subject is a current smoker, $D_1 = 1$ and $D_2 = 0$; if an ex-smoker, $D_1 = 0$ and $D_2 = 1$; if a non-smoker, $D_1 = 0$ and $D_2 = 0$. Notice that in the last situation that the smoking status variable effectively disappears from the model.

This coding scheme can be extended to deal with nominal variables with any reasonable number of categories, depending on the sample size.[6] The simplest situation is a nominal variable with only *two* categories, such as sex, which can be represented by one design variable with values 0 (if male) or 1 (if female).

Exercise 21.12. Suppose that the first three subjects in the study of SBP and its relationship with age and smoking habit are, a 50-year old smoker, a 55-year-old non-smoker and a 35-year-old ex-smoker, respectively. Fill in the first three rows of the data sheet shown in Figure 21.17 as appropriate.

Building your model. Which variables to include?

At the beginning of this chapter, we chose mother's weight and/or mother's height to explain birthweight. In practice, researchers may or may not have an idea about which independent variables they think are relevant in explaining the variation in their dependent variable. Whether they do or they don't will influence their decision as to which variables to include in their model, that is, their *variable selection procedure*. There are two main approaches to the model-building process:

- First, *automated* variable selection – the computer does it for you. This approach is perhaps more appropriate if you have little idea about which variables are likely to be relevant in the relationship.

Subject	Age	D_1	D_2
1			
2			
3			

Figure 21.17   Data sheet for systolic blood pressure against age and smoking status

---

[6]As a rule of thumb, you need at *the very least* 15 subjects for each independent variable in your model. If you have got, say, five ordinal and/or metric independent variables in your model, you would need a minimum of 75 subjects. If you want also to include a single nominal variable with five categories (i.e. four design variables), you would need another 60 subjects. In these circumstances, it might help to amalgamate some categories.

- Second, *manual* selection – *you* do it! This approach is more appropriate if you have a particular hypothesis to test, in which case you will have a pretty good idea which independent variable is likely to be the most relevant in explaining your dependent variable. However, you will almost certainly want to include other variables to control for confounding (more on confounding in regression models below)

Both of these methods have a common starting procedure, as follows[7]:

- Identify a list of independent variables that you think might possibly have some role in explaining the variation in your dependent variable. Be as broad-minded as possible here.

- Draw a scatterplot of each of these candidate variables (if it is not a nominal variable), against the dependent variable. Examine for linearity. If any of the scatterplots show a strong, but not a linear relationship with the dependent variable, you will need to code them first before entering them into the computer data sheet. For example, you might find that the relationship between the dependent variable and 'age' is strong but not linear. One approach is to group the *age* values into four groups, using its three quartile values to define the group boundaries and then code the groups with three design variables.

- Perform a series of univariate regressions, that is, regress each candidate independent variable in turn against the dependent variable. Note the p-value in each case.

- At this stage, all variables that have a p-value of ≤ 0.25 should be considered for inclusion in the model. Using a p-value less than this may fail to identify variables that could subsequently turn out to be important in the final model.

With this common starting procedure out of the way, we can briefly describe the two variable selection approaches, starting with automated methods.

Automated variable selection methods

- *Forwards selection*: The program starts with the variable that has the lowest p-value from the univariate regressions. It then adds the other variables one at a time, in lowest p-value order, regressing each time, retaining all variables with p-values <0.05 in the model.

- *Backwards selection*: The reverse of forwards selection. The program starts with *all* of the candidate variables in the model, then the variable that has the highest p-value >0.05, is removed. Then, the next highest p-value variable and so on, until only those variables with a p-value <0.05 are left in the model and all other variables have been discarded.

- *Forwards or backwards stepwise selection*: After each variable is added (or removed), the variables which were already (or are left) in the model are re-checked for statistical significance; if no longer significant they are removed. The end result is a model where all variables have a p-value <0.05.

---

[7]Note that the criteria used by the different computer regression programs to select and de-select variables differ.

These automated procedures have a number of disadvantages, including misleadingly narrow confidence intervals and exaggerated coefficient values (and thus their effect size), although they may be useful when researchers have little idea about which variables are likely to be relevant. As an example of the automated approach, the authors of a study into the role of arginase in sickle cell disease, in which the outcome variable was $\log_{10}$ arginase activity comment:

> This modelling used a stepwise procedure to add independent variables, beginning with the variables most strongly associated with $\log_{10}$ arginase with P $\leq$0.15. Deletion of variables after initial inclusion in the model was allowed. The procedure continued until all independent variables in the final model had P $\leq$0.05, adjusted for other independent variables, and no additional variables had P $\leq$0.05.
>
> *Morris* et al. *(2005)*

Manual variable selection methods

Manual, DIY methods, are often more appropriate if the investigators know in advance which is likely to be their principal independent variable. They will include this variable in the model, together with any other variables that they think may be potential confounders. The identity of potential confounders will have been established by experience, a literature search, discussions with colleagues and patients and so on (see more below on confounders).

Manual variable selection will sometimes offer insights into variable behaviour and importance as the model building process develops, which the automatic selection of variables cannot. Besides which, there is a feeling of being more in control of the process. There are two alternative manual selection procedures:

- *Backward elimination*: The main variable plus all of the potentially confounding variables are entered into the model at the start. A regression analysis will then reveal which variables are statistically significant (*p*-value <0.05). Non-significant variables can then be dropped from the model, one at a time, in decreasing *p*-value order, with a fresh regression analysis after each variable exit. However, if the coefficient of any of the remaining variables changes markedly[8] when a variable is dropped, the variable should be retained as this may indicate that it is a confounder.

- *Forward elimination*: The main explanatory variable of interest is put in the model, and the other (confounding) variables are added one at a time in order of (lowest) *p*-value (from the univariate regressions).

The regression analysis is repeated each time a variable is added. If the added variable is statistically significant, it is retained, if not it is dropped, unless any of the coefficients of the existing variables change noticeably, suggesting that the new variable may be a confounder. The end result of either of these manual approaches should be a model containing the same

---

[8]There is no rule about how big a change in a coefficient should be considered noteworthy. A value of 10 per cent has been suggested, but this seems on the small side.

variables (although this model may differ from a model derived using one of the automated procedures).

In any case, the overall objective is *parsimony*, that is, having as few explanatory variables in the model as possible, while at the same time explaining the maximum amount of variation in the dependent variable. Parsimony is particularly important when sample size is on the small side. As a rule of thumb, researchers will need at least 15 observations for each independent variable to ensure mathematical stability, and at least 20 observations to obtain reasonable statistical reliability (e.g. narrow-ish confidence intervals).

As an example of the manual backwards selection approach, the authors of a study of birthweight and cord serum EPA concentration knew that cord serum EPA was their principal independent variable, but they wanted to include possible confounders in their model. They commented:

> Multiple regression analysis was used to determine the relevant importance of predictors of the outcome (variable). Potential confounders were identified on the basis of previous studies, and included maternal height and weight, smoking during pregnancy, diabetes, parity, gestational length, and sex of the child. Covariates[9] were kept in the final regression equation if statistically significant (p < 0.01) after backwards elimination.
>
> *Grandjean* et al. *(2000)*

Incidentally, the main independent variable, cord serum concentration, was found to be statistically significant (p-value $= 0.037$), as were all of the confounding variables.

Exercise 21.13.　Briefly outline the two main approaches to variable selection in multiple linear regression models. What are the advantages and shortcomings of each approach?

Adjustment and confounding

One of the most attractive features of the multiple regression model is its ability to *adjust* for the effects of possible association between the independent variables. It is quite possible that two or more of the independent variables will be associated. For example, mother's weight and mother's height (used in the example mentioned earlier) are significantly positively associated ($r = 0.383$ and p-value <0.000). The consequence of such association is that increases in mother's weight are likely to be accompanied by increases in mother's height. The increase in mother's weight will cause birthweight to increase directly, but also indirectly via mother's height. In these circumstances, it is difficult to tell how much of the increase in birthweight is due *directly* to an increase in mother's weight and how much to the *indirect* effect of an associated increase in mother's height.

---

[9]That is, independent variables.

The beauty of the multiple regression model is that each regression coefficient measures only the *direct* effect of its independent variable on the dependent variable and controls or adjusts for any possible interaction from any of the other variables in the model. In terms of the results in Figures 21.10 and 21.11, an increase in mother's weight of 1 kg will cause mean birthweight to increase by 8.6 g (the value of b_1), and *all* of this increase is caused by the change in mother's weight (plus the inevitable random error). Any effect that a concomitant change in mother's height might have is discounted.

We can use the adjustment property to deal with confounders in just the same way. You will recall that a confounding variable has to be associated with one of the independent variables *as well as* the dependent variable (see the discussion in Chapter 7). Notice that when mother's weight was the only independent variable in the model, the coefficient b_1 was 11.010 but decreases to 8.613 with two independent variables. A marked change like this in the coefficient of a variable already in the model when a new variable is added, is an indication that one of the variables is a potential confounder. As you have already seen in the model building section described earlier, in these circumstances both variables should be retained in the model.

An example from practice

Figure 21.18 is from a cross-sectional study into the relationship between bone lead and blood lead levels and the development of hypertension in 512 individuals selected from a cohort study (Cheng *et al.* 2001). The table shows the outcome from three multiple linear regression models with SBP as the dependent variable. The first model includes blood lead as an independent variable, along with six possible *confounding* variables.[10] The second and third models were the same as the first model, except tibia and patella lead, respectively, were substituted for blood lead. The results include 95 per cent confidence intervals and the R^2 for each model.

As the table shows, the tibia lead model has the best goodness-of-fit ($R^2 = 0.1015$) but even this model only explains 10 per cent of the observed variation in SBP. However, this is the only model that supports the relationship between hypertension and lead levels; the 95 per cent confidence interval for tibia lead (0.02 to 2.73) does not include zero. The only confounders statistically significant in all three models are age, family history of hypertension and calcium intake.

Exercise 21.14.   From the results shown in Figure 21.18 (a) which independent variables are statistically significant in all three models? (b) Explain the 95 per cent confidence interval of (0.28 to 0.64) for *age* in the blood lead model. (c) In which model does a unit increase in age (age is measured in units of 1 year) change SBP the most?

---

[10]The inclusion of Age^2 in the model is probably an attempt to establish the linearity of the relationship between systolic blood pressure and age. If the coefficient for Age^2 is not statistically significant then the relationship is probably linear.

Variable	Baseline model + blood lead		Baseline model + tibia lead		Baseline model + patella lead	
	Parameter estimate	95% CI	Parameter estimate	95% CI	Parameter estimate	95% CI
Intercept	128.34		125.90		127.23	
Age (years)	0.46*	0.28, 0.64	0.39*	0.20, 0.58	0.44*	0.26, 0.63
Age squared (years^2)	−0.02*	−0.04, −0.00	−0.02*	−0.04, −0.00	−0.02*	−0.04, −0.00
Body mass index	0.36*	0.01, 0.72	0.33	−0.02, 0.69	0.35	−0.00, 0.71
Family history of hypertension (yes/no)	4.36*	1.42, 7.30	4.36*	1.47, 7.25	4.32*	1.42, 7.22
Alcohol intake (g/day)	0.08*	0.00, 0.149	0.07	−0.00, 0.14	0.07	−0.00, 0.14
Calcium intake (10 mg/day)	−0.04*	−0.08, −0.00	−0.04*	0.07, −0.00	−0.04*	−0.07, −0.00
Blood lead (SD)[†]	−0.13	−1.35, 1.09				
Tibia lead (SD)[†]			1.37*	0.02, 2.73		
Patella lead (SD)[†]					0.57	−0.71, 1.84
Model R^2	0.0956		0.1015		0.0950	

*$p < 0.05$
[†]based on one standard deviation (SD) in lead levels

Figure 21.18 Multiple regression results from a cross-section study into the relationship between bone lead and blood lead levels and the development of hypertension in 512 individuals selected from a cohort study. The figure shows the outcome from three multiple linear regression models, with systolic blood pressure as the dependent variable. Source: Cheng *et al.* (2001). Reproduced by permission of Oxford University Press

Diagnostics – checking the basic assumptions of the multiple linear regression model

The ordinary least squares method of coefficient estimation will only produce the best estimators if the basic assumptions of the model are satisfied. That is, a metric continuous dependent variable, a linear relationship between the dependent and each independent variable, error terms with constant spread and Normally distributed, and the independent variables not perfectly correlated with each other. Checking that the first two assumptions are satisfied is reasonably straightforward (see below) but checking the others is too complicated to cover in this book. The first two assumptions can be checked as follows:

- *A metric continuous dependent variable.* Refer to Chapter 1 if you are unsure how to identify a metric continuous variable.

- *A linear relationship between the dependent variable and each independent variable.* Easiest to investigate by plotting the dependent variable against each of the independent variables; the scatter should lie approximately around a straight line.[11]

Multiple linear regression is popular in clinical research. Much more popular though, for reasons which will become clear in the next chapter, is logistic regression.

Analysis of variance

Analysis of variance (ANOVA) is a procedure that aims to deal with the same problems as that of linear regression analysis, and many medical statistics books contain at least one chapter describing ANOVA. It has a history in the social sciences, particularly psychology. However, regression and ANOVA are simply two sides of the same coin – the *generalised linear model.* As Field (2013) says:

> Anova is fine for simple designs, but becomes impossibly cumbersome in more complex situations. The regression model extends very logically to these more complex designs, without getting bogged down in mathematics. Finally, the method (Anova) becomes extremely unmanageable in some circumstances, such as unequal sample sizes. The regression method makes these situations considerably more simple.

In view of the fact that anything ANOVA can do, regression can also do, and for me anyway, do it in a way that is conceptually easier, I am not going to discuss ANOVA in this book. If you are interested in exploring ANOVA in more detail, you could do worse than read Andy Field's book or that of Altman (1991).

---

[11]Notice that we only have to establish this property of linearity for the metric-independent variables in the model. Any binary variables are linear by default – they only have two points, which can be joined with a straight line. Any ordinal independent variables will have to be expressed as binary dummies – again linear by default for the same reason.

22
Curvy models: Logistic regression

A second health warning!

The logistic regression model is much more popular and appears much more frequently in research papers than the linear regression model. The reason for this will become apparent as we work through the chapter. Although the maths underlying the logistic regression model is perhaps more complicated than that in linear regression, once more a brief description of the

Medical Statistics from Scratch: An Introduction for Health Professionals, Third Edition. David Bowers.
© 2014 John Wiley & Sons, Ltd. Published 2014 by John Wiley & Sons, Ltd.

underlying idea is necessary if you are to gain some understanding of the procedure and be able to sensibly interpret logistic computer outputs.

Binary-dependent variables

In linear regression, the dependent or outcome variable must be metric continuous. In clinical research, however, the outcome variable will more often be dichotomous (or *binary*), that is, it is able to take only *two* different values: alive or dead, malignant or benign, stillborn or not stillborn, and so on. In addition, variables that are not naturally binary can often be made so. For example, birthweight might be coded 'less than 2500 g' and '2500 g or more', and Apgar scores coded 'less than 7' and '7 or more'. In this chapter, I want to describe the logistic regression model and how it is suited to a binary-dependent variable and how it can take the place of the inappropriate linear regression model.

Finding an appropriate model when the outcome variable is binary

If you are trying to find an appropriate model to describe the relationship between two variables, let us say hypertension (the metric-dependent variable) and salt intake, you can draw a scatterplot of the two variables (Figure 21.5 is a good example) and if this has a linear shape, you can model the relationship with a linear regression model. However, when the outcome variable is binary, this graphical approach is not particularly helpful.

For example, suppose you are interested in using the breast cancer/stress data from the study referred to in Figure 1.7 to investigate the relationship between the outcome variable 'Diagnosis', and the independent variable 'Age'. Diagnosis is, of course, a binary variable with two values: $Y = 1$ (malignant) or $Y = 0$ (benign). If we plot *Diagnosis* against *Age*, we get the scatterplot as shown in Figure 22.1, from which it is pretty well impossible to draw any definite conclusions about the nature of the relationship.

The problem is that the large variability in age, in both the malignant and benign groups, obscures the difference in age (if any) *between* them (see the discussion in Chapter 14 on within-subject and between-subject variation). However, if you *group* the age data: 40–49, 50–59, and so on and then calculate the *proportion* of women with a malignant diagnosis (i.e. with $Y = 1$) in each group, this will reduce the variability but preserve the underlying relationship between the two variables. The results of doing this are shown in Figure 22.2.

Notice that I have labelled the first column as the probability that $Y = 1$ (the lump is malignant), written as $p(Y = 1)$. Here is why. In linear regression, you will recall that the dependent variable is the *mean* of the Y values for a given X value. But what about a binary-dependent variable? Can we find something analogous to the mean? As it happens, the mean of a set of binary (zero or one) values is the same as the *proportion* of ones,[1] so an appropriate equivalent version of the binary-dependent variable would seem to be the proportion of $(Y = 1)$s.

But proportions can be interpreted as probabilities (see Chapter 11). So the dependent variable becomes the 'Probability that $Y = 1$', or $p(Y = 1)$, for a given value of X. For example, we

---

[1] For example, the mean of the five values: 0, 1, 1, 0, 0 is $2/5 = 0.4$, which is the same as the proportion of 1s, that is, 2 in 5.

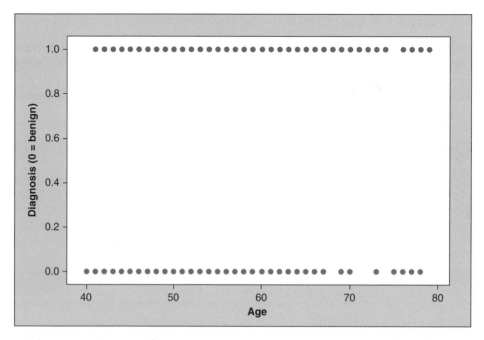

Figure 22.1 Scatter plot of Diagnosis against age for the 332 women in the stress and breast cancer study referred to in Table 1.1

Probability of malignant lump in each age group, i.e. $p(Y=1)$	Midpoint of age group
0.140	45
0.226	55
0.635	65
0.727	75

Figure 22.2 Proportion of women with malignant lump in each age group

can write the probability of a malignant diagnosis ($Y=1$) for all of those women aged 40, as $p(Y=1)$ given $X=40$[2].

You can see in the table of Figure 22.2 that the proportion with malignant breast lumps (the probability that $Y=1$) increases with age, but does it increase linearly? A scatterplot of the proportion with malignant lumps, $Y=1$, against group age midpoints is shown in Figure 22.3, which does suggest *some* sort of relationship between the two variables. But it is definitely *not* linear, so a *linear* regression model will not work. In fact, the curve has more of an elongated S shape, so what we need is a mathematical equation that will give such an S-shaped curve.

---

[2]Statisticians would write this as: $p(Y=1|X=40)$. The|sign means 'given that'.

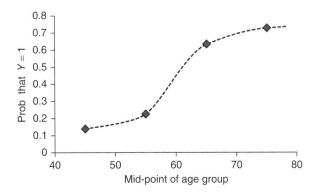

Figure 22.3 Scatter plot of the proportion of women with a malignant diagnosis, that is, the proportion for whom $Y = 1$, or the probability that $Y = 1$, against mid-points of age groups (data from Figure 1.7). The curve is certainly *not* linear but perhaps more like a very stretched 'S'

There are several possibilities, but the *logistic* model is the model of choice. Not only because it produces an S-shaped curve, which we want, but, critically, it has a meaningful clinical interpretation. Moreover, the value of $p(Y = 1)$ is restricted by the maths of the logistic model to lie between zero and one, which is also what we must have, because it is a probability. Although the linear regression model is based on a continuous metric-dependent variable, the binary logistic model is based on a dependent variable, which has a binomial distribution.

The logistic regression model

I know that not all of my readers will want to know the mathematical details of the logistic regression model, and if you are one of those, you might want to skip the next page. If you are still with me . . . the simple[3] *population* logistic regression equation is:

$$p(Y = 1) = \frac{(e^{\beta_0 + \beta_1 X})}{1 + e^{\beta_0 + \beta_1 X}} \qquad (22.1)$$

where the dependent variable is the probability that $Y = 1$, X is the independent variable, which may be nominal, ordinal or metric, and β_0 and β_1 are the population regression constant and slope parameters, respectively. Note that e is the exponential operator, equal to 2.7183, and has nothing to do with the residual term in linear regression. You use a suitable computer program (with your data) to get the values of the sample regression coefficients b_0 and b_1, and hence the *sample* logistic regression equation:

$$p(Y = 1) = \frac{(e^{b_0 + b_1 X})}{1 + e^{b_0 + b_1 X}} \qquad (22.2)$$

---

[3]'Simple' because there is only one independent variable – so far.

We will come back to getting values for the sample coefficients shortly. As you can see, the logistic regression model is mathematically a bit more complicated than the linear regression model.

Exercise 22.1. In linear regression we can plot Y against X to determine whether the relationship between the two variables is linear. Explain why this approach is not particularly helpful when Y is a binary variable. What approach might be more useful?

To illustrate the idea, let us return to our stress and breast cancer study (Figure 1.7). We want to know whether the use of the oral contraceptive pill (OCP is a risk factor for breast cancer, i.e. getting a malignant diagnosis. Our outcome variable is *diagnosis*, where $Y = 1$ (malignant) or $Y = 0$ (benign). We will start with one independent variable – *Ever used an oral contraceptive pill* (OCP), Yes = 1 or No = 0. We are going to treat OCP use as a possible risk factor for receiving a malignant diagnosis. This gives us the sample regression model:

$$P(Y = 1) = \frac{(e^{b0+b1 \times OCP})}{1 + e^{b0+b1 \times OCP}} \tag{22.3}$$

So all we have got to do to determine the probability that a woman picked at random from the sample will get a malignant diagnosis ($Y = 1$), with and without OCP use, is to determine the values of b_0 and b_1 and then put them in the logistic regression equation, with OCP = 0 or OCP = 1.

Estimating the parameter values

Although the linear regression models commonly use the method of ordinary least squares (OLS) to estimate the regression parameters β_0 and β_1, logistic regression models use what is called *maximum likelihood estimation*. Essentially, this means choosing the population which is *most likely* to have generated the sample results observed. Figures 22.4 and 22.5, respectively, show the output from SPSS's and Minitab's logistic regression program for the above OCP model.

Note that SPSS uses something called the Wald statistic and its associated p-value to measure the significance of the parameters, whereas Minitab uses what is known as the z distribution (I have omitted this from Figure 22.4).

You will also see a term called the *Log-Likelihood* in the Minitab output in Figure 22.4. (The log-likelihood is also provided in the SPSS output but I have not shown it here). The likelihood is the *probability* that you will get the observed results *given* the parameter estimates. Any further explanation of the log-likelihood would be a step too far for this book, so I will simply say that the closer the value of the log-likelihood to 0, the better is the model. The initial value for the log-likelihood is for a model in which only the constant is included. This is used as the baseline against which models with independent variables are judged. As we successively add independent variables to the initial model, we hope to see the log-likelihood value get

Binary Logistic Regression: Diagnosis(1 = malignant) versus Ever OCP?

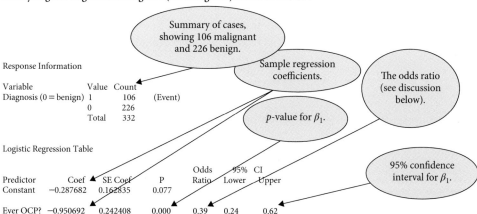

Figure 22.4 Output (abridged) from Minitab for logistic regression of diagnosis, $p(Y=1)$, lump is malignant, against Ever used the oral contraceptive pill (OCP). Data from Figure 1.7

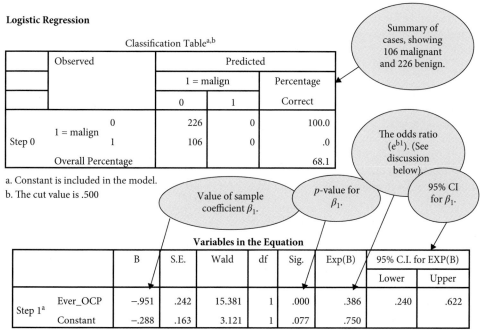

Figure 22.5 Output (abridged) from SPSS for logistic regression of diagnosis $p(Y=1)$, lump is malignant, against Ever used the oral contraceptive pill (OCP). Data from Figure 1.7

progressively closer to zero (i.e. less and less negative). You can see from Figure 22.4 that with just OCP use in the model, the log-likelihood value is -200.009.

SPSS's and Minitab's logistic regression program both give $b_0 = -0.288$ and $b_1 = -0.951$. If we substitute these values into the logistic regression model of Equation (22.3), we get:

$$P(Y = 1) = \frac{(e^{-0.288 + -0.951 \times OCP})}{(1 + e^{-0.288 + -0.951 \times OCP})} \tag{22.4}$$

If you now substitute the two values for oral contraceptive use, $OCP = 0$ and $OCP = 1$, we get[4]:

$$\text{if } OCP = 0 \text{ (has never used OCP), then } P(Y = 1) = 0.4286$$

$$\text{if } OCP = 1 \text{ (has used OCP), then } P(Y = 1) = 0.2247$$

So a woman who has never used an oral contraceptive pill has a probability of getting a malignant diagnosis nearly twice than that of a woman who *has* used an oral contraceptive pill. Rather than being a risk factor for a malignant diagnosis, in this sample the use of oral contraceptives seems to confer some protection against a breast lump being malignant.

The odds ratio

The great and glowing attraction of the logistic regression model is that it readily produces odds ratios. But how? There's quite a lot of maths involved, but eventually we can get to the following result[5]

$$\text{Odds ratio} = \frac{e^{b0+b1}}{e^{b0}} = e^{b1}$$

Thus to find the odds ratio for any variable on the right-hand side of the equation all you need to do is raise e to the power b_1, or b_2, or b_3 and so on, which is easily done on a decent calculator, but SPSS and Minitab do it for you anyway. It is this ability to produce odds ratios that has made the logistic regression model so popular in clinical studies.

For example, in our Diagnosis/OCP model, $b_1 = -0.9507$, so the odds ratio for a malignant diagnosis for woman using OCP compared to women not using OCP is:

$$\text{Odds ratio} = e^{-0.9507} = 0.386$$

In other words, a woman who has used OCP has only about a third of the odds of getting a malignant diagnosis as a woman who has not used OCP. This result seems to confirm our earlier result that use of OCP provides some protection against a malignancy. Minitab and SPSS both

---

[4]You'll first need to work out the values of $(b_0 + b_1 \times OCP)$, then $(b_0 + b_1 \times OCP)$, then raise e to each of these powers. Then, divide the former by the latter, first adding 1 to the denominator. And do this for $OCP = 0$ and $OCP = 1$. Phew!

[5]Making use of the rule that $X^a/X^b = X^{a-b}$.

produce the odds ratio for OCP as a risk factor for a malign diagnosis – I have pointed them out in both Figures 22.4 and 22.5.

Of course, we do not know whether this result is due to chance or whether this represents a real statistically significant relationship in the population. To answer this question, we will need either a confidence interval for β_1 or a p-value, and I will deal with this significance issue very shortly.

> **Exercise 22.2.** Explain why, in terms of the risk of using OCP and the probability of getting a malignant diagnosis, that the values $p(Y=1)=0.4286$ when OCP $=0$ and $p(Y=1)=0.2247$, when OCP $=1$, are compatible with an odds ratio $=0.386$ for a malignant diagnosis, among women using OCP compared to women not using OCP.

Interpreting the regression coefficient

In linear regression, the coefficient b_1 represents the increase in Y for a unit increase in X. In the logistic regression model, we are not so much interested in the meaning of b_1, except to note that if the independent variable is ordinal or metric, then you might be more interested in the effect on the odds ratio of changes of *greater* than one unit. For example, if the independent variable is age, then the effect on the odds ratio of an increase in age of one year may not be as interesting as say a change of 10 years. In these circumstances, if the change in age is c years, then the change in the odds ratio is e^{cb_1}. In addition, note that antilog$_e$ of the coefficient of b_1 is equal to the odds ratio. So in the OCP example seen earlier, $b_1 = -0.9507$, so the odds ratio $=$ antilog$_e$ $(-0.9507) = 0.386$.

> **Exercise 22.3.** If we use Minitab to regress Diagnosis against Age for the data in Figure 1.7 we get the output shown in Figure 22.6. (a) Is age significant? (b) Use the Minitab values to write down the estimated logistic regression model. (c) Calculate the probability that the diagnosis will be malignant, that is, $p(Y=1)$, for women aged: (i) 45 and (ii) 50. (d) Calculate $[1 - p(Y=1)]$ in each case, and hence calculate the odds ratio for a malignant diagnosis in women aged 45 compared to women aged 50. Explain your result. (e) Confirm that the antilog$_e$ of the coefficient on *Age* is equal to the odds ratio. (f) What effect does an increase in *Age* of 10 years have on the odds ratio?

Statistical inference in the logistic regression model

As you saw in Chapter 15, if the population odds ratio is equal to 1, then the risk factor in question has no effect on the odds for any particular outcome; that is, the variable concerned is *not* a statistically significant risk (or benefit). We can use either the p-value or the confidence interval to decide whether any departures from a value of 1 for the odds ratio is merely due to chance or is it an indication of statistical significance.

Logistic Regression

Predictor	Coef	SE Coef	P	Odds Ratio	95% CI Lower	95% CI Upper
Constant	−6.46725	0.763193	0.000			
Age	0.102306	0.0132579	0.000	1.11	1.08	1.14

Figure 22.6 Output from Minitab for the logistic regression of *Diagnosis* on *Age*, using the data from Figure 1.7

In fact, in Figure 22.4, the 95 per cent confidence interval for the odds ratio of 0.39 for OCP use (the odds of a malignant diagnosis for women who had used an oral contraceptive compared to the odds for women who had not used an oral contraceptive) is (0.24 to 0.62), and as this does not include 1, the odds ratio is statistically significant. In addition, the *p*-value is <0.000 (so a lot less than 0.05). However, we still need to be cautious about this result because it represents only a crude odds ratio, which, in reality, would need to be adjusted for other possible confounding variables, such as age. We can make this adjustment in logistic regression just as easily as in the linear regression model, simply by including the variables we want to adjust for on the right-hand side of the model.

> **Exercise 22.4.** Figure 22.7 shows the output from SPSS for the regression of Diagnosis on Body Mass Index (BMI) using the data from Figure 1.7. Comment on the statistical significance of BMI as a risk factor for receiving a malignant diagnosis.

		B	S.E.	Wald	df	Sig.	Exp(B)	95% C.I. for EXP(B) Lower	95% C.I. for EXP(B) Upper
Step 1[a]	BMI	.085	.024	12.268	1	.000	1.089	1.038	1.141
	Constant	−2.924	.635	21.169	1	.000	.054		

Variables in the EQUATION

[a]Variable(s) entered on step 1: BMI.

Figure 22.7 Output from SPSS for the regression of Diagnosis on Body Mass Index (BMI) (Data from Figure 1.7.)

The multiple logistic regression model

In my explanation of the odds ratio above, I used a simple logistic regression model, that is, one with a single independent variable (OCP), because this offers the simplest explanation.

However, the result we got, that the odds ratio is equal to e^{b_1}, applies to *each* coefficient if there is more than one independent variable, that is, e^{b_2}, e^{b_3} and so on. The usual situation is to have a risk factor variable plus a number of confounder variables (the usual suspects – age, sex, etc.). Suppose, for example, that you decided to include *age* and BMI along with OCP as independent variables. Equation (22.3) would then become:

$$p(Y = 1) = \frac{(e^{\beta 0 + \beta_1 \times OCP + \beta_2 \times age + \beta_3 \times BMI})}{(1 + e^{\beta 0 + \beta_1 \times OCP + \beta_2 \times age + \beta_3 \times BMI})}$$

$p(Y=1)$ is still, of course, the probability that the woman will receive a malignant diagnosis, $Y=1$. The odds ratio for *age* is e^{b_2}; the odds ratio for BMI is e^{b_3}. Moreover, as with linear regression, each of these odds ratios is *adjusted* for any possible interaction between the independent variables.

As an example, output from Minitab for the above multiple regression model of Diagnosis against use of oral contraceptives (OCP), Age and BMI, is shown in Figure 22.8.

Exercise 22.5. Comment on what is revealed in the output in Figure 22.8 about the relationship between the probability of a malignant diagnosis [$p(Y=1)$] and the three potential risk factor variables shown. What does the value of log-likelihood, compared to its value in the model with only OCP use, (see Figure 22.4) tell you?

Logistic Regression Table

Predictor	Coef	SE Coef	P	Odds Ratio	95% CI Lower	95% CI Upper
Constant	−9.24814	1.30391	0.000			
Ever OCP?	0.356767	0.329147	0.278	1.43	0.75	2.72
Age	0.111670	0.0164348	0.000	1.12	1.08	1.15
BMI	0.0812739	0.0275908	0.003	1.08	1.03	1.14
Log-Likelihood = −165.645						

Figure 22.8 Output (abridged) from Minitab for multiple logistic regression of Diagnosis against oral contraceptive use (OCP), Age, and body mass index (BMI). Data from Figure 1.7

Building the model

The strategy for model building in the logistic regression model is similar in many respects to that for linear regression (see the section on variable selection in Chapter 21). Once again, there are two possible approaches, automatic or manual variable selection. And within these two approaches, we can use either forwards or backwards variable elimination. I would favour manual selection for the reasons I gave in Chapter 21.

As a reminder, in the forwards elimination approach, the main independent variable of interest is entered into the model, and the other variables (potential confounders) are then entered one at a time in the order of the p-value obtained from a preliminary series of univarate regressions or other statistical tests (lowest p-value variable first). This is the best approach if you have a good candidate for the main relationship with your chosen dependent variable. You enter this into the model first and then add the likely confounders.

The backwards elimination approach starts with all of the variables included in the model (including the main independent variable). Variables are then dropped one at a time if not significant. In both approaches you need to watch out for changes in a variable coefficient when a variable is added or subtracted from the model – this indicates possible confounding. The variable selection process can be summed up as follows:

- Make a list of candidate-independent variables.

- For any nominal or ordinal variables in the list, construct a contingency table and perform a chi-squared test.[6] Make a note of the p-value.

- For any metric variables, perform either a two-sample t test or a univariate logistic regression; note the p-value in either case.

- Identify those variables in the list whose p-value is 0.25 or less.[7] Then, either start with *all* of the variables on this list included in the model and drop them one at a time (backwards elimination) or select your prime candidate variable (forwards elimination) then add the other variables (potential confounders) one at a time.

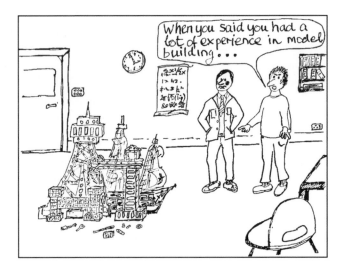

---

[6]Provided the number of categories is not too big for the size of your sample: you do not want any empty cells or low expected values (see Chapter 17).
[7]Remember from Chapter 21 that using a p-value less than this may fail to identify variables that could subsequently turn out to be important in the final model

As an example of a backwards stepwise approach, the following extract is from a cross-sectional study to develop and validate a prognostic model for early death in patients with traumatic bleeding. The authors write:

> We used a backward stepwise approach. Firstly, we included all potential prognostic factors and interaction terms that users considered plausible. These interactions included all potential predictors with type of injury, time since injury, and age. We then removed, one at a time, terms for which we found no strong evidence of an association, judged according to the P values (<0.05) from the Wald test. Each time, we calculated a log likelihood ratio test to check that the term removed did not have a big effect in the model. Eventually, we reached a model in which all terms were statistically significant.
>
> *Perel* et al. *(2012)*

A second example, this time using the forward variable selection process, is from a study to assess the risk of adverse perinatal events of vaccination of pregnant women with an MF59 adjuvanted vaccine:

> Logistic regression analysis
> After assessing the association of several covariates with both the exposure of interest and the outcome, we entered those potential confounders one by one into the model already containing the monovalent MF59 vaccine. We retained variables that changed the crude estimated effect of the vaccine on the outcome by at least 10% in the final model as confounders (number of antenatal visits, maternal age, and smoking). We considered others, such as educational and income level and parity, although the change was between 5% and 10%, on the basis of the bivariate association with both exposure and outcome and their clinical and or epidemiological significance.
>
> *Rubinstein* et al. *(2013)*

The results shown in Figure 22.9 are from the same study and show the crude and adjusted odds ratios from the logistic regression of three separate outcomes, and a composite outcome, on vaccination (yes or no) and seven possible confounding variables (see table footnote). As you can see, the crude odds ratios for vaccination compared to non-vaccination are significant for all three separate outcomes, as well as for the the composite outcome and only perinatal mortality becomes non-significant when the odds ratios are adjusted for the variables shown in the table footnote.

Exercise 22.6. What does Figure 22.9 tell you about the odds (adjusted) for vaccinated women compared to non-vaccinated women, of delivering pre-term or having babies with low birthweight?

Exercise 22.7. Summarise briefly the alternative methods available for variable selection in logistic regression.

Outcome	No (%)		Odds ratio (95% CI)	
	Vaccinated H1N1 ($n=7293$)	Non-vaccinated H1N1 ($n=23\ 195$)	Crude	Multiple logistic regression adjusted*
Preterm + low birth weight + perinatal mortality	513 (7.0)	2160 (9.3)	0.74 (0.67 to 0.81)	0.80 (0.72 to 0.89)
Preterm (<37 weeks)	354 (4.9)	1505 (6.5)	0.73 (0.65 to 0.83)	0.79 (0.69 to 0.90)
Low birth weight	357 (4.9)	1606 (6.9)	0.69 (0.61 to 0.78)	0.74 (0.65 to 0.83)
Perinatal mortality	54 (7.4)	257 (11.0)	0.63 (0.46 to 0.86)	0.68 (0.42 to 1.06)

*Adjusted for number of antenatal visits, level of education, maternal age, income, parity, smoking, and history of pregnancy-induced hypertension.

Figure 22.9   Crude and adjusted perinatal outcomes in vaccinated and non-vaccinated women. The table shows the results from the logistic regression of three separate outcomes, and a composite outcome, on vaccination (yes or no), together with seven possible confounding variables. Data from a study to assess the risk of adverse perinatal events of vaccination of pregnant women with an MF59 adjuvanted vaccine (Rubinstein *et al.* 2013).

Goodness-of-fit

In the linear regression model, we can use R^2 to measure goodness-of-fit. In the logistic regression model, measuring goodness-of-fit is more complicated and can involve graphical as well as numeric measures. Minitab presents three goodness-of-fit measures (all based on chi-square): *Pearson*, *Deviance*, and *Hosmer-Lemeshow*. The null hypothesis is that the model *provides a good fit*, and we can use the resulting *p*-value to reject or not reject this hypothesis. The graphical methods are quite complex and you should consult more specialist sources for further information on this and other aspects of this complex procedure. Hosmer and Lemeshow (2013) is an excellent source.

As an example, Figure 22.10 shows the output from Minitab for a multiple regression of Diagnosis on OCP use, Age and BMI, giving the three goodness-of-fit statistics. As you can see, all three have *p*-values >0.05, so we cannot reject the good fit hypothesis. Good fit = good news! SPSS provides a Hosmer-Lemeshow value.

Poisson regression (just to say 'Hello')

I do not intend to discuss *Poisson* regression in this book (at least not in this edition anyway) other than very briefly. To summarise the method, Poisson regression is appropriate when the data is a *count* of events, particularly rare events. For example, the number of stillbirths in a year in a particular hospital or region, or the number of road traffic accident victims presenting at an Emergency Department in a month, or the number of new cases of HIV in a city in a year. The data is thus clearly discrete.

Binary Logistic Regression: Diagnosis(1=malignant) versus Ever OCP?, Age, BMI

				Odds	95% CI	
Predictor	Coef	SE Coef	P	Ratio	Lower	Upper
Constant	−9.24814	1.30391	0.000			
Ever OCP?	0.356767	0.329147	0.278	1.43	0.75	2.72
Age	0.111670	0.0164348	0.000	1.12	1.08	1.15
BMI	0.0812739	0.0275908	0.003	1.08	1.03	1.14

Log-Likelihood = −165.645

Goodness-of-Fit Tests

Method	Chi-Square	DF	P
Pearson	329.603	321	0.358
Deviance	328.516	321	0.374
Hosmer-Lemeshow	2.581	8	0.958

Figure 22.10 Output from Minitab for a multiple regression of Diagnosis on OCP use, Age and BMI, showing the three goodness-of-fit statistics. As you can see, all three have p-values >0.05, so we cannot reject the good-fit hypothesis

The Poisson model takes the form:

$$\log_e Y = \beta_0 + \beta_1 X_1 + \beta_2 X_2 + \ \dots$$

which means that:

$$Y = (e^{\beta 0})\,(e^{\beta 1 X 1})\,(e^{\beta 2 X 2}) \ \dots \ \text{etc}$$

Incidentally, if the counts are categorical (i.e. you have a contingency table with counts in the cells), the convention is to call this approach *log-linear* modelling, whereas, if the counts are numerical/continuous, it is usual to refer to the method as a Poisson regression.

Estimation of the parameter values (β_0, β_1, β_2, etc) is done using *maximum likelihood*, as with the logistic regression. Most statistical computer programmes will do a Poisson regression, including Stata, SPSS and Minitab.

And that's all I intend to say on Poisson (thin rations!!!)

However, we are not finished with regression just yet. In the next chapter, I will discuss the application of another regression technique – in the context of survival analysis.

X

Three More Chapters

23

Measuring survival

Learning objectives

When you have finished this chapter, you should be able to:

- Explain what censoring means.

- Calculate Kaplan–Meier survival probabilities.

- Draw a Kaplan–Meier survival curve.

- Use the Kaplan–Meier curve to estimate median survival time.

- Explain the use of the log-rank test to determine whether the survival experience of two or more groups is significantly different.

- Explain the role of the hazard ratio in comparing the relative survival experience of two groups.

- Outline the general idea behind Cox proportional hazards regression and interpret the results from such a regression.

Medical Statistics from Scratch: An Introduction for Health Professionals, Third Edition. David Bowers.
© 2014 John Wiley & Sons, Ltd. Published 2014 by John Wiley & Sons, Ltd.

Preamble

Imagine that you have a patient who has overdosed on paracetamol. Their partner asks you what their chances of 'coming through it' are. Or suppose a patient with breast cancer wants to know which of two possible treatments offers them the best chance of survival. You can answer questions like these with the help of a procedure known as *survival analysis*. The basis of this method is the measurement of the time from some *intervention* or *procedure* to some *event of interest*.

For example, if you were studying survival after mastectomy for breast cancer (the 'procedure'), you would want to know how long each woman survived following surgery. Here, the event of 'interest' would be death. For practical reasons, you usually have to limit the duration of the study, for example, to six months, or a year or whatever.

Very often you will want to compare the survival experiences of two groups of patients; for example, women having a mastectomy with women having a lumpectomy. I should emphasise that 'survival' in this context does not necessarily mean not dying. The event of interest can be death, but it can also be one of a number of things; for example, cancer-free survival, relapse, re-admission to hospital, return to work, or giving birth. Survival is the useful portmanteau word we use.

Censored data

One particular problem which makes this type of analysis tricky is that you often don't observe the event of interest in *all* of the subjects. For example, if you are looking at long-term survival after mastectomy and your study period is five years, many of the women involved will still be alive at the five-year point. We do not know how long these women will live after the end of the study period, only that they are still alive when the study period ends. In addition, some patients may withdraw from the study during the study period; they may move away, or simply refuse further participation, or die from a cause unrelated to the study. These types of incomplete data are said to be *censored*.

A final problem is that not all patients may enter the study at the same time. So all in all, analysis of survival in these circumstances is tricky. Fortunately, methods have been developed to deal with these difficulties. One of these, the *Kaplan–Meier method*, gives us a table of survival probabilities, which can be charted as the Kaplan–Meier chart. The two questions that are often of the greatest interest are:

- What is the probability of a patient surviving for some given period of time?

- What is the *comparative* survival experience of two or more groups of patients?

A simple example of survival in a single group

See the data in Figure 23.1. This shows survival data (in months) for a group of 12 patients diagnosed with a brain tumour, who were followed up for 12 months. You can see that seven

Patient	Month of entry to study (0 indicates present at beginning of study)	Time after study start date to death or censoring (months)	Outcomes: Died (D), Survived (S) or left study prematurely (P)	Survival times
1	0	12	S*	12
2	0	12	S*	12
3	0	11	D	11
4	0	8	D	8
5	1	6	P*	5
6	2	12	S*	10
7	2	4	D	2
8	2	5	D	3
9	2	9	D	7
10	3	9	P*	6
11	3	8	D	5
12	3	7	D	4

Figure 23.1 Survival times (months) over a 12-month study period, of 12 patients diagnosed with brain tumour. *Indicates censored data – patient survived (S) or left study prematurely (P). The *actual* survival time for these patients is not known

patients died, two left the study prematurely and three survived. This means that you have seven definite and five censored survival times. We can represent the survival times in the last column graphically, as in Figure 23.2, where the survival times are arranged in *ascending* order.

Calculating survival probabilities and the proportion surviving: the Kaplan–Meier table

The Kaplan–Meier method requires a Kaplan–Meier table like Figure 23.3, with, strictly speaking, rows *only* for time periods when a death occurs (shown in bold in the table). However, I have included all 12 rows in the table to help illustrate the method more clearly.

- The first column indicates the time period (t)

- The second column tells us how many people (n), were still alive at the beginning of each month t.

- Column 3 (w) is the number of premature withdrawals during month t.

- Column 4 is the number of deaths (d) in month t.

- Column 5 is the total number at risk (r) during the month.

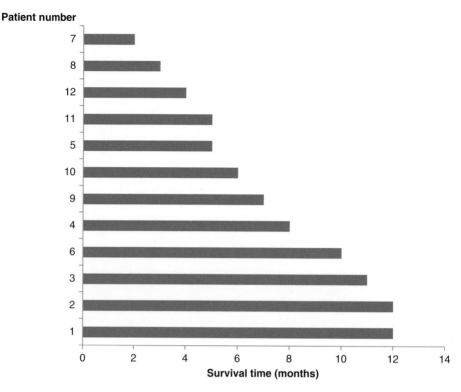

Figure 23.2   Chart of survival times (in ascending order) from table in Figure 23.1

- Column 6 is the result of dividing column 4 by column 5, to get d/r. This is the probability that a patient still alive at the beginning of the month will die during that month (which is equivalent to the *proportion* of patients dying in that month).

As d/r is the probability of dying during a time period, then $(1 - d/r)$ must be the probability of surviving to the end of the time period. This survival probability is shown in column 7. To calculate the probability of surviving *all* of the preceding time periods *and* the current time period, you must successively multiply the probabilities in column 7 together. The resultant cumulative probabilities, labelled S, are shown in column 8. For example, the value for S of 0.818 in row 5 is $1 \times 1 \times 1 \times 0.909 \times 0.900$. These column 8 values are the *Kaplan – Meier survival probabilities*.

The results in Figure 23.3 indicate that the probability of a patient surviving to the end of the third month is 1, to the end of the fourth month is 0.909 and so on, and for the full 12 months after the diagnosis is 0.239.

We can also interpret these values as *proportions*. For example, 0.909 of the patients (or 90.9 per cent) will survive to the end of the fourth month. About a quarter (23.9 per cent) will survive the full 12 months. We can generalise these results to the *population* of patients of whom this sample is representative, and who have the same type of brain tumour, at the same

1	2	3	4	5	6	7	8
Month	Number still in study at start of month t	Withdrawn prematurely during month t	Deaths in month t	Number at risk in month t	Probability of death in month t	Probability of surviving month t	Cumulative probability of surviving to month t
t	n	w	d	r	d/r	$p = 1 - d/r$	S
1	12	0	0	12	0	1	1
2	12	0	0	12	0	1	1
3	12	0	0	12	0	1	1
4	12	0	1	11	$1/11 = 0.091$	0.909	0.909
5	11	0	1	10	$1/10 = 0.100$	0.900	0.818
6	10	1	0	9	0	1	0.818
7	9	0	1	8	$1/8 = 0.125$	0.875	0.716
8	8	0	2	6	$2/6 = 0.333$	0.667	0.478
9	6	1	1	4	$1/4 = 0.250$	0.750	0.358
10	4	0	0	4	0	1	0.358
11	4	0	1	3	$1/3 = 0.333$	0.667	0.239
12	3	0	0	3	0	1	0.239

Figure 23.3   Calculation of Kaplan–Meier survival probabilities

stage of development, and receive the same level of care. In addition, we may want to adjust for possible confounding variables such as age, sex and so on. We will deal with this later.

The Kaplan–Meier curve

If you plot the cumulative survival probabilities in the last column of Figure 23.3 against time, you get the *Kaplan–Meier curve*, as shown in Figure 23.4. Notice that the survival 'curve' looks like a staircase, albeit with uneven steps. Every time there is a death, the curve steps down. As there are seven deaths, there are seven steps down.[1]

> **Exercise 23.1.**   The data in Figure 23.5 shows the survival times (in days) of eight patients with acute myocardial infarction, treated with a new reperfusion drug Explase as part of a fibrinolytic regimen. Patients were followed up for 14 days. Calculate the survival probabilities and plot Kaplan–Meier survival curves. Comment on your results.

---

[1] Notice there is a double step down at period 8 because of the two deaths.

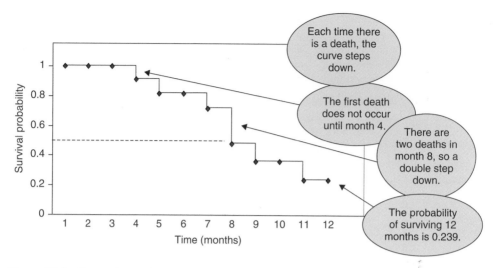

Figure 23.4 The Kaplan–Meier survival curve drawn from the data in Figure 23.3 (the dotted line indicates median proportion surviving – see text below)

Patient	Day of entry to study (0 indicates present at beginning of study)	Time after study start date to death or censoring (days)	Outcomes: Died (D), Survived (S) or Left study prematurely (P)
1	0	3	D
2	0	14	S
3	0	8	D
4	0	12	P
5	1	14	S
6	2	13	D
7	2	14	S
8	2	14	S

Figure 23.5 The survival times (in days) of eight patients with acute myocardial infarction. Patients were followed up for 14 days

Determining median survival time

One of the consequences of not knowing the actual survival times of all of those subjects who survive beyond the end of the study period is that we cannot calculate the mean survival time of the whole group. However, if you interpret the probabilities on the vertical axis of a Kaplan–Meier chart as proportions or percentages, you can often determine *median* survival times. It is that value which corresponds to a probability of 0.5 (i.e. 50 per cent). In Figure 23.4, the median survival time is eight months (at this time, the probability is that half of the patients still survived). Obviously, the survival time of any proportion of the sample can be determined in this same way, including the interquartile range values, *provided that* the Kaplan–Meier curve goes down far enough (unfortunately, it often does not).

> **Exercise 23.2.** The Kaplan–Meier curve in Figure 23.6 is from a cohort study in which the authors stated, 'We aimed to establish the natural history of oral HPV infection in men.' The curve shows the cumulative probability of the time to clearance of infection of incident oncogenic oral HPV. What is the median time to clearance of infection?

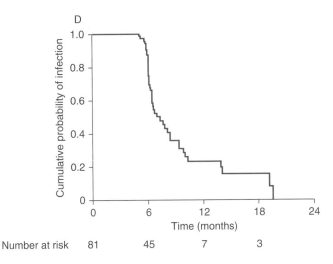

Figure 23.6 Kaplan–Meier curve of the cumulative incidence and time to clearance of incident oncogenic oral HPV. Source: Kreimer *et al.* (2013). Reproduced by permission of Elsevier

Comparing survival with two groups

Although the survival curve for a single group may sometimes be of interest, we are usually much more interested in comparing the 'survival experience' of two or more groups. For example, Figure 23.7 is from a randomized controlled trial to investigate whether the insertion of a cervical pessary in women with a short cervix reduces the rate of early pre-term delivery. One group of women were randomly allocated to either the cervical pessary or expectant management group (no cervical pessary). (We encountered this study in connection with Figures 5.1 and 15.7.)

As you can see, the cumulative percentage of women who did not give birth spontaneously before 34 weeks (238 days) was higher in the pessary group than in the non-pessary (expectant management) group. In fact, the authors provide information in their paper, that this difference was significant: six per cent of women in the pessary group had a spontaneous delivery before

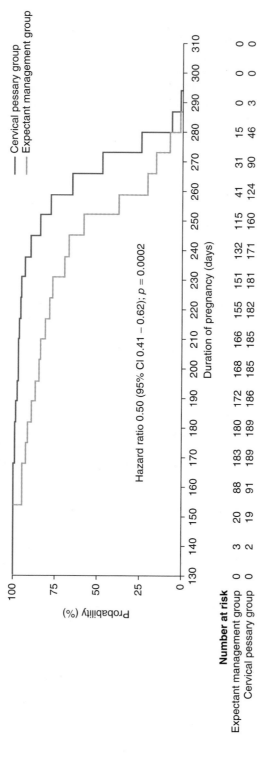

Figure 23.7 Kaplan–Meier plot of the probability of continued pregnancy without delivery in the cervical pessary group (top curve) and expectant management group (bottom curve). Source: Goya *et al.* (2012). Reproduced by permission of Elsevier

34 weeks compared to 27 per cent in the non-pessary group: odds ratio 0.18, with a 95 per cent confidence interval of (0.08 – 0.37).

Notice that the authors have provided information under their figure showing the numbers at risk at each time interval. This is to remind us that the smaller numbers of 'survivors' towards the end of a trial produce less reliable results. As a direct consequence of this effect, you should not assume that just because the gap between two survival curves gets progressively larger (as it is often seen to do, but not in this example) that this is *necessarily* due to an actual divergence in the survival experiences in the two groups. It might well be caused simply by the low numbers of subjects still at risk. This can make the ends of the curves unreliable.

> **Exercise 23.3.**   Using Figure 23.7, half of the women in each group gave birth sponta-
> neously before how many days?

The log-rank test

If you want to compare the *overall* survival experience of two (or more) groups of patients rather than, say, comparing just the median survival times as we did above, then one possible approach is to use the non-parametric *log-rank test*. The log-rank test assesses if any difference exists between the two groups of patients in survival times *at any point during the study period*. Essentially, the null hypothesis to be tested is that the two samples (the two groups) are from the same population as far as their survival experience is concerned. In other words, there is *no difference* in the survival experiences.

The log-rank test of this hypothesis uses a comparison of observed with expected events (say, deaths), given that the null hypothesis is true.[2] If the *p-value* is less than 0.05, you can reject the null hypothesis and conclude that there is a statistically significant difference between the survival experiences of the groups. You can then use the Kaplan – Meier curves to decide which group had the significantly better survival. A limitation of the log-rank test is that it cannot be used to explore the influence on survival of more than one variable, that is, the possibility of confounders – for this you need Cox's proportional regression, which we will come to shortly.

An example of the log-rank test in practice

Figure 23.8 is from a randomised trial to compare early surgery with initial conservative treatment in patients with spontaneous supratentorial lobar intracerebral haematomas.

---

[2]You may have spotted the similarity with the chi-squared test considered earlier in the book. In fact, the calculations are exactly the same.

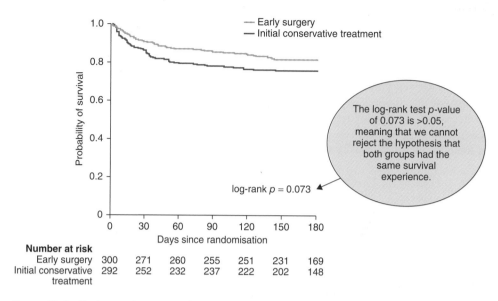

Figure 23.8 Kaplan–Meier curves of percentage surviving early surgery (top curve) versus Initial conservative treatment (bottom curve). Note that the log-rank p-value of 0.073 is >0.05, meaning that we cannot reject the hypothesis of equal survival experience between the two groups. Source: Mendelow *et al.* (2013). Reproduced by permission of Elsevier

---

Exercise 23.4. In women with a multiple pregnancy, spontaneous pre-term delivery is the leading cause of perinatal morbidity and mortality. Interventions to reduce pre-term birth in these women have not been successful. The Kaplan–Meier curves in Figure 23.9 are from a randomised controlled trial to assess whether a cervical pessary could effectively prevent poor perinatal outcomes. The women, with a multiple pregnancy between 12 weeks' and 20 weeks' gestation, were randomly assigned to pessary or control groups. The top curves are for women with a cervical length of less than 38 mm, the bottom curves for women with a cervical length of at least 38 mm. What does the log-rank test indicate about the comparable survival experience of the women with shorter and longer cervixes?

The hazard ratio

You may remember that I only introduced the hazard ratio quite briefly in Chapter 15. Now, I want to deal with it in a bit more detail. Essentially, the hazard is a *risk* (or probability); the risk of some particular clinical outcome (e.g. death), at any point in some specified time, usually during a follow-up period. The hazard ratio is typically used to compare the experience of two (or more) groups in terms of their time to the outcome in question, for example, a treatment group and a placebo group.

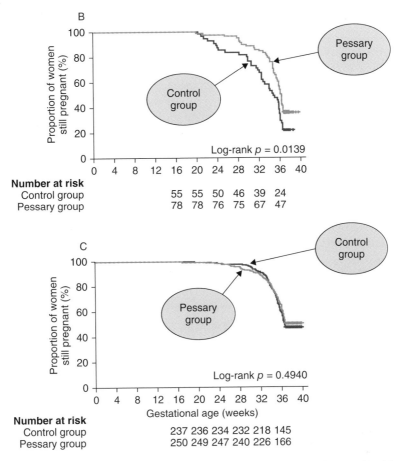

Figure 23.9 Kaplan–Meier curves of proportion of continued pregnancies in: women with a cervical length of less than 38 mm (top graph) and women with a cervical length of at least 38 mm (bottom graph). The women, with a multiple pregnancy between 12 and 20 weeks' gestation, were randomly assigned to pessary or control groups. All curves censored at 37 weeks' gestation. 38 mm is the 25th percentile of cervical length. Source: Liem *et al.* (2013). Reproduced by permission of Elsevier

As you saw in Chapter 15, the interpretation of confidence intervals for the hazard ratios is the same as that for odds and risk ratios. If the interval contains 1, the risk factor concerned is not a statistically significant hazard in the population. If it does not contain 1, the factor is a statistically significant hazard. If a hazard ratio is less than 1, it means that the hazard is decreased and if greater than 1, it means that the hazard is increased. For example, if, in a comparison of death in a treatment group compared to a placebo group, the hazard ratio is 0.80, this means that the hazard (the risk) of death in the treatment group was 0.80 times than that in the placebo group. In other words, there was a reduction in the risk of 0.20 or 20 per cent. Whether this was significant would depend on whether the confidence interval contained 1 or not.

The proportional hazards (Cox's) regression model

Although researchers can use the log-rank test to distinguish survival between two groups, the test only provides a *p-value*: it will tell you if there is a significant difference between the survival experiences of two groups, but it does not *quantify* any difference, that is, it does not tell us how big that difference might be. It would be more useful to have an estimate of a difference in survival (if any), along with the corresponding confidence interval.

For example, a hazard ratio of 0.50, with a 95 per cent confidence interval of (0.41 to 0.62), is shown in Figure 23.7. As this confidence interval does not include 1, the hazard ratio is significant in the population. We can interpret this as meaning that the women in the cervical pessary group have a hazard (a risk) of only 0.50 of pre-term delivery compared to the expectant management (non-pessary) group.

The hazard ratio mentioned above provides the confidence interval, but neither the log-rank test nor the simple hazard ratio allow for adjustment for possible confounding variables which may significantly affect survival. For this, we can use an approach known as *proportional hazards (or Cox's) regression*. This procedure will provide both estimates and confidence intervals for variables that affect survival and enable researchers to adjust for confounders. I will discuss, briefly, the principle underlying the method and the meaning of some of the terms used, before giving a few examples.

The focus of *proportional hazards regression* is the *hazard*. The hazard is akin to a failure rate. For example, if the end-point is death, then the hazard is the rate at which individuals die at some point during the course of a study. The hazard can go up or down over time, and the distribution of hazards over the length of a study is known as the *hazard function*. You will not see authors quote the hazard regression function or equation but for those interested it looks like this:

$$\text{Hazard} = h_0 + e^{(\beta_1 X_1 + \beta_2 X_2 + \dots)}$$

h_0 is the baseline hazard and is of little importance – like the constant coefficient β_0 in linear and logistic regressions. The explanatory or independent variables can be any mixture of nominal, ordinal or metric, and nominal variables can be 'dummied', as described in Chapters 21 and 22. The same variable selection procedures as in linear or logistic regression models can also be used, that is, either automated or by hand.

The most interesting property of this model is that e^{β_1}, e^{β_2} and so on give us the *hazard ratios* (or HRs) for the variables X_1, X_2 and so on (notice the obvious similarity with the odds ratios in logistic regression). The hazard ratios are essentially *risk ratios* but called hazard ratios in the context of survival studies. For example, in a study of the survival of women with breast cancer, the variable X_1 might be 'micrometastases present (Y/N)'. In which case, the hazard ratio HR_1, represents the risk of death for a patient when micrometastases are present compared to that for a patient when they are absent and is equal to e^{b1}.

All of this is true only if the relative effect (essentially the *ratio*) of the hazard in the two groups remains constant over the whole course of the study. Note that the hazard rate for either group may not be constant throughout the whole study period, but the *ratio* of the hazard rates in the two groups is assumed to be constant throughout. For example, if a person has a risk of death at some initial time point that is twice as high as that of another person, then at all subsequent points, the risk of death remains twice as high. In other words, they are *proportional*.

An example of proportional hazards regression

Figure 23.10 is from a randomized controlled trial in which the authors stated, 'Enteral nutrition (EN) is recommended for patients in the intensive-care unit (ICU), but it does not consistently achieve nutritional goals. We assessed whether delivery of 100% of the energy target from days 4–8 in the ICU with EN plus supplemental parenteral nutrition (SPN) could optimise clinical outcome.' Patients were randomly assigned to receive EN or SPN. The primary outcome was the occurrence of nosocomial infection after cessation of intervention (day 8), measured until the end of follow-up (day 28). The figure shows the hazard ratios derived from a Cox regression (crude and adjusted) for a number of demographic and clinical risk factors.

As you can see, only two of the univariable crude hazard ratios had p-values <0.05 (SAPS II score and Study intervention) and were thus likely to be significant in the population. Note however that the 95 per cent confidence interval for the SAPS II score included 1. This may be due to some sort of rounding error. The remaining confidence intervals contained 1 (and

	Univariable analysis		Multivariable analysis*	
	Hazard ratio (95% CI)	p-value	Hazard ratio (95% CI)	p-value
Sex (women vs men)	1.02 (0.66–1.58)	0.9265	..	..
Age (1-year increase)	0.99 (0.98–1.00)	0.1934	..	..
SAPS II score (1-point increase)	1.01 (1.00–1.03)	0.0491	..	..
Body-mass index (1-kg/m² increase)	1.04 (0.99–1.08)	0.1205	..	..
Hospital (Geneva vs Lausanne)	1.18 (0.78–1.78)	0.4377	..	..
Study intervention (SPN vs EN)	0.62 (0.42–0.93)	0.0200	0.65 (0.43–0.97)	0.0338†
Admission category (surgery vs medicine)	1.01 (0.68–1.50)	0.9488	..	..
Antibiotics before day 9 (yes vs no)	1.20 (0.70–2.05)	0.5048	..	..
Infections before day 9 (yes vs no)	0.84 (0.56–1.26)	0.3958	..	..
Mechanical ventilation before day 9 (yes vs no)	1.53 (0.94–2.50)	0.0897	..	..

SPN, supplemental parenteral nutrition; EN, enteral nutrition.

*Variables in the multivariable analysis were SAPS II score, hospital, study intervention, admission category, previous antibiotic use before day 9, and mechanical ventilation before day 9.

†Statistically significant with Benjamini–Hochberg correction.

Figure 23.10 Univariable and multivariable hazard ratios from a Cox regression model for first nosocomial infection during follow-up (primary end-point). Taken from a randomized controlled trial to compare enteral nutrition (EN) versus EN plus supplemental parenteral nutrition (SPN) in patients in ICU. Data from Heidegger *et al.* (2013)

the p-values were all >0.05). However, the multivariable regression (adjusted for the variables listed in the table footnote) was significant, and the hazard ratio was 0.65 with a 95 per cent confidence interval of (0.43 to 0.97). This implies that patients fed with EN plus SPN had only a 65 per cent chance of acquiring a nosocomial infection compared to the EN only patients.

Exercise 23.5.   Figure 23.11 is from a study into the relative survival of two groups of patients with non-metastatic colon cancer; one group having open colectomy (OC) and the other laparoscopy-assisted colectomy (LAC). The table shows the hazard ratios and their confidence intervals after the patients were stratified according to tumour stage for the probability: of being free of recurrence, for overall survival, and for cancer-related survival. What do you conclude from these results about the survivability with OC surgery versus LAC surgery?

	Hazard ratio (95% CI)	p
Probability of being free of recurrence		
Lymph-node metastasis (presence vs absence)	0.31 (0.16–0.60)	0.0006
Surgical procedure (OC vs LAC)	0.39 (0.19–0.82)	0.012
Preoperative serum CEA concentrations (≥ 4 ng/ml vs <4 ng/ml)	0.43 (0.22–0.87)	0.018
Overall survival		
Surgical procedure (OC vs LAC)	0.48 (0.23–1.01)	0.052
Lymph-node metastasis (presence vs absence)	0.49 (0.25–0.98)	0.044
Cancer-related survival		
Lymph-node metastasis (presence vs absence)	0.29 (0.12–0.67)	0.004
Surgical procedure (OC vs LAC)	0.38 (0.16–0.91)	0.029

OC, open colectomy; LAC, laparoscopy-assisted colectomy; CEA, carcinoembryonic antigen.

Figure 23.11 Results of a Cox proportional hazards regression analysis comparing the survival of patients with open colectomy versus laparoscopy-assisted colectomy, for the treatment of non-metastatic colon cancer. Source: Lacy *et al.* (2002). Reproduced by permission of Elsevier

Checking the proportional hazards assumption

The *proportional* hazards assumption can be checked graphically using what is known as the *log–log* plot. However, a description of this procedure is again a step too far for an introductory book.

24

Systematic review and meta-analysis

Learning objectives

When you have finished this chapter you should be able to:

- Provide a broad outline of the idea of systematic review.

- Outline a typical search procedure.

- Describe what is meant by publication bias and its implications.

- Describe how we can use the funnel plot to examine for the presence of publication bias.

- Explain the importance of heterogeneity across studies and how the I^2 statistic can be used to detect this condition.

- Explain the meaning of meta-analysis.

- Outline the role of the Mantel-Haenszel procedure in combining studies.

- Describe what a forest plot is and how it is used.

Medical Statistics from Scratch: An Introduction for Health Professionals, Third Edition. David Bowers.
© 2014 John Wiley & Sons, Ltd. Published 2014 by John Wiley & Sons, Ltd.

Introduction

If you have a patient with atrial fibrillation and you want to know the current consensus on the most effective treatment, then you could perhaps ask the opinions of colleagues (although they may know no more than you) or maybe look through some pharmaceutical promotional materials, or read all the relevant journals lying around your clinic or office. Better still, if you have access to one of the clinical databases such as PubMed, then the job will be that much easier; in fact, anything like an adequate search is almost impossible otherwise. If you want your search to capture everything written on your topic then you will need a systematic approach. This process of searching for all relevant studies (or trials) is known as a *systematic review*.

However, when you do your systematic review, you are likely to encounter some difficulties:

- Many of the studies you turn up will be based on smallish samples. As you know, small samples may well produce unreliable results.

- Partly as a consequence of the above problem, many of the studies come to different and conflicting conclusions.

- There will be some studies that you simply do not find. Perhaps because they are published in obscure and/or non-English-language journals or are not published at all (e.g. internal pharmaceutical company reports or research dissertations). This shortfall may lead to what is known as *publication bias* (I will come back to publication bias again shortly).

To some extent, you can address the first two of these problems by combining all of these individual studies into one large study, a process called *meta-analysis* (as you will see later), and you will also want to deal with the potential for publication bias. But let's start with a brief description of systematic review.

Systematic review

The basis of a systematic review is a comprehensive search that aims to identify all similar and relevant studies that satisfy a pre-defined set of *inclusion and exclusion criteria*. As an example, the authors, Chopra *et al.* (2013), of a study into the possible risk of venous thromboembolism from peripherally inserted catheters, first stated the background of their study:

> *Background*
> Peripherally inserted central catheters (PICCs) are associated with an increased risk of venous thromboembolism. However, the size of this risk relative to that associated with other central venous catheters (CVCs) is unknown. We did a systematic review and meta-analysis to compare the risk of venous thromboembolism associated with PICCs versus that associated with other CVCs.

They then described their search strategy as follows:

Methods

Search strategy and selection criteria

We followed the Preferred Reporting Items for Systematic Reviews and Meta-Analyses (PRISMA) recommendations for this meta-analysis. With the assistance of a medical research librarian, we did serial literature searches for English and non-English articles (between Jan 12, 2012, and Dec 31, 2012). We searched Medline (1950–present, via Ovid), Embase (1946–present), Biosis (1926–present), the Cochrane Central Register of Controlled Trials (1960–present, via Ovid), and Evidence-Based Medicine Reviews (various coverage dates, via Ovid). We used Boolean logic with search terms including "peripherally inserted central catheter", "PICC", "deep vein thrombosis", "pulmonary embolism", and "venous thromboembolism". Controlled vocabularies (eg, Medical Subject Heading terms) were used to identify synonyms.

The appendix provides a more detailed search strategy. All studies in human beings that were published in full text, abstract, or poster form were eligible for inclusion, with no restrictions on publication date, language, or status. Conference posters and abstracts were electronically searched through the Conference Papers Index provided by ProQuest (1982–present), Biosis (1926–present), and Scopus (1996–present). Ongoing clinical trials were identified from the clinicaltrials.gov website, and additional studies of interest were found through internet searches and hand searches of bibliographies.

The authors thus described their inclusion and exclusion:

Three authors (VC, SA, and AH) independently established study eligibility; any difference in opinion about eligibility was resolved by consensus. We **included** studies if they included participants 18 years of age or older; included patients with a PICC placed in the arm; and reported the development of deep vein thrombosis, pulmonary embolism, or both after PICC insertion. We **excluded** studies if they involved neonates or patients younger than 18 years; compared complications between different types of PICCs (eg, varying PICC gauge or lumens); reported catheter lumen thrombosis, superficial phlebitis, or thrombophlebitis but not venous thromboembolism; involved PICCs inserted into the leg; or were case reports of unusual complications.

The end result of a systematic review then, is a list of studies, each one of which provides a value for the specified outcome measure. In the above example, this outcome measure was the occurrence of venous thromboembolism (deep vein thrombosis or pulmonary embolism) after peripherally inserted central catheter (PICC) insertion. Examination of this list of outcome values may provide the required insights into treatment effectiveness.

> **Exercise 24.1.**   What is the purpose of a systematic review? Briefly outline the procedure and some of the problems that may arise.

The forest plot

The list of studies produced by the systematic review is often accompanied by what is known as a *forest plot*. This plot has study outcome on the vertical axis, usually arranged by the size of study (i.e. by sample size) and the outcome measure on the horizontal axis. The outcome measure might be odds or risk ratios, means or proportions, or their differences and so on. There are a number of ways of displaying the data. For example, by using a box-shape or a lozenge-shape, with a horizontal line through it whose length represents the width of the 95 per cent confidence interval for whatever outcome measure is being used. Or with a diamond shape, whose width represents the 95 per cent confidence interval. The area of each box or diamond should be proportional to its sample size.

As an example, the sytematic review for the catheter study referred to earlier discovered 11 suitable studies, and the forest plot for these studies is shown in Figure 24.1. Each study is represented by a black diamond (not proportional in size to the study sample size in this example) with a horizontal black line through it indicating the extent of its 95 per cent confidence interval. The overall result is shown by a large open diamond shape at the bottom of the plot. I will return to the meaning of this in the meta-analysis section.

As you can see, for eight of the studies, the 95 per cent confidence interval line crosses the odds ratio $= 1$ vertical axis, implying that the PICC offers no greater or lesser odds of venous thromboembolism than a central venous catheter. But three of the studies have significant odds

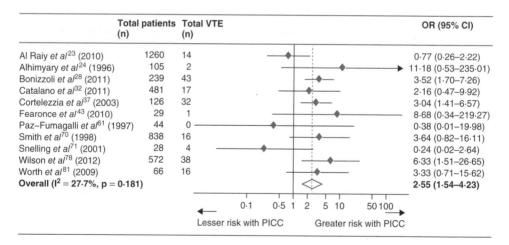

Figure 24.1   Forest plot of risk (measured by odds ratio and 95 per cent confidence intervals) of venous thromboembolism (VTE) between peripherally inserted central catheters (PICC) and central venous catheters (CVT) in studies with a comparison group. Source: Chopra *et al.* (2013). Reproduced by permission of Elsevier

ratios, all showing a greater risk with a PICC, odds ratios of: 3.52, 3.04 and 6.33. All with confidence intervals that do not contain 1.

Exercise 24.2.   The results shown in Figure 24.2 show the outcomes (relative risk for proportion of subjects with side effects) from each of six randomised trials comparing antibiotic with placebo for treating acute cough in adults (Fahey *et al.* 1998). Draw a forest plot of this data and comment briefly on what it shows. Note: relative risks greater than 1 favour the placebo (i.e. fewer side effects).

Study	Sample size	Relative risk (95 % CI)
Briskfield *et al.*	50	0.51 (0.20 to 1.32)
Dunlay *et al.*	57	7.59 (0.43 to 134.81)
Franks and Gleiner	54	3.48 (0.39 to 31.38)
King *et al.*	71	2.30 (0.93 to 5.70)
Stott and West	207	1.49 (0.63 to 3.48)
Verheij *et al.*	158	1.71 (0.80 to 3.67)
Total	597	1.51 (0.86 to 2.64)

Figure 24.2   The outcomes (relative risk for proportion of subjects with side effects), from each of six randomised trials comparing antibiotic with placebo for treating acute cough in adults. Source: Fahey *et al.* (1998). Reproduced by permission of BMJ Publishing Group Ltd

Publication and other biases

The success of any systematic review depends critically on how thorough and wide-ranging the search for relevant studies is. One frequently quoted difficulty is that of *publication bias*, which can arise from a number of sources:

- The tendency for journals to favour the acceptance of studies showing *positive* outcomes at the expense of those with negative outcomes.

- The tendency for authors to favour the submission of studies to journals showing *positive* outcomes at the expense of those with negative outcomes.

- Studies with positive results are more likely to be published in English language journals giving them a better chance of capture in the search process.

- Studies with positive results are more likely to be cited, giving them a better chance of capture in the search process.

- Studies with positive results are more likely to be published in more than one journal, giving them a better chance of capture in the search process.

- Some studies are never submitted for publication. For example, those that fail to show a positive result, those by pharmaceutical companies (particularly if the results are unfavourable), graduate dissertations and so on.

In addition to these biases, a number of other potential biases exist. For example, *inclusion bias* is the consequence of setting inclusion and exclusion criteria so that the studies with particularly 'helpful' outcomes are favoured over non-helpful studies. Furthermore, smaller studies can be methodologically less sound, with wider variability in their outcomes, and are thus less reliable. Besides which, studies of lower *quality* have a tendency to show larger effects. These issues need to be addressed.

With respect to the quality of the studies identified by the search process, the authors of the catheter study mentioned earlier state:

> Two authors (VC and MB) assessed the risk of bias independently. Since all the included studies were non-randomised and had a cohort or case-control design, the Newcastle–Ottawa scale was used to judge study quality, as recommended by the Cochrane Collaboration. This scale uses a star system to assess the quality of a study in three domains: selection of study groups; comparability of groups; and ascertainment of outcomes. Studies that received a star in every domain were judged to be of high quality.

The possible presence of publication bias can be investigated with what is known as a *funnel plot*.

The funnel plot

A funnel plot is a scatter plot, with the estimates of the effect from individual studies on the horizontal axis (e.g. as measured by an odds or risk ratio or a difference in means) against some measure of the *size* of the study (e.g. number of patients or standard error) on the vertical axis, which is usually plotted with a reversed scale that puts the larger, most powerful studies towards the top. Larger studies shown at the top of the funnel will be more precise (their results will not be so spread out); smaller studies, shown towards the bottom will be less precise and therefore more spread out.

In the absence of bias, the funnel plot should have the shape of a *symmetric* upturned cone or funnel. (Note that sometimes funnel plots are drawn horizontally) However, if the funnel is asymmetrical, for example, if its parts are missing or poorly represented – and this will usually be near the bottom of the funnel where the smaller studies are located – then this is suggestive of bias of one form or another.[1]

As an example, Figure 24.3 is a funnel plot from a systematic review of the effectiveness of topically applied non-steroidal anti-inflammatory drugs in acute and chronic pain conditions.

---

[1] There are a number of other possible causes of bias in systematic reviews. Those interested should look, for example, at Egger and Davey Smith (1998), where other possible biases are discussed.

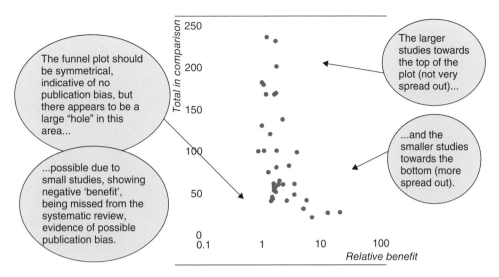

Figure 24.3 Funnel plot used to check for publication bias in a systematic review of the effectiveness of topically applied non-steroidal anti-inflammatory drugs. The asymmetry of the funnel is an indication of publication bias. Reproduced from BMJ, Jan 1998; 316: 333–338, courtesy of BMJ Publishing Group

Relative benefit (risk ratio) is shown on the horizontal axis (Moore *et al.* 1998) and the number of patients in the studies on the vertical axis. Each point in the figure represents one of the studies. Values to the left of the value of 1 on the horizontal axis show negative 'benefit' and values to the right show positive benefit.

The asymmetry in the funnel is quite marked, with a noticeable absence of small studies showing negative 'benefit' (risk ratio less than 1). The authors comment:

> The funnel plot might be interpreted as showing publication bias. The tendency for smaller trials to produce a larger analgesic effect might be construed as supporting the absence of trials showing no difference between topical non-steroidal and placebo. We made strenuous efforts to unearth unpublished data and contacted all pharmaceutical companies in the United Kingdom that we identified as producing non-steroidal products. One company made unpublished data available to us, but the others did not feel able to do so.

Exercise 24.3. (a) Outline the major sources of publication bias. (b) Figure 24.4 shows a funnel plot from a systematic review of trials to investigate the link between a low estimated glomerular filtration rate (eGFR) at baseline and risk of future stroke. The plot has odds ratio (horizontal axis) against the standard error of the log RR. Comment on the evidence for publication bias.

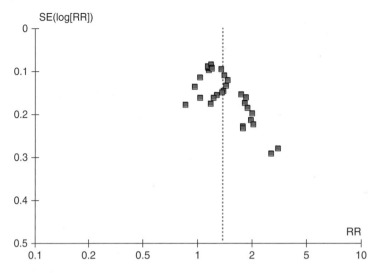

Figure 24.4   Funnel plot from a systematic review of trials to investigate the link between a low estimated glomerular filtration rate (eGFR <60 ml/min/1.73 m^2) at baseline and risk of future stroke. The horizontal axis shows relative risk (RR). High relative risks indicate a greater chance of stroke. The vertical dotted line represents the aggregate relative risk. Source: Lee *et al.* (2010). Reproduced by permission of BMJ Publishing Group Ltd

Combining the studies: meta-analysis

Meta-analysis is the process of combining a number of separate studies to produce one 'super-study'. So, for example, we might have three separate studies, with sample sizes of 40, 80 and 150. When combined, we get a super-study with a sample size of 270. The assumption of the meta-analysis is that this super-study will provide a more reliable and a precise overall result for the output variable in question than any of the smaller individual studies. The underlying assumption (i.e. the null hypothesis) of meta-analysis is that all of the studies measure the same effect in the same population, and that any differences between them is due to chance alone. When the results are combined the chance element cancels out, and we are left with the true effect.

How do we combine the studies? By using the *Mantel–Haenszel* procedure[2] (which I am not going to describe). However, before studies can be combined, they must satisfy the *homogeneity* criterion. A few words about that first, before we look at an example of meta-analysis.

The problem of heterogeneity

Even when a set of apparently similar studies has been identified, researchers have to make sure that they are similar enough to be combined. We call this property of being 'similar enough',

---

[2]Note that this is not to be confused with the Mantel–Haenszel test for heterogeneity – of which more in a moment.

homogeneity. For example, they should have similar subjects, have the same type and level of intervention, the same output measure and the same treatment effect. It is safe to combine them only if studies are *homogeneous* in this way.

For example, the forest plot shown in Figure 24.4 shows studies for which the outcome is relative risk (RR). If these studies were homogenous then these relative risk values would all be similar in size – any variation in these values would be no more than you might expect when you take repeated samples from a population – differences due to sampling error. Studies which do not have this quality of homogeneity are said to suffer from *heterogeneity*. Needlesss to say, we should test for heterogeneity. Two tests are commonly used – the Cochrane Q test and the I^2 statistic, both of which are based on the chi-squared distribution.[3] The null hypothesis for both tests is that the studies are homogeneous. *p*-values <0.05 would cause us to reject the null hypothesis and conclude that the studies suffered from heterogeneity and thus were not similar enough to be combined.

Because Cochrane's Q test is not always successful at detecting heterogeneity when the number of studies is small (often the case) and because it has a tendency to overestimate heterogeneity when the number of studies is small, Higgins I^2 statistic is often used as well. I^2, which can vary between 0 per cent (no heterogeneity) and 100 per cent (complete heterogeneity), represents the percentage of variation between the sample estimates. If I^2 has a value above 50 per cent, then heterogeneity is considered significant.

The homogeneity assumption can also be tested graphically using what is known as a *L' Abbé plot*, but this is not often seen these days to justify any further discussion.

An example of the tests for heterogeneity is shown in the forest plot of Figure 24.5 which compares outcome from trials using the Peto odds ratios.[4] The authors of this study stated:

> The balance of risk and benefit from early neurosurgical intervention for conscious patients with superficial lobar intracerebral haemorrhage of 10–100 mL and no intraventricular haemorrhage admitted within 48 h of ictus is unclear. We therefore tested the hypothesis that early surgery compared with initial conservative treatment could improve outcome in these patients.

As you can see, the overall outcome has a *p*-value = 0.0002, so we can reject the null hypothesis of outcomes for not being significantly better with early surgery. The overall odds of 0.74 confirm this result. However, there is evidence of significant heterogeneity among the trials as the *p*-value of 0.002 for the Q statistic and the value of $I^2 = 66.9$ per cent strongly suggest that heterogeneity is present. The authors of this study concluded:

> The result shows a significant advantage of surgery with an odds ratio of 0.74 (95% CI 0.64–0.86; p < 0.001), although there is significant heterogeneity (p = 0.002) because the studies included different patient groups and different types of surgery.

---

[3] The I^2 statistic is due to Higgins and Thompson (2002).

[4] Peto odds ratios are better than the other approaches at estimating odds ratios in trials where treatment effects are small. It was developed for use in trials in cancer and heart disease where small effects are likely, yet very important.

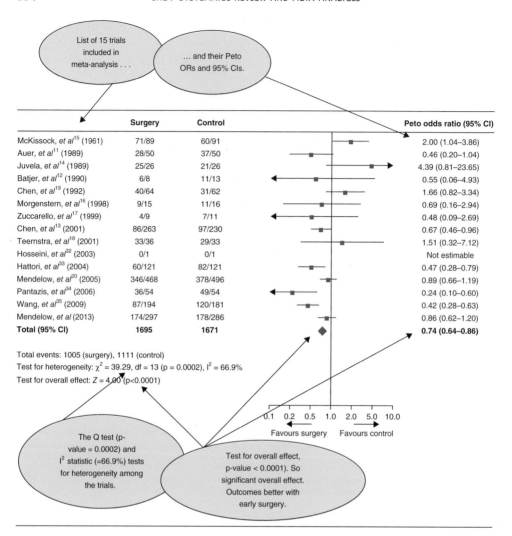

Figure 24.5 Forest plot of trials measuring Peto odds for improved outcome with early surgery compared with initial conservative treatment in patients with superficial lobar intracerebral haemorrhage. The I^2 test for heterogeneity among the trials has a value of 66.9 per cent, indicative of heterogeneity. Source: Mendelow *et al.* (2013). Reproduced by permission of Elsevier

Exercise 24.4. (a) Outline the problem with heterogeneity among samples in a meta-analysis. (b) Do you think there is evidence of heterogeneity in the forest plot of Figure 24.1?

Finally I must mention the *Cochrane Library*. This is an electronic database of a huge number of published systematic reviews. It is an excellent source of information on best (and not so good) treatments for a wide variety of illnesses and conditions. It is also a very useful source if you are contemplating a systematic review of your own as it provides a comprehensive guidance as to the best ways of searching, reviewing, combining and appraising research.

25

Diagnostic testing

Learning objectives

When you have finished this chapter, you should be able to:

- Explain sensitivity, specificity, positive predictive value, and negative predictive value.

- Explain the necessity for a trade-off between sensitivity and specificity.

- Interpret a receiver operating characteristic (ROC) curve.

Preamble

Making an accurate diagnosis is crucial in health care. The measures used to attempt a correct diagnosis vary, ranging from simple observation to quite complex procedures or tests. In this chapter, we are going to discuss some of the important characteristics of these diagnostic measures as an aid to understanding what you may see in clinical papers.

Medical Statistics from Scratch: An Introduction for Health Professionals, Third Edition. David Bowers.
© 2014 John Wiley & Sons, Ltd. Published 2014 by John Wiley & Sons, Ltd.

The measures

Researchers generally use four separate but interconnected measures when they examine the accuracy of a diagnostic test:

- *Sensitivity*: the percentage of those patients *with* the condition whom the test correctly identifies as having it. In other words, the percentage of true positives.

- *Specificity*: the percentage of those patients *without* the condition whom the test correctly identifies as not having it. In other words, the percentage of true negatives.

- *Positive predictive value (PPV)*: the percentage of patients whom the test identifies as having the condition who do have it.

- *Negative predictive value (NPV)*: the percentage of patients whom the test does not identify as having the condition who do not have it.

For example, suppose that you were using fasting plasma glucose (FPG) as a test for diagnosing diabetes and using a cut-off value of 7.0 mmol/l. Let us say that in a sample of 80 individuals, 10 have diabetes of whom two had an FPG below 7 mmol/l and 70 do not have diabetes, of whom five have an FPG > 7 mmol/l. From this, we can say that:

The sensitivity of the test = 8/10 = 0.80 or 80 per cent. So eight true positives. But two individuals are *incorrectly* diagnosed as not having diabetes. In other words, two false negatives.

The specificity of the test = 65/70 = 0.93 or 93 per cent. So 65 true negatives. But five individuals are identified as *having* diabetes when they do not have, that is, five false positives.

We can display this situation schematically in Figure 25.1.

Calculation of the PPV and the NPV is a little bit complicated. Expressed in probabilities, the formulae are:

$$\text{PPV} = \frac{(\text{sensitivity} \times \text{prevalence})}{[(\text{sensitivity} \times \text{prevalence}) + (1 - \text{specificity}) \times (1 - \text{prevalence})]}$$

$$\text{NPV} = \frac{[\text{specificity} \times (1 - \text{prevalence})]}{[\text{specificity} \times (1 - \text{prevalence}) + \text{prevalence} \times (1 - \text{sensitivity})]}$$

So, in our diabetes/FPG example, eight individuals have diabetes out of a total of 80; therefore, the prevalence is 8/80 = 0.10. Thus:

$$\text{PPV} = \frac{(0.80 \times 0.10)}{[(0.80 \times 0.10) + (1 - 0.93) \times (1 - 0.10)]}$$

$$= \frac{0.08}{(0.08 + 0.07 \times 0.90)} = 0.56$$

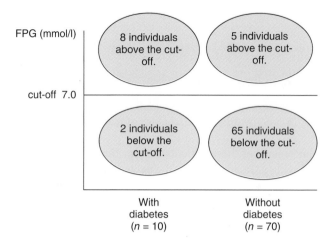

Figure 25.1 Schematic diagram of individuals with and without diabetes with fasting plasma glucose (FPG) using 7.0 mmpl/l as a cut-off for a diagnosis of diabetes. Bear in mind that the numbers with and without diabetes is unknown to the diagnoser

This means that 56 per cent of those who test positive (FPG > 7.0 mmol/l) will have diabetes.

Note that the calculation of PPV and NPV depends on knowing the prevalence of the condition in question. In this example, with a single group, we can work out the prevalence of diabetes, but this will not always be the case.

Clearly, the positive and negative predictive diagnostics are clinically more useful. As a clinician, you want to know, typically, the chances of a patient having the condition if they return a positive test result (PPV), rather than whether they will give a positive test result if they are known to have the condition (sensitivity). Notice that as the sensitivity of a test depends on the condition being present, and the specificity depends on the condition being absent then both of these measures are unaffected by the prevalence of the condition. This is not true for PPV and NPV which, as you have seen earlier, is affected by prevalence.

In an ideal world, we would like a test which had 100% sensitivity and 100% specificity, but sadly this is not possible in practice. There is an optimal (but never perfect) value for the cut-off between sensitivity and specificity, which gives the best results for both measures, although this will also be influenced by the nature of the condition. For example, a diagnostic test for acute myocardial infarction (AMI) using serum CK-BB concentration needs as high a sensitivity as possible so that immediate thrombolytic action can be taken for those individuals actually experiencing an AMI.[1] A high specificity is not so crucial, as counter-measures are not likely to harm those not having an AMI (although it might alarm them). Choosing an appropriate cut-off value of CK-BB is thus fairly crucial.

---

[1] You have a better chance of surviving and recovering from a heart attack if you receive a thrombolytic drug within 12 hours after the heart attack starts, but ideally, you should receive thrombolytic medications within the first 90 minutes after arriving at the hospital for treatment.

Exercise 25.1. In a four-week period, 28 patients arrive at an emergency department with chest pain. Each has their serum CK-BB (µg/l) level measured as a diagnostic test for a possible acute myocardial infarction (AMI). Twenty of these individuals are in fact experiencing an AMI but eight are not (although the clinicians do not know who is and who is not). As an indicator of probable AMI, the clinicians decide to use as a cut-off, a particular value of serum CK-BB. Above this cut-off, the individual concerned is judged likely to be experiencing an AMI and will be treated accordingly, and below this value, it is not.

The levels of serum CK-BB among the 28 individuals are shown in Figure 25.2. What is the sensitivity and specificity of the test, if the cut-off value is (a) 12 µg/l and (b) 8 µg/l?

With AMI ($n = 20$)	7.5, 7.7, 11.0, 14.0, 21.0, 24.0, 26.0, 32.0, 41.0, 47.0, 62.0, 71.0, 83.0, 85.0, 91.0, 105.0, 145.0, 172.0, 195.0, 310.0
Without AMI ($n = 8$)	1.0, 3.0, 5.0, 6.0, 6.5, 7.5, 21.0, 32.0

Figure 25.2 Serum CK-BB levels (µg/l) among 35 individuals attending an emergency department with chest pain. Unknown to the clinicians, but known to us, 20 of the individuals are experiencing an acute myocardial infarction (AMI) but eight are not

The sensitivity versus specificity trade-off: the ROC curve

I now want to return to the sensitivity versus specificity trade-off question. As I said earlier, what we would really like is a test which gives only true positives, that is, no false negatives, implying a sensitivity of 1 (or 100%), and only true negatives, that is, no false positives; in other words (1 − specificity) = 0.

One common method for finding the optimum cut-off point is to draw a *receiver operating characteristic* curve or ROC curve. For each cut-off point, this plot has sensitivity (i.e. the true positive rate) on the vertical axis and on the horizontal axis plots (1 − specificity) – the false positive rate. The only plot of cut-off points which will give us a sensitivity of 1 (no false negatives) and no false positives (1 − specificity = 0), is a line which goes up the vertical axis to the top left-hand corner (corresponding to a sensitivity of 1) and then across the top of the graph to where (1 − specificity) = 1.

The total area of this rectangular shape is then $1 \times 1 = 1$. We call this the *area under the curve*, or *AUC* for short. Note that a test which produces as many false positives as true positives, that is, a test with no discriminatory power would give a ROC curve which lay on the 45 degree diagonal from the origin.

The optimal cut-off thus corresponds to that point on the curve which lies closest to the top left corner because this is the cut-off value with a sensitivity of 1 (no false negatives) and for which (1 − specificity) = 0 – no false positives. This is also the value which maximises the AUC. If we are choosing between more than one available test (e.g. we might want to compare the performance of a new test with a 'gold standard' test which is assumed to give the correct result), we will be looking for the test with the largest AUC. When you are reading a paper which contains one or more ROC curves, you will want to see a value for each AUC, together with its confidence interval.

To see how this works, in practice, consider the ROC curves in Figure 25.3. This is from a study to validate the Glasgow-Blatchford Bleeding Scale (GBS) as a possible instrument for deciding whether a patient with upper-gastrointestinal haemorrhage should be admitted to hospital or might be suitable for outpatient management.

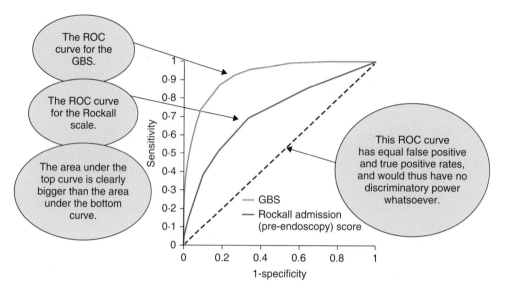

Figure 25.3 ROC curve comparison of Glasgow-Blatchford Bleeding Scale (GBS) and admission Rockall score, for the prediction of the need for intervention or death for 647 patients suffering from upper-gastrointestinal haemorrhage. Source: Stanley *et al.* (2009). Reproduced by permission of Elsevier

The authors proposed to compare the GBS with the widely used Rockall score, which includes endoscopic findings. The problem with this is that many patients are kept in hospital until this procedure is undertaken. Although many hospitals in the UK have an emergency endoscopy rota, this facility is usually for individuals with major haemorrhage only, with others waiting until the next day or longer for a semi-elective procedure. The advantage of the GBS does not depend on endoscopy findings, so decisions can be made more quickly, without a possible unnecessary admission.

The authors conclude that the ROC curve comparison of the 647 patients with full data for both scores, showed that GBS was superior to the admission Rockall score for the prediction of intervention or death. The respective AOC (and their 95 per cent confidence intervals) are GBS, 0.92, (0.88 to 0.93); Rockall, 0.72 (0.65 to 0.75).

Exercise 25.2.   Using the data in Figure 25.4, draw a ROC curve for cut-offs for prostate specific antigen (PSA). What is the optimal cut-off value?

PSA cut-off (ng/ml)	Sensitivity	Specificity
0.5	0.99	0.13
1.0	0.96	0.44
2.0	0.78	0.75
3.0	0.59	0.87
4.0	0.44	0.92
5.0	0.33	0.95
10.0	0.13	0.99
20.0	0.05	1.00

Figure 25.4   Cut-off values for prostate specific antigen (PSA). Holmström *et al.* (2009)

As a final point, note that if a test uses a nominal (yes/no) measure – for example, blood in stool (Y/N), pain when urinating (Y/N), then there can be no trade-off between sensitivity and specificity.

Appendix

Table of random numbers

23157	54859	01837	25993	76249	70886	95230	36744
05545	55043	10537	43508	90611	83744	10962	21343
14871	60350	32404	36223	50051	00322	11543	80834
38976	74951	94051	75853	78805	90194	32428	71695
97312	61718	99755	30870	94251	25841	54882	10513
11742	69381	44339	30872	32797	33118	22647	06850
43361	28859	11016	45623	93009	00499	43640	74036
93806	20478	38268	04491	55751	18932	58475	52571
49540	13181	08429	84187	69538	29661	77738	09527
36768	72633	37948	21569	41959	68670	45274	83880
07092	52392	24627	12067	06558	45344	67338	45320
43310	01081	44863	80307	52555	16148	89742	94647
61570	06360	06173	63775	63148	95123	35017	46993
31352	83799	10779	18941	31579	76448	62584	86919
57048	86526	27795	93692	90529	56546	35065	32254
09243	44200	68721	07137	30729	75756	09298	27650
97957	35018	40894	88329	52230	82521	22532	61587
93732	59570	43781	98885	56671	66826	95996	44569
72621	11225	00922	68264	35666	59434	71687	58167
61020	74418	45371	20794	95917	37866	99536	19378
97839	85474	33055	91718	45473	54144	22034	23000
89160	97192	22232	90637	35055	45489	88438	16361
25966	88220	62871	79265	02823	52862	84919	54883
81443	31719	05049	54806	74690	07567	65017	16543
11322	54931	42362	34386	08624	97687	46245	23245

Medical Statistics from Scratch: An Introduction for Health Professionals, Third Edition. David Bowers.
© 2014 John Wiley & Sons, Ltd. Published 2014 by John Wiley & Sons, Ltd.

References

Aiken, L.H., Sermeus, W., Van den Heede, K. *et al.* (2012) Patient safety, satisfaction, and quality of hospital care: cross sectional surveys of nurses and patients in 12 countries in Europe and the United States. *BMJ*, **344**, e1717.

Altman, D.G. (1991) *Practical Statistics for Medical Research*. Chapman & Hall, London.

Antoniou, T., Gomes, T., Mamdani, M.M. *et al.* (2011) Trimethoprim-sulfamethoxazole induced hyperkalaemia in elderly patients receiving spironolactone: nested case–control study. *BMJ*, **343**, d5228.

ASSENT-2 (Assessment of the Safety and Efficacy of a New Thrombolytic) investigators (1999) *Lancet*, **354**, 716–721.

Barr, B., Taylor-Robinson, D., Whitehead, M. & Duncan, W.H. (2012) Impact on health inequalities of rising prosperity in England 1998–2007, and implications for performance incentives: longitudinal ecological study. *BMJ*, **345**, e7831.

Bath, S.C., Steer, C.D., Golding, J., Emmett, P. & Rayman, M.P. (2013) Effect of inadequate iodine status in UK pregnant women on cognitive outcomes in their children: results from the Avon Longitudinal Study of Parents and children (ALSPAC). *Lancet*, **382**, 331–337.

Bhatnagar, S., Wadhwa, N., Aneja, S. *et al.* (June 2012) Zinc as adjunct treatment in infants aged between 7 and 120 days with probable serious bacterial infection: a randomised double-blind, placebo-controlled trial. *Lancet*, **379**, 2–8.

Blackberry, I.D., Furler, J.S., Best, J.D. *et al.* (2013) Effectiveness of general practice based, practice nurse led telephone coaching on glycaemic control of type 2 diabetes: the Patient Engagement And Coaching for Health (PEACH) pragmatic cluster randomised controlled trial. *BMJ*, **347**, f5272.

Blanchard, J.F., Bernstein, C.N., Wajda, A. & Rawsthorne, P. (2001) Small-area variations and sociodemographic correlates for the incidence of Crohn's disease and ulcerative colitis. *American Journal of Epidemiology*, **154**, 328–333.

Bland, J.M. & Altman, D.G. (1986) Statistical methods for assessing agreement between two clinical measurements. *Lancet*, **1**, 307–310.

Bland, M. (1995) *An Introduction to Medical Statistics*. Oxford University Press, Oxford.

Born in Bradford, 2012.

Boyle, E.M., Poulsen, G., Field, D.J. *et al.* (2012) Effects of gestational age at birth on health outcomes at 3 and 5 years of age: population based cohort study. *BMJ*, **344**, e896.

Medical Statistics from Scratch: An Introduction for Health Professionals, Third Edition. David Bowers.
© 2014 John Wiley & Sons, Ltd. Published 2014 by John Wiley & Sons, Ltd.

Brueren, M.M., Schouten, H.J.A., de Leeuw, P.W., van Montfrans, G.A. & van Ree, J.W. (1998) A series of self-measurements by the patient is a reliable alternative to ambulatory blood pressure measurement. *British Journal of General Practice*, **48**, 1585–1589.

Buekens, P., Notzon, F., Kotelchuck, M. & Wilcox, A. (1999) Why do Mexican Americans give birth to few low-birth-weight infants? *American Journal of Epidemiology*, **152** (4), 347–351.

Byrne, R.A., Neumann, F.-J., Mehilli, J. *et al.*, for the ISAR-DESIRE 3 investigators (2013) Paclitaxel-eluting balloons, paclitaxel-eluting stents, and balloon angioplasty in patients with restenosis after implantation of a drug-eluting stent (ISAR-DESIRE 3): a randomised, open-label trial. *Lancet*, **381**, 46–47.

Carr, A.J., Robertsson, O., Graves, S. *et al.* (2012) Knee replacement. *Lancet*, **379**, 1331–1340.

Chang, S.-S., Stuckler, D., Yip, P. & Gunnell, D. (2013) Impact of 2008 global economic crisis on suicide: time trend study in 54 countries. *BMJ*, **347**, f5239.

Chapman, K.R., Kesten, S. & Szalai, J.P. (1994) Regular vs as-needed inhaled salbutamol in asthma control. *Lancet*, **343**, 1379–1383.

Cheng, Y., Schartz, J., Sparrow, D. *et al.* (2001) Bone lead and blood lead levels in relation to baseline bloodpressure and the prospective development of hypertension. *American Journal of Epidemiology*, **153**, 164–171.

Chi-Ling, C., Gilbert, T.J. & Daling, J.R. (1999) Maternal smoking and Down syndrome: the confounding effect of maternal age. *American Journal of Epidemiology*, **149**, 442–446.

Chopra, V., Anand, S., Hickner, A. *et al.* (2013) Risk of venous thromboembolism associated with peripherally inserted central catheters: a systematic review and meta-analysis. *Lancet*, **382**, 311–325.

Chosidow, O., Chastang, C., Brue, C. *et al.* (1994) Controlled study of Malathion and d-phenothrin lotions for Pediculus humanus var capitas-infested schoolchildren. *Lancet*, **344**, 1724–1726.

Christiansen, E.V., Jensen, L.O., Thayssen, P. *et al.*, for the Scandinavian Organization for Randomized Trials with Clinical Outcome (SORT OUT) V investigators (2013) Biolimus-eluting biodegradable polymer-coated stent versus durable polymer-coated sirolimus-eluting stent in unselected patients receiving percutaneous coronary intervention (SORT OUT V): a randomised non-inferiority trial. *Lancet*, **381**, 661–669.

Cockman, P., Dawson, L., Mathur, R. & Hull, S. (2011) Improving MMR vaccination rates: herd immunity is a realistic goal. *BMJ*, **343**, d5703.

Collins, M.G., Teo, E., Cole, S.R. *et al.* (2012) Screening for colorectal cancer and advanced colorectal neoplasia in kidney transplant recipients: cross sectional prevalence and diagnostic accuracy study of faecal immunochemical testing for haemoglobin and colonoscopy. *BMJ*, **345**, e4657.

Conley, L.J., Ellerbrock, T.V., Bush, T.J. *et al.* (2002) HIV-1 infection and risk of vulvovaginal and perianal condylomata acuminate and intraepithelial neoplasia: a prospective cohort study. *Lancet*, **359**, 108–114.

Conter, V., Cortinovis, I., Rogari, P. & Riva, L. (1995) Weight growth in infants born to mothers who smoked during pregnancy. *BMJ*, **310**, 768–771.

Crescenti, A., Borghi, G., Bignami, E. *et al.* (2011) Intraoperative use of tranexamic acid to reduce transfusion rate in patients undergoing radical retropubic prostatectomy: double blind, randomised, placebo controlled trial. *BMJ*, **343**, d5701.

Coupland, C., Dhiman, P., Morriss, R., Arthur, A., Barton, G. & Hippisley-Cox, J. (2011) Antidepressant use and risk of adverse outcomes in older people: population based cohort study. *BMJ*, **343**, d4551.

De Matteis, S., Consonni, D., Pesatori, A.C. *et al.* (2013) Are women who smoke at higher risk for lung cancer than men who smoke? *American Journal of Epidemiology*, **177** (7), 601–612.

De, S., Williams, G.J., Hayen, A. *et al.* (13 February 2013) Accuracy of the "traffic light" clinical decision rule for serious bacterial infections in young children with fever: a retrospective cohort study. *BMJ*, **346**, f866.

DeStafano, F., Anda, R.F., Kahn, H.S., Williamson, D.F. & Russell, C.M. (1993) Dental disease and risk of coronary heart disease and mortality. *BMJ*, **306**, 688–691.

de Vet, H.C.W., Mokkink, L.B., Terwee, C. & Hoekstra, O.S. (2013) Clinicians are right not to like Cohen's *κ*. *BMJ*, **346**, f2125.

Doll, R. & Hill, A.B. (1956) Lung cancer and other causes of death in relation to smoking: a second report on the mortality of British doctors. *BMJ*, **ii**, 1071–1081.

Dunne, M.W., Bozzette, S., McCutchan, J.A., Kemper, C.A., Havlir, D. *et al.*, for the California Collaborative Treatment Group (1999) Efficacy of azithromycin in prevention of pneumocystis carinii pneumonia: a randomised trial. *Lancet*, **354**, 891–895.

Durán-Cantolla, J., Aizpuru, F., Montserrat, J.M. *et al.* (2010) Continuous positive airway pressure as treatment for systemic hypertension in people with obstructive sleep apnoea: randomised controlled trial. *BMJ*, **341**, c5991.

Egger, M. & Davey Smith, G. (1998) Bias in location and selection of studies. *BMJ*, **316**, 61–66.

EURODIAB ACE Study Group (11 March 2000) Variation and trends in incidence of childhood diabetes in Europe. *Lancet*, **355**, 873–876.

Fahey, T., Stocks, N. & Thomas, T. (1998) Quantitative systematic review of randomised controlled trials comparing antibiotic with placebo for acute cough in adults. *BMJ*, **316**, 906–910.

Fall, C.H.D., Vijayakumar, M., Barker, D.J.P., Osmond, C. & Duggleby, S. (1995) Weight in infancy and prevalence of coronary heart disease in adult life. *BMJ*, **310**, 17–19.

Feder, G., Davies, R.A., Baird, K. *et al.* (2011) Identification and Referral to Improve Safety (IRIS) of women experiencing domestic violence with a primary care training and support programme: a cluster randomised controlled trial. *Lancet*, **378**, 1788–1795.

Field, A. (2013) *Discovering Statistics Using SPSS for Windows*. Sage, London.

Fleten, C., Nystad, W., Stigum, H. *et al.* (2012) Parent-offspring body mass index associations in the Norwegian Mother and Child Cohort Study: a family-based approach to studying the role of the intrauterine environment in childhood adiposity. *American Journal of Epidemiology*, **176**, 83–92.

FRISC II (FRagmin and Fast Revascularisation during InStability in Coronary artery disease) investigators (1999) Long-term low-molecular-mass heparin in unstable coronary-artery disease: FRISC II prospective randomised multicentre study. *Lancet*, **354**, 701–707.

Gardosi, J., Madurasinghe, V., Williams, M., Malik, A. & Francis, A. (2013) Maternal and fetal risk factors for stillbirth: population based study. *BMJ*, **346**, f108.

Gebre, T., Ayele, B., Zerihun, M. *et al.* (2013) Comparison of annual versus twice-yearly mass azithromycin treatment for hyperendemic trachoma in Ethiopia: a cluster-randomised trial. *Lancet*, **379**, 143–151.

Goel, V., Iron, K. & Williams, J.I. (1997) Enthusiasm or uncertainty: small area variations in the use of the mammography services in Ontario, Canada. *Journal of Epidemiology and Community Health*, **51**, 378–382.

Goldhaber, S.Z., Visani, L. & De Rosa, M. (1999) Acute pulmonary embolism: clinical outcomes in the International Cooperative Pulmonary Embolism Registry (ICOPER). *Lancet*, **353**, 1386–1389.

Goya, M., Pratcorona, L., Merced, C. *et al.* (2012) Cervical pessary in pregnant women with a short cervix (PECEP): an open-label randomised controlled trial. *Lancet*, **379**, 1800–1806.

Grampian Asthma Study of Integrated Care (1994) Integrated care for asthma: a clinical, social, and economic evaluation. *BMJ*, **308**, 559–564.

Grandjean, P., Bjerve, K.S., Weihe, P. & Steuerwald, U. (2000) Birthweight in a fishing community: significance of essential fattey acids and marine food contaminants. *International Journal of Epidemiology*, **30**, 1272–1277.

Greenhalgh, T. (1997) How to read a paper: statistic for the non-statistician. II: "Significant" relations and their pitfalls. *BMJ*, **315**, 422.

Gregory, I.N. (2009) Comparisons between geographies of mortality and deprivation from the 1900s and 2001: spatial analysis of census and mortality statistics. *BMJ*, **339**, b3454.

Griffin, S. (1998) Diabetes care in general practice: a meta-analysis of randomised control trials. *BMJ*, **317**, 390–396.

Gronbaek, M., Deis, A., Sorensen, T.I.A. *et al.* (1994) Influence of sex, age, body mass index, and smoking on alcohol intake and mortality. *BMJ*, **308**, 302–306.

Grun, L., Tassano-Smith, J., Carder, C. *et al.* (1997) Comparison of two methods of screening for genital chlamydia infection in women attending in general practice: cross sectional survey. *BMJ*, **315**, 226–230.

Guyatt, G., Jaeschke, R., Heddle, N., Cook, D., Shannon, H. & Walter, S. (1995) Basic statistics for clinicians: 2. Interpreting study results: confidence intervals. *Journal of the Canadian Medical Association*, **152** (2), 169–173.

Hackshaw, A. & Kirkwood, A. (2011) Interpreting and reporting clinical trials with results of borderline significance. *BMJ*, **343**, d3340.

Harrison, E.M., O'Neill, S., Meurs, T.S. *et al.* (2012) Hospital volume and patient outcomes after cholecystectomy in Scotland: retrospective, national population based study. *BMJ*, **344**, e3330.

He, Y., Lam, T.H., Li, L.S. *et al.* (1994) Passive smoking at work as a risk factor for coronary heart disease in Chinese women who have never smoked. *BMJ*, **308**, 380–384.

Hearn, J., Higinson, I.J. & on behalf of the Palliative Care Core Audit Project Advisory Group (1999) Development and validation of a core outcome measure for palliative care: the palliative care outcome scale. *Quality in Health Care*, **8**, 219–227.

Heart Protection Collaborative Group (2011) C-reactive protein concentration and the vascular benefits of statin therapy: an analysis of 20,536 patients in the Heart Protection Study. *Lancet*, **377**, 469–476.

Heidegger, C.M., Berger, M.M., Graf, S. *et al.* (2013) Optimisation of energy provision with supplemental parenteral nutrition in critically ill patients: a randomised controlled clinical trial. *Lancet*, **381**, 385–393.

Hettiaratchy, S. & Dziewulski, P. (2004) ABC of burns: introduction. *BMJ*, **328**, 1366.

Higgins, J.P.T. & Thompson, S.G. (2002) Quantifying heterogeneity in a meta-analysis. *Statistics in Medicine*, **21**, 1539–1558.

Hill, A.B. (1965) The environment and disease: association or causation? *Proceedings of the Royal Society of Medicine*, **58**, 295–300.

Holmström, B., Johansson, M., Bergh, A., Stenman, U.K., Hallmans, G. & Stattin, P. (2009) Prostate specific antigen for early detection of prostate cancer: longitudinal study. *BMJ*, **339**, b3537.

Hosmer, D.W. & Lemeshow, S. (2013) *Applied Logistic Regression Analysis*. John Wiley & Sons, Ltd., Chichester.

Hollands, G.J., Whitwell, S.C.L., Parker, R.A. *et al.* (2012) Effect of communicating DNA based risk assessments for Crohn's disease on smoking cessation: randomised controlled trial. *BMJ*, **345**, e4708.

Hovorka, R., Kumareswaran, K., Harris, J. *et al.* (2011) Overnight closed loop insulin delivery (artificial pancreas) in adults with type 1 diabetes: crossover randomised controlled studies. *BMJ*, **342**, d1855.

Hu, F.B., Wand, B., Chen, C. *et al.* (2000) Body mass index and cardiovascular risk factors in a rural Chinese population. *American Journal of Epidemiology*, **151**, 88–97.

Imperial Cancer Fund OXCHECK Study Group (1995) Effectiveness of health checks conducted by nurses in primary care: final results of the OXCHECK study. *BMJ*, **310**, 1099–1104.

Inskip, H.M., Dunn, N., Godfrey, K.M., Cooper, C. & Kendrick, T., and the Southampton Women's Survey Study Group (2008) Is birth weight associated with risk of depressive symptoms in young women? Evidence from the Southampton Women's Survey. *American Journal of Epidemiology*, **167**, 164–168.

Inzitari, D., Eliasziw, M., Gates, P. *et al.* (2000) The causes and risk of stroke in patients with asymptotic internal-carotid-artery stenosis. *New England Journal of Medicine*, **342**, 1693–1699.

Islami, F., Pourshams, A., Nasrollahzadeh, D. *et al.* (2009) Tea drinking habits and oesophageal cancer in a high risk area in northern Iran: population based case–control study. *BMJ*, **338**, b929.

Janson, C., Chinn, S., Jarvis, D. *et al.*, for the European Community Respiratory Health Survey (2001) Effect of passive smoking on respiratory symptoms, bronchial responsiveness, lung function, and total serum IgE in the European Community Respiratory Health Survey: a cross-sectional study. *Lancet*, **358**, 2103–2109.

Jolly, K., Lewis, A., Beach, J. *et al.* (2011) Comparison of range of commercial or primary care led weight reduction programmes with minimal intervention control for weight loss in obesity: lighten up randomised controlled trial. *BMJ*, **343**, d6500.

Kadri, S.R., O'Donovan, M., Debiram, I. *et al.* (2010) Acceptability and accuracy of a non-endoscopic screening test for Barrett's oesophagus in primary care: cohort study. *BMJ*, **341**, c4372.

Kavanagh, S. & Knapp, M. (1998) The impact on general practitioners of the changing balance of care for elderly people living in an institution. *BMJ*, **317**, 322–327.

Kirby, M.J., Ameh, D., Bottomley, C. *et al.* (2009) Effect of two different house screening interventions on exposure to malaria vectors and on anaemia in children in The Gambia: a randomised controlled trial. *Lancet*, **374**, 998–1009.

Knaus, W.A., Draper, E.A., Wagner, D.P. & Zimmerman, J.E. (1985) APACHE II: a severity of disease classification system. *Critical Care Medicine*, **13**, 818–829.

Kobayashi, T., Otani, T.S.T., Takeuchi, K. *et al.* (2012) Efficacy of immunoglobin plus prednisolone for prevention of coronary artery abnormalities in severe Kawasaki disease (RAISE study): a randomized, open- label, blinded-endpoints trial. *Lancet*, **379**, 1613–1620.

Kokkinos, P.F., Faselis, C., Myers, J., Panagiotakos, D. & Doumas, M. (2013) Interactive effects of fitness and statin treatment on mortality risk in veterans with dyslipidaemia: a cohort study. *Lancet*, **381**, 394–399.

Kreimer, A.R., Campbell, C.M.P., Lin, H.-Y. *et al.* (2013) Incidence and clearance of oral human papillomavirus infection in men: the HIM cohort study. *Lancet*, **382**, 877–887.

Lacy, A.M., Garcia-Valdecasas, J.C., Delgado, S. *et al.* (2002) Laparoscopy-assited colectomy versus open colectomy for treatment of non-metastatic colon cancer: a randomised trial. *Lancet*, **359**, 2224–2230.

Ladwig, K.H., Roll, G., Breithardt, G., Budde, T. & Borggrefe, M. (1994) Post-infarction depression and incomplete recovery 6 months after acute myocardial infarction. *Lancet*, **343**, 20–23.

Lamb, S.E., Gates, S., Williams, M.A. *et al.* (2013) Emergency department treatments and physiotherapy for acute whiplash: a pragmatic, two-step, randomised controlled trial. *Lancet*, **381**, 546–556.

Langan, S.M., Smeeth, L., Hubbard, R., Fleming, K.M., Smith, C.J.P. & West, J. (2008) Bullous pemphigoid and pemphigus vulgaris – incidence and mortality in the UK: population based cohort study. *BMJ*, **337**, a180.

Lasalvia, A., Zoppei, S., Van Bortel, T. *et al.* (2013) Global pattern of experienced and anticipated discrimination reported by people with major depressive disorder: a cross-sectional survey. *Lancet,* **381**, 55–62.

Lee, M., Saver, J.L., Chang, K.-H., Liao, H.-W., Chang, S.-C. & Ovbiagele, B. (2010) Low glomerular filtration rate and risk of stroke: meta-analysis. *BMJ,* **341**, c4249.

Lefaucheur, C., Loupy, A., Vernerey, D. *et al.* (2013) Antibody-mediated vascular rejection of kidney allografts: a population-based study. *Lancet,* **381**, 313–319.

Leeson, C.P.M., Kattenhorn, J.E. & Lucas, A. (2001) Duration of breast feeding and arterial distensibility in early adult life: a population based study. *BMJ,* **322**, 643–647.

Liem, S., Schuit, E., Hegeman, M. *et al.* (2013) Cervical pessaries for prevention of preterm birth in women with a multiple pregnancy (ProTWIN): a multicentre, open-label randomised controlled trial. *Lancet,* **382**, 1341–1349.

Lindberg, G., Bingefors, K., Ranstam, J. & Rastam, A.M. (1998) Use of calcium channel blockers and risk of suicide: ecological findings confirmed in population based cohort study. *BMJ,* **316**, 741–745.

Lindelow, M., Hardy, R. & Rodgers, B. (1997) Development of a scale to measure symptoms of anxiety and depression in the general UK population: the psychiatric symptom frequency scale. *Journal of Epidemiology and Community Health,* **51**, 549–557.

Lindqvist, P., Dahlback, M.D. & Marsal, K. (1999) Thrombotic risk during pregnancy: a population study. *Obstetrics and Gynecology,* **94**, 595–599.

Little, P., Barnett, J., Barnsley, L., Marjoram, J., Fitzgerald-Barron, A. & Mant, D. (3 August 2002) Comparison of agreement between different measures of blood pressure in primary care and daytime ambulatory blood pressure. *BMJ,* **325**, 254.

Lowe, A.J., Carlin, J.B., Bennett, C.M. *et al.* (2010) Paracetamol use in early life and asthma: prospective birth cohort study. *BMJ,* **341**, c4616.

Ludwig, D.S. & Currie, J. (2010) The association between pregnancy weight gain and birthweight: a within-family comparison. *Lancet,* **376**, 984–990.

Luke, A., Durazo-Arvizu, R., Rotimi, C. *et al.* (1997) Relations between body mass index and body fat in black population samples from Nigeria, Jamaica, and the United States. *American Journal of Epidemiology,* **145**, 620–628.

Machin, D., Campbell, M.J., Fayers, P.M. & Pinol, A.P.Y. (1987) *Sample Size Tables for Clinical Studies.* Blackwell Scientific, Oxford.

Mackenbach, J.P., Karanikolos, M. & McKee, M. (2013) The unequal health of Europeans: successes and failures of policies. *Lancet,* **381**, 1125–1134.

Maughan, T.S., James, R.D., Kerr, D.J. *et al.*, for the British MRC Colorectal Cancer Working Party (2002) *Lancet,* **359**, 1555–1563.

McCreadie, R., Macdonald, E., Blacklock, C. *et al.* (1998) Dietary intake of schizophrenic patients in Nithsdale, Scotland: case–control study. *BMJ,* **317**, 784–785.

McKee, M. & Hunter, D. (1995) Mortality league tables: do they inform or mislead? *Quality in Health Care,* **4**, 5–12.

Medical Research Council Advanced Bladder Working Party (1999) Neoadjuvant cisplatin, methotrexate, and vinblastine chemotherapy formuscle-invasive bladder cancer: a randomised controlled trial. *Lancet,* **354**, 533–539.

Mendelow, A.D., Gregson, B.A., Rowan, E.N., Murray, G., Gholkar, A. & Mitchell, P.M. (2013) Early surgery versus initial conservative treatment in patients with spontaneous supratentorial lobar intracerebral haematomas (STICH II): a randomised trial. *Lancet,* **382**, 397–408.

Metzelthin, S.F., van Rossum, E., de Witte, L.P. *et al.* (2013) Effectiveness of interdisciplinary primary care approach to reduce disability in community dwelling frail older people: cluster randomised controlled trial. *BMJ*, **347**, f5264.

Michaëlsson, K., Melhus, H., Warensjö Lemming, E., Wolk, A. & Byberg, L. (2013) Long term calcium intake and rates of all cause and cardiovascular mortality: community based prospective longitudinal cohort study. *BMJ*, **346**, f228.

Michelson, D., Stratakis, C., Hill, L. *et al.* (1995) Bone mineral density in women with depression. *New England Journal of Medicine*, **335**, 1176–1181.

Miller, G., Luo, R., Zhang, L. *et al.* (2012) Effectiveness of provider incentives for anaemia reduction in rural China: a cluster randomised trial. *BMJ*, **345**, e4809.

Moore, R.A., Tramer, M.R., Carroll, D., Wiffen, P.J. & McQuay, H.J. (1998) Quantitative systematic review of topically applied non-steroidal anti-inflamatory drugs. *BMJ*, **316**, 333–338.

Morris, C.R., Kato, G.J., Poljakovic, M. *et al.* (2005) Dysregulated arginine metabolism, hemolysis-associated pulmonary hypertension, and mortality in sickle cell disease. *JAMA*, **294**, 81–91.

Myers, M.G., Godwin, M., Dawes, M. *et al.* (2011) Conventional versus automated measurement of blood pressure in primary care patients with systolic hypertension: randomised parallel design controlled trial. *BMJ*, **342**, d286.

Nikolajsen, L., Ilkjaer, S., Christensen, J.H., Kroner, K. & Jensen, T.S. (1997) Randomised trial of epidural bupivacaine and morphine in prevention of stump and phantom pain in lower-limb amputation. *Lancet*, **350**, 1353–1357.

Nordentoft, M., Breum, L., Munck, L.K., Nordestgaard, A.H. & Bjaeldager, P.A.L. (1993) High mortality by natural and unnatural causes: a 10 year follow up study of patients admitted to a poisoning treatment centre after suicide attempts. *BMJ*, **306**, 1637–1641.

Norman, G., Monteiro, S. & Salama, S. (2012) Sample size calculations: should the emperor's clothes be off the peg or made to measure? *BMJ*, **345**, e5278.

Nüesch, E., Dieppe, P., Reichenbach, S., Williams, S., Iff, S. & Jüni, P. (2011) All cause and disease specific mortality in patients with knee or hip osteoarthritis: population based cohort study. *BMJ*, **342**, d1165.

Oakeshott, P., Aghaizu, A., Reid, F. *et al.* (2012) Frequency and risk factors for prevalent, incident, and persistent genital carcinogenic human papillomavirus infection in sexually active women: community based cohort study. *BMJ*, **344**, e4168.

Olson, J.E., Shu, X.O., Ross, J.A., Pendergrass, T. & Robison, L.L. (1997) Medical record validation of maternity reported birth characteristics and pregnancy-related events: a report from the Children's Cancer Group. *American Journal of Epidemiology*, **145**, 58–67.

Perel, P., Prieto-Merino, D., Shakur, H. *et al.* (2012) Predicting early death in patients with traumatic bleeding: development and validation of prognostic model. *BMJ*, **345**, e5166.

Prevots, D.R., Watson, J.C., Redd, S.C. & Atkinson, W.A. (1997) Re: Outbreak in highly vaccinated populations: implications for studies of vaccine performance. *American Journal of Epidemiology*, **146**, 881–882.

Priest, P., Yudkin, P., McNulty, C. & Mant, D. (2001) Antibacterial prescribing and antibacterial resistance in English general practice: cross sectional study. *BMJ*, **323**, 1037–1041.

Protheroe, D., Turvey, K., Horgan, K. *et al.* (1999) Stressful life events and difficulties and onset of breast cancer: case–control study. *BMJ*, **319**, 1027–1030.

Pursehouse, R.C., Meier, P.S., Brennan, A. & Taylor, K.B. (2010) Estimated effect of alcohol pricing policies on health and health ecominc outcomes in England: an epidemiological model. *Lancet*, **375**, 1355–1364.

Rai, D., Lee, B.K., Dalman, C., Golding, J., Lewis, G. & Magnusson, C. (2013) Parental depression, maternal antidepressant use during pregnancy, and risk of autism spectrum disorders: population based case-control study. *BMJ*, **346**, f2059.

Rainer, T.H., Jacobs, P., Ng, Y.C. *et al.* (2000) Cost effectiveness analysis of intravenous ketorolac and morphine for treating pain after limb injury: double blind randomised controlled trail. *BMJ*, **321**, 1247–1251.

Relling, M.V., Rubnitz, J.E., Rivera, G.K. *et al.* (1999) High incidence of secondary brain tumours after radiotherapy and antimetabolites. *Lancet*, **354**, 34–39.

Riddoch, C.J., Leary, S.D., Ness, A.R. *et al.* (2009) Prospective associations between objective measures of physical activity and fat mass in 12–14 year old children: the Avon Longitudinal Study of Parents and Children (ALSPAC). *BMJ*, **339**, b4544.

Roberts, I., Perel, P., Prieto-Merino, D. *et al.* (2012) Effect of tranexamic acid on mortality in patients with traumatic bleeding: prespecified analysis of data from randomised controlled trial. *BMJ*, **345**, e5839.

Robinovitch, S.N., Feldman, F., Yang, Y. *et al.* (2013) Video capture of the circumstances of falls in elderly people residing in long-term care: an observational study. *Lancet*, **381**, 47–54.

Rodgers, M. & Miller, J.E. (1997) Adequacy of hormone replacement therapy for osteoporosis prevention assessed by serum oestradiol measurement, and the degree of association with menopausal symptoms. *British Journal of General Practice*, **47**, 161–165.

Rogers, A. & Pilgrim, D. (1991) Service users views of psychiatric nurses. *British Journal of Nursing*, **3**, 16–17.

Roig, E., Castaner, A., Simmons, B., Patel, R., Ford, E. & Cooper, R. (1987) In-hospital mortality rates from acute myocardial infarction by race in U.S. hospitals: findings from the National Hospital Discharge Survey. *Circulation*, **76** (2), 280–288.

Rowan, K.M., Kerr, J.H., Major, E. *et al.* (1993) Intensive Care Society's APACHE II study in Britain and Ireland – I: Variations in case mix of adult admissions to general intensive care units and impact on outcome. *BMJ*, **307**, 972–981.

Rubinstein, F., Micone, P., Bonotti, A. *et al.*, on behalf of "EVA" Study Research Group (Estudio "Embarazo y Vacuna Antigripal") (2013) Influenza A/H1N1 MF59 adjuvanted vaccine in pregnant women and adverse perinatal outcomes: multicentre study. *BMJ*, **346**, f393.

Sachedina, N. & Donaldson, L.J. (2011) Paediatric mortality related to pandemic influenza A H1N1 – infection in England: an observational population-based study. *Lancet*, **376**, 1846–1852.

Sainio, S., Jarvenpaa, A.-L. & Kekomaki, R. (2000) Thrombocytopenia in term infants: a population-based study. *Obstetrics and Gynecology*, **95** (3), 441–444.

Schoeman, S.A., Stewart, C.M.W., Booth, R.A., Smith, S.D., Wilcox, M.H. & Wilson, J.D. (2012) Assessment of best single sample for finding chlamydia in women with and without symptoms: a diagnostic test study. *BMJ*, **345**, e8013.

Schrader, H., Stovner, L.J., Helde, G., Sand, T. & Bovin, G. (2001) Prophylactic treatment of migraine with angiotensin converting enzyme inhibitor (lisinopril): randomised, placebo-controlled, cross-over study. *BMJ*, **322**, 19–22.

Shinton, R. & Sagar, G. (1993) Lifelong exercise and stroke. *BMJ*, **307**, 231–234.

Sharwood, L.N., Elkington, J., Meuleners, L., Ivers, R., Boufous, S. & Stevenson, M. (2013) Use of caffeinated substances and risk of crashes in long distance drivers of commercial vehicles: case–control study. *BMJ*, **346**, f1140.

Smits, P.C., Hofma, S., Togni, M. *et al* (2013) Abluminal biodegradable olymer biolimus-eluting stent versus durable polymer everolimis-eluting stent (COMPARE II): a randomised, controlled trial. *Lancet*, **381**, 661–669.

Smolina, K., Wright, F.L., Rayner, M. & Goldacre, M.J. (2012) Determinants of the decline in mortality from acute myocardial infarction in England between 2002 and 2010: linked national database study. *BMJ*, **344**, d8059.

Staessen, J.A., Byttebier, G., Buntinx, F. *et al.* (1997) Antihypertensive treatment based on conventional or ambulatory blood pressure measurement. *JAMA*, **278**, 1065–1072.

Stanley, A.J., Ashley, D., Dalton, H.R. *et al.* (2009) Outpatient management of patients with low-risk upper-gastrointestinal haemorrhage: multicentre validation and prospective evaluation. *Lancet*, **373**, 42–47.

Sterry, W., Ortonne, J.P., Kirkham, B. *et al.* (2010) Comparison of two etanercept regimens for treatment of psoriasis and psoriatic arthritis: PRESTA randomised double blind multicentre trial. *BMJ*, **340**, c147.

Sutter, R.W., John, T.J., Jain, H. *et al.* (2010) Immunogenicity of bivalent types 1 and 3 oral poliovirus vaccine: a randomised, double-blind, controlled trial. *Lancet*, **376**, 1682–1688.

Tang, J.L., Armitage, J.M., Lancaster, T. *et al.* (1998) Systematic review of dietary intervention trials to lower blood total cholesterol in free-living subjects. *BMJ*, **316**, 1213–1220.

Thomson, A.B., Campbell, A.J., Irvine, D.S. *et al.* (2002) Semen quality and spermatozoal DNA integrity in survivors of childhood cancer: a case–control study. *Lancet*, **360**, 361–366.

Thomson, C.S., Woolnough, S., Wickenden, M., Hiom, S. & Twelves, C.J. (2010) Sunbed use in children aged 11–17 in England: face to face quota sampling surveys in the National Prevalence Study and Six Cities Study. *BMJ*, **340**, c877.

Toren, P., Margel, D., Kulkarni, G., Finelli, A., Zlotta, A. & Fleshner, N. (2013) Effect of dutasteride on clinical progression of benign prostatic hyperplasia in asymptomatic men with enlarged prostate: a post hoc analysis of the REDUCE study. *BMJ*, **346**, f2109.

Tripathy, P., Nair, N., Barnett, S. *et al.* (2010) Effect of a participatory intervention with women's groups on birth outcomes and maternal depression in Jharkhand and Orissa, India: a cluster-randomised controlled trial. *Lancet*, **375**, 1182–1192.

Tsai, J.N., Uihlein, A.V., Lee, H. *et al.* (2013) Teriparatide and denosumab, alone or combined, in women with postmenopausal osteoporosis: the DATA study randomised trial. *Lancet*, **382**, 50–56.

Turnbull, D., Holmes, A., Shields, N. *et al.* (1996) Randomised, controlled trial of efficacy of midwife-managed care. *Lancet*, **348**, 213–219.

Vadillo-Ortega, F., Perichart-Perera, O., Espino, S. *et al.* (2011) Effect of supplementation during pregnancy with L-arginine and antioxidant vitamins in medical food on pre-eclampsia in high risk population: randomised controlled trial. *BMJ*, **342**, d2901.

Vamos, E.P., Harris, M., Millett, C. *et al.* (2012) Association of systolic and diastolic blood pressure and all cause mortality in people with newly diagnosed type 2 diabetes: retrospective cohort study. *BMJ*, **345**, e5567.

Vanderpump, M.P.J., Lazarus, J.H., Smyth, P.P. *et al.*, on behalf of the British Thyroid Association UK Iodine Survey Group (2011) Iodine status of UK schoolgirls: a cross-sectional survey. *Lancet*, **377**, 2007–2012.

van Es, R., Jonker, J.J., Verheught, F.W.A., Deckers, J.W. & Grobbee, D.E., for the Antithrombotics in the Secondary Prevention of Events in Coronary Thrombosis-2 (ASPECT-2) Research Group (2002) Aspirin and coumadin after acute coronary syndromes (the ASPECT-2 study): a randomised controlled trial. *Lancet*, **360**, 109–114.

van Nimwegen, M., Speelman, A.D., Overeem, S. *et al.* (2013) Promotion of physical activity and fitness in sedentary patients with Parkinson's disease: randomised controlled trial. *BMJ*, **346**, f576.

Vickers, A.J., Ulmert, D., Sjoberg, D.D. *et al.* (2013) Strategy for detection of prostate cancer based on relation between prostate specific antigen at age 40–55 and long term risk of metastasis: case-control study. *BMJ*, **346**, f2023.

Vuillermin, P.J., Robertson, C.F., Carlin, J.B., Brennan, S.L., Biscan, M.I. & South, M. (2010) Parent initiated prednisolone for acute asthma in children of school age: randomised controlled crossover trial. *BMJ*, **340**, c843.

Wannamethee, S.G., Lever, A.F., Shaper, A.G. & Whincup, P.H. (1997) Serum potassium, cigarette smoking, and mortality in middle-aged men. *American Journal of Epidemiology*, **145**, 598–607.

Watson, J.M., Kang'ombe, A.R., Soares, M.O. *et al.* (2011) Use of weekly, low dose, high frequency ultrasound for hard to heal venous leg ulcers: the VenUS III randomised controlled trial. *BMJ*, **342**, d1092.

Yeung, E.H., Saudek, C.D., Jahren, A.H. *et al.* (2010) Evaluation of a novel isotope biomarker for dietary consumption of sweets. *American Journal of Epidemiology*, **172**, 1045–1052.

Yong, L.-C., Brown, C.C., Schatzkin, A. *et al.* (1997) Intake of vitamins E, C, and A and risk of lung cancer. *American Journal of Epidemiology*, **146**, 231–243.

Zinman, B., Harris, S.B., Neuman, J. *et al.* (2010) Low-dose combination therapy with rosiglitazone and metformin to prevent type 2 diabetes mellitus (CANOE trial): a double-blind randomised controlled study. *Lancet*, **376**, 103–111.

Zoltie, N., de Dombal, F.T. & on behalf of the Yorkshire Trauma Audit Group (1993) The hit and miss of ISS and TRISS. *BMJ*, **307**, 906–909.

Solutions to Exercises

Note: Although I have provided complete solutions to the calculating parts of the exercises, I have provided only brief comments (if at all) where a commentary is required. This is deliberate, firstly, because I do not want to write the book again in terms of the solutions and secondly, because tutors might want to tease these answers from the students themselves, perhaps as part of a wider discussion.

Chapter 1

1.1 Because the values are taken from a larger population (from the Born in Bradford cohort study).

1.2 16%

1.3 Ethnicity, sex, marital status, type of operation, smoking status, etc.

1.4 Apgar, Waterlow, Edinburgh Post-natal Depressions, Rankin, SF36, Beck Depression Inventory, etc.

1.5 GCS produces ordinal data, which are not real numbers, so cannot be added or divided.

1.6 Height, temp., cholesterol, body mass index, age, time, etc.

1.7 Number of deaths, number of angina attacks, number of operations performed, number of stillbirths, etc.

1.8 A continuous metric variable has an infinite or an uncountable number of possible values. A discrete metric variable has a limited, countable number of possible values. (a) 7 (0, 1, 2, ... 6). (b) Not possible to do this as the number of possible weights is infinite.

1.9 VAS data is ordinal because these data are subjective judgements, which are not measured but assessed and will probably vary from patient to patient and from moment to moment. So it's not possible to calculate *average* if by this is meant adding up four values and dividing by four because ordinal data are not real numbers.

1.10 Age, MC. Social class, O. No. of children, MD. Age at 1st child, MC. Age at menarche, MC. Menopausal state, O. Age at menopause, MC. Lifetime use of oral contraceptives, N. No.

Medical Statistics from Scratch: An Introduction for Health Professionals, Third Edition. David Bowers.
© 2014 John Wiley & Sons, Ltd. Published 2014 by John Wiley & Sons, Ltd.

years taking oral contraceptives, MC. No. months breastfeeding, MC. Lifetime use of hrt, MC. Years of hrt, MC. Family history of ovarian cancer, N. Family history of breast cancer, N. Units of alcohol, MD. No. cigs per day, MD. Body mass index, MC. (key: N = nominal, O = ordinal, MD = metric discrete, MC = metric cont.).

1.11 Maternal age, MC, but given here in ordinal groups. Parity, MD. No. cigs daily, MD. Multiple pregnancy, N. Pre-eclampsia, N. Caesarean, N.

1.12 Age, MC. Sex, N. Number of rooms in home, MD. Length of hair, O. Colour of hair, N. Texture of hair, N. Pruritus, N. Excoriations, N. Live lice, O. Viable nits, O.

Chapter 2

2.1

Smoked?	Frequency
Yes	16
No	84

Order not important with nominal variables.

2.2

Smoked?	Frequency	Per cent
Yes	16	16.00
No	84	84.00

2.3

Cause of injury	Number of patients $n = 75$	Relative (%) frequency
Falls	46	61.3
Crush	20	26.7
Motor vehicle crash	6	8.0
Other	3	4.0

% Crush = $(20/75) \times 100 = 26.67$

2.4

Satisfaction with nursing care	Number of patients ($n = 475$)	Relative (%) frequency
Very satisfied	121	25.5
Satisfied	161	33.9
Neutral	90	18.9
Dissatisfied	51	10.7
Very dissatisfied	52	10.9

Very dissatisfied = 10.9%

2.5 Much better: 26.3 and 30.3

Much worse: 0.6 and 0.5

Missing values, if there are a sizeable number can lead to inaccurate conclusions. There are a number of methods to deal with them.

2.6 ParkFit = 73.9, Control = 77.7. So not the same.

2.7 67%.

2.8 B-e stent: 1 stent = 68.4. 2 stents = 20.9.

E-e stent: 1 stent = 68.3. 2 stents = 21.6

2.9

Self-rated benefit	Usual care group $n = 1094$	% freq	% cum freq	Active management group $n = 1543$	% freq	% cum freq
Much better	288	26.3	26.3	468	30.3	30.3
Better	297	27.1	53.4	479	31.0	61.3
Same	429	39.2	92.6	491	31.8	93.1
Worse	73	6.7	99.3	98	6.4	99.5
Much worse	7	0.6	100.0	7	0.5	100.0

Same or Worse, or Much worse. Usual care group = 1 − 53.4 = 46.6%.

Same or Worse, or Much worse. Active management group = 1 − 61.3 = 38.7%.

2.10 Because ordering is arbitrary.

2.11

Mortality	No. ICUs
10.0 – 14.9	9
15 – 19.9	8
20 – 24.9	5
25 – 29.9	3
30 – 34.9	1

Most ICUs have % mortality between 10 and 20, then progressively fewer and fewer. Minimum mortality is >10% and maximum is <35%.

2.12

		Smoked while pregnant?	
		Yes ($n = 77$)	No ($n = 423$)
Birthweight (g)	<2500	3 (3.9)	37 (8.7)
	2500 g – 3999	65 (84.4)	353 (83.5)
	≥4000	9 (11.7)	33 (7.8)

No significant differences in birthweights.

2.13

		Mother's weight		
		≤60 kg	>60 kg	All
Birthweight	≤3000 g	9	2	11
		81.82	18.18	100.00
		75.00	11.11	36.67
	>3000 g	3	16	19
		15.79	84.21	100.00
		25.00	88.89	63.33
All		12	18	30

It looks like heavier mothers have heavier babies and lighter mothers lighter babies.

2.14 The percentage figures in each cell are the percentage of the whole table, which is not very helpful. More helpful would be the percentage that each cell is of that cell's column total.

Those who anticipate discrimination are likely to experience it and those who don't, don't.

2.15 Ranks

2240	2	4110	3.5	3590	10	2880	20	2850	23.5
2660	23.5	4040	22	3580	11	1960	21	3550	5
3050	18	3130	16.5	2660	3.5	3150	9	3220	6
3990	8	4020	1	3040	12	3460	14	4230	19
4110	7	2780	15	2840	13	3660	25	3580	16.5

Chapter 3

3.1 Those in Figure 3.2, but completely a personal choice I think.

3.2

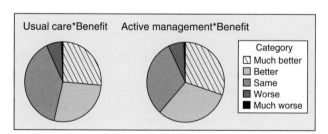

3.3

Blood group	Kidney recipients without rejection ($n=1777$)	Kidney recipients with rejection ($n=302$)
Type A	42	40
Type B	10	16
Type O	41	34
Type AB	5	9

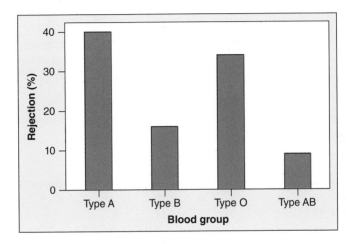

3.4 Type AB.

3.5

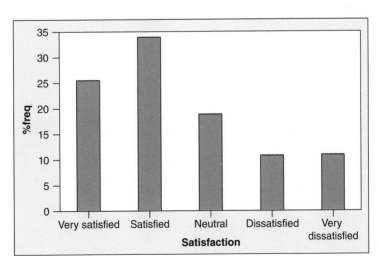

3.6 Level of physical activity is generally higher in those groups taking ≥ 1400 mg/day calcium, except for the lowest.

3.7   Two possible formats depending on what you want to focus on.

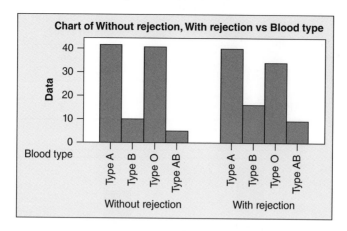

3.8   More developed diabetes in placebo group, more developed NGT with treatment group. No difference for IGT, IFG or both.

3.9   Attendance was highest (≥50%) in the free Choice group and lowest in the General Practice and Pharmacy groups (<25%)

3.10

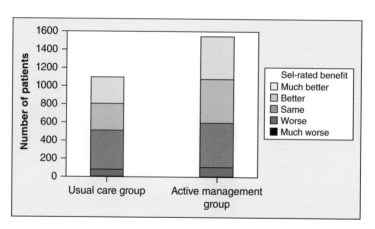

3.12

Weight (kg)	Frequency	% frequency	Cumulative % frequency
40–59.9	12	40.0	40.0
60–79.9	12	40.0	80.0
80–99.9	4	13.3	93.3
100–119.9	1	3.3	96.9
120–190	1	3.3	100.0

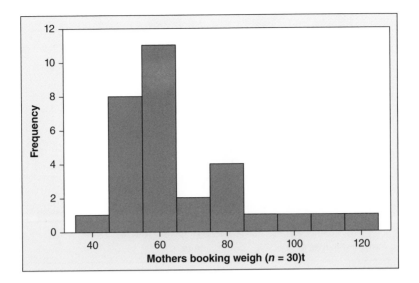

3.13

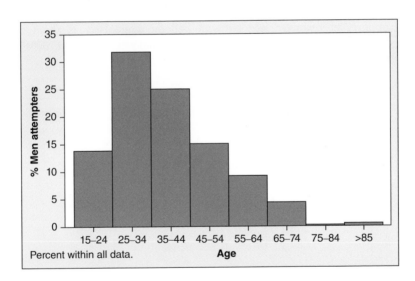

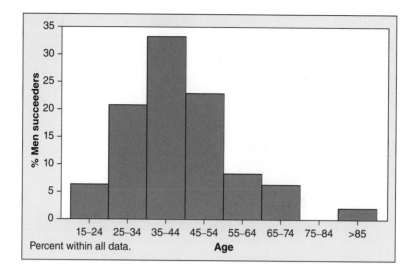

3.14 Median iodine levels are similar across centres – a bit less than 100 (µg/l), but the spread varies widely.

3.15 Median level of diameter stenosis with balloon angioplasty is about 57%. With paclitaxel-eluting stent and balloon, the diameter stenoses are about 30% and 32%, respectively.

3.16

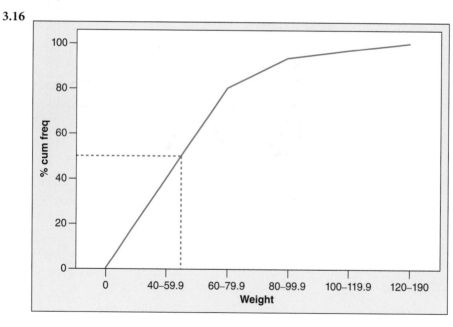

About 55 kg.

3.17 3.17. There appears to be a notable falling off from 1997 to 1998 (what a coincidence!). Numbers did not start to recover until 2003–2004.

Chapter 4

4.1 70–79; <15.

4.2 Positive

4.3 Slightly negatively skewed.

4.4 Almost symmetrical.

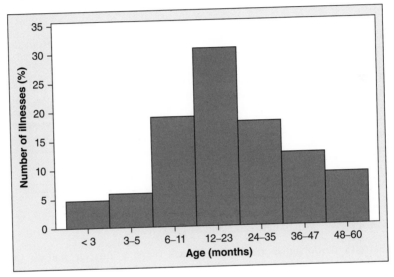

4.5 About 3300 g. Long tails possible because of small numbers of very low and very high birthweight babies.

4.6 All appear to be positively skewed.

4.7 From about $25 \times 10^6/\text{l}$ to $575 \times 10^6/\text{l}$, although there appears to be an outlier at about $725 \times 10^6/\text{l}$.

Chapter 5

5.1 19.5%. 20.0%.

5.2 (a) $67/149 = 0.4496$ or 44.96%; (b) $93/182 = 0.5110$ or 51.1%.

5.3 Spontaneous vaginal delivery and Emergency Caesarean Section both have eight occurrences. So two modes.

5.4 (a) Social class: cases mode = II; control mode = II; (b) level of satisfaction mode = 'Satisfied'; (c) self-rated benefit scores mode = 'Same', in both groups. (d) Parity mode = 0 (49 mothers).

5.5 Because it is nominal data and ordering is arbitrary.

5.6 5

5.7 (a) median mortality =17.95%. (b) All 35–44. (c) both 'Better'.

5.8 (a) Mean > median. (b) Mean > median. (c) The same.

5.9 Mean mortality = 18.66%, which is > median of 17.95%.

5.10 (a) With outliers, mean = 720.4, median = 500. Without outliers, mean = 610.6, median = 500.

5.11 25th percentile is value in $(25/100) \times (30 + 1)$th position = $0.25 \times 31 = 7.75$th position. The 7th value is 2740, the 8th is 2780, so the 7.75th value is 3/4 of the way from 2740 to 2780, which is 2770 g.

The 75th percentile is the value in the $75/100 \times 31$th position, that is, the 23.25th position. The 23rd position value is 3500, the 24th value is 3540, so the 23.25th value is 3510 g. Half the babies weighed between 2770 g and 3510 g. A quarter weighed <2770 g and a quarter >3510 g.

Chapter 6

6.1 (0–9)

6.2 With Barrett's oesophagus: median pack-years = 23; a quarter had <3 pack-years, a quarter had >31 pack-years. A half between 3 and 31 pack-years.

Without Barrett's oesophagus: median = 0.3 pack-years; a quarter had <0 (actually =) pack-years; a quarter >19.2 pack-years. Half between 0 and 19.2 pack-years.

6.3 IQR = (2770–3510)g

6.4 (a) about 2600 g. (b) about 8%.

6.5 Median is about 6.2; IQR is about (5.3 to 7.0).

6.6 Minimum birthweight = 2170 g; maximum birthweight = 4140 g; Q1 = 2770 g; median = 3310 g; Q3 = 3510 g.

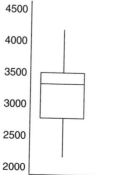

6.7   It means (approx) that the values of cord platelet count are on average 69 away from the mean of 308.

6.8   Values of LDL cholesterol are on average 0.88 from the mean of 2.71. C of $V = 0.88/2.71 = 0.325$.

Values for HDL cholesterol are on average 0.25 from their mean of 1.18. C of $V = 0.25/1.18 = 0.219$.

So, relatively speaking, LDL values are further away.

6.9   2.5%. 0.5%.

6.10   (a) For a variable to be Normally distributed, it should be possible to fit three standard deviations on either side of the mean; in particular, without straying into negative values. For none of these variables would it be possible to fit three standard deviations less than the mean without getting a negative value. For example, for days with headache: $19.7 - 3 \times 14 = -22.3$ hours. So none of them can be Normally distributed.

Chapter 7

7.1   (a) Exposure variable is BMI. (b) Outcome variable is myocardial infarction. (c) See below. (d) Hypertension (the confounder) is associated with obesity and causally related to myocardial infarction.

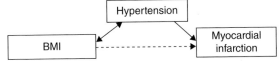

7.2   Could randomly allocate babies (and parents) into three groups according to sleeping arrangements, then follow-up to see outcomes and compare.

Chapter 8

8.4   (a) Participants were followed up from 'Today' into the future. (b) Risk factor is smoke (active or passive). (c) The proportion of stillbirths among those inhaling smoke is $167/32864 = 0.00508$ and among no smoke $= 166/52473 = 0.00316$. So there is smaller proportion of stillbirths among the non-smoke inhalers.

8.5   (a) Retrospective means forward from a start point sometime in the past. (b) Cardiovascular disease. (c) Proportion of deaths in the study period among those with cardiovascular disease was $3535/12379 = 0.286$, among the no cardiovascular disease proportion $= 21\,906/113\,713 = 0.193$, which is (as you might expect), smaller.

8.6   (a) The cases were chosen from those drivers who had had a crash. The controls were drivers with similar characteristics except that they had not had a crash. (b) Caffeine. (c) Age, gender, years driving, etc. (d) Thirty per cent of those who crashed used caffeine compared to 56% who did not had a crash. Looks like caffeine helps avoid crashes.

Chapter 9

9.1 To share out the known and unknown characteristics (including potential confounders) between the groups, thereby making the groups much the same – except for the treatment.

9.3 (b) Any solution to this problem will of course depend on the particular set of random numbers used. My random numbers were 2 3 1 5 (7) 5 4 (8) 5 (9) (0) 1 (8) 3 (7) 2. Since we have only six blocks, we can't use the random numbers in ( ). With blocks of four:

Block 1, CCTT;	Block 2, CTCT;	Block 3, CTTC;
Block 4, TCTC;	Block 5, TCCT;	Block 6, TTCC

The first number is 2, so the first four subjects are allocated as block 2: C, T, C and T. The next number is 3, so the next four subjects are allocated as: C, T, T and C. Continue this same procedure until there are 20 in each group.

Chapter 10

10.2 Needs a sampling frame.

Chapter 11

11.1 (a) Probability $= 121/475 = 0.255$; (b) $52/475 = 0.109$

Satisfaction with nursing care	Number of patients $n = 475$
Very satisfied	121
Satisfied	161
Neutral	90
Dissatisfied	51
Very dissatisfied	52

11.2 $0.7 \times 0.7 = 0.49$ or 49 in 100.

11.3 P (satisfied or very satisfied) $= (161/475 + 121/475) = 0.339 + 0.255 = 0.593$.

11.4

Outcome	Probability
HH	0.25
HT	0.25
TH	0.25
TT	0.25

11.5 Looks a bit like a Normal curve.

7	0.0888952
8	0.114823
9	0.130416
10	0.131865
11	0.119878
12	0.0987880
13	0.0743021

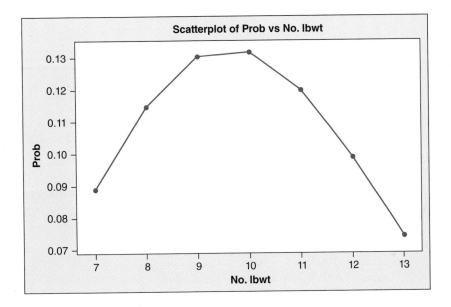

11.6 0.0418103

11.7 ≤ 225 0.115

≥ 425 $(1-0.955) = 0.045$

Chapter 12

12.1 (a) Zinc: absolute risk of failure $= 34/332 = 0.1024$. Placebo: absolute risk of failure $= 0.2052$.

(b) absolute risk reduction $= 0.2052 - 0.1024 = 0.1028$ or 10.28%.

12.2 Relative risk $= 0.1024/0.2052 = 0.499$. So risk of failure in zinc group is almost half of what it is in the placebo group.

12.3 Relative risk reduction $= (1 - RR) = (1 - 0.499) = 0.501$. So the zinc treatment reduces the risk of treatment failure compared to the placebo group by 50.1%.

12.4 NNT = 1/absolute risk reduction = 1/0.1028 = 9.73 or 8 (always round up). So we would need to treat nine children with zinc to avoid one child experiencing treatment failure.

12.5 The most economic is an IPSS score increase by >4 pts. The least economic is urinary tract infection.

12.6 (a) Odds for depression of mothers of cases = 7/9 = 0.7778. Odds for controls = 14/360 = 0.3889. Odds for depression among mothers of cases are twice the odds for mothers of controls.

12.7 (a) Under 35.

	Down syndrome baby	
Smoked	Yes	No
Yes	112	1411
No	421	5214
Totals	533	6625

(i) The odds that a woman having a Down syndrome baby, smoked = 112/421 = 0.2660.

(ii) The odds that a woman having a healthy baby, smoked = 1411/5214 = 0.2706.

(b) ≥35

	Down syndrome baby	
Smoked	Yes	No
Yes	15	108
No	186	611
Totals	201	719

(i) The odds that a woman having a Down syndrome baby, smoked = 15/186 = 0.0806. (ii) The odds that a woman having a healthy baby, smoked = 108/611 = 0.1768.

Interpretation. Among the under 35 mothers, there is little difference in the odds for Down syndrome between smoking and non-smoking mothers (0.2660 vs. 0.2706). Among mothers ≥35, the odds for Down syndrome among smoking mothers is about a half the odds for non-smoking mothers (0.0806 vs. 0.1768).

12.8 Age ≥35. (a) $p = 0.0806/(1 + 0.806) = 0.0746$; (ii) $p = 0.1768/(1 + 0.1768) = 0.1502$.

12.9 Odds of having stroke among those who had exercised = 55/130 = 0.4231. Odds among the non-exercisers = 70/68 = 1.0294.

12.10 (a) Mothers <35. Odds ratio for a woman with a Down syndrome baby having smoked, compared to a woman with a healthy baby = 0.2660/0.2706 = 0.9830. (b) Mothers ≥35. Odds ratio = 0.0806/0.1768 = 0.4558.

Interpretation. In younger mothers, the odds ratio close to 1 (0.9830) implies that smoking neither increases nor decreases the odds ratio for Down syndrome. In older mothers, the odds ratio of 0.4558 implies that mothers who smoked during pregnancy have under half the odds of having a Down syndrome baby compared to non-smoking mothers.

12.11 Hint: if a is small (a rare disease) then $(a + c) \approx c$

Chapter 13

13.1 The smaller the s.e. of the sample mean, the more precise the estimate of the population mean. In this case, the sample mean vitamin E intake of 6.30 mg (non-cases), has an s.e. of 0.05 mg, so we can be 95% confident that the *population* mean vitamin E intake (non-cases) is no further than 2 s.e.s from this mean, that is, within ± 0.10 mg. The largest s.e., 5.06 mg, and therefore the least precise estimate of the population mean, is that for vitamin C (cases).

13.2 (a) Cases. Sample mean age $= 61.6$ years, sample s.d. $= 10.9$ years, $n = 106$. Thus, s.e.$(\bar{x}) = 10.9/\sqrt{106} = 1.059$. The 95% confidence interval is therefore $(61.6 \pm 2 \times 1.059)$ or (59.582 to 63.718) years. (b) Controls. Sample mean age $= 51.0$ years, sample s.d. $= 8.5$ years, $n = 226$. Thus, s.e.$(\bar{x}) = 8.5/\sqrt{226} = 0.565$. The 95% confidence interval is therefore $(51.0 \pm 2 \times 0.565)$ or (49.870 to 52.13) years. The fact that the two CIs do not overlap means that we can be 95% confident that the two population mean ages are significantly different.

13.3 For the integrated care group, over 12 months the sample mean number of admissions is 0.15. The 95% confidence interval means we can be 95% confident that the interval from 0.11 to 0.19 will contain the population mean number of visits for the population of which this is a representative sample. For the conventional care group, the sample mean number of visits is lower, 0.11 and the 95% confidence interval implies that we can be 95% confident that the interval from 0.08 to 0.15 will contain the population mean number of visits.

13.4
$$\text{s.e.}(\bar{x}) = \text{s.d.}/\sqrt{n} = 564.2/\sqrt{3251.8} = 9.8940$$

95% CI for population mean (μ), is $(3251.8 - 2 \times 9.8940$ to $3251.8 + 2 \times 9.8940)\text{g} = (3232.01$ to $3271.59)\text{g}$

13.5 $p = 77/500 = 0.154$. s.e.$(p) = \sqrt{\frac{0.154(1-0.154)}{500}} = 0.0161$

95% CI for π is: $(0.154 - 1.96 \times 0.0161$ to $0.154 + 1.96 \times 0.0161) = (0.1224$ to $0.1856)$ or $(12.24$ to $18.56)\%$

13.6 66.4% and 60.8%. Etanercept 50 mg. Once weekly then once weekly.

13.7 Age 45 – 49.

$$\text{For death : proportion} = 44\%, 95\% \text{ CI is } (34 \text{ to } 53)\%$$

$$\text{For metastases : proportion} = 40\%; 95\% \text{ CI is } (33 \text{ to } 48)$$

Age 51–55.

$$\text{For death : proportion} = 44\%, 95\% \text{ CI is} (32 \text{ to } 56)\%$$

$$\text{For metastases : proportion} = 42\%; 95\% \text{ CI is} (32 \text{ to } 52)$$

Not much difference in widths (therefore precision) of confidence intervals.

13.8 Included practices have (a) a noticeably larger average number of patients (median of 7142 vs 5524) with a slightly narrower interquartile range, than declined practices; (b) slightly smaller percentage of median numbers of female doctors (median 45.3 vs 47.9) but wider, and lower, interquartile ranges. From box plots, distribution of percentage of female doctors in randomised practices is quite negatively skewed. Among Declined practices it is very slightly positively skewed.

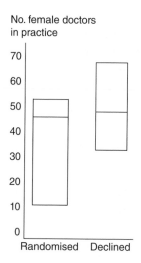

Chapter 14

14.1 Much smaller sample.

14.2 (a) All except diurnal systolic, diurnal diastolic and diurnal mean. (b) 1.6, 1.1. (c) See figure below. The upper limit of all the confidence intervals cross the clinically useful 2 mmHg line, so all are potentially useful.

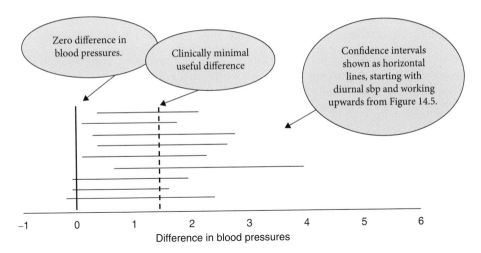

14.3 (a) 202, 29, 232. (b) Too difficult for me to draw Normal curves I am afraid. Suctioned blood loss is positive and definitive (significant and conclusive). Gauze blood loss is negative but not definitive (not significant and inconclusive). Intraoperative blood loss is positive and not definitive (significant but inconclusive).

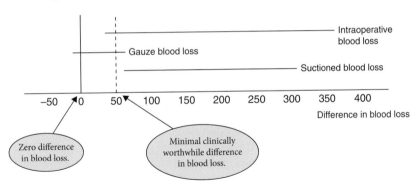

14.4 When repeated measurements (of say heart rate) are made on the same person, the variation in these measurements is called within-subject variation. When a single measurement is made on each of a number of people, the variation in these values is called between-subject variation. The between-subject variability can cloud differences of the within-subject variation. We would like to be rid of between-subject variation, which we can do with paired measurements (e.g. before and after on the same individual).

14.5 All differences are significant in the population because none of the confidence intervals include 0.

14.6 For the primary outcome (number of quit attempts at 6 months), the difference in the number of quit attempts is given as −1. This means that the knowledge of the DNA risk *reduced* the number of quit attempts by 1. Not what we might have hoped for. For the three secondary outcomes, the number of seven-day abstinences was more by 3 when measured at one week but less at six months by 3. The biochemical validation confirmed that the situation was worse among the group who were given information on their DNA, by -1 7-day abstinence.

14.7 Of the five procedures, the only significant difference in median times between the two groups is that between receiving the analgesia and leaving the emergency department. The median difference is 20 minutes with a 95% confidence interval of (4.0 to 39.0) minutes. The confidence intervals for median difference for the other four procedures all include 0.

14.8 (a) This confidence interval includes 0, so we can be 95% confident that there is no difference between the patients and controls in the population. But note the point estimate value of 15.9, which is the best guess for the difference. (b) But we can be 95% confident that is there is a difference in the population for alcohol intake as the confidence interval does not contain 0.

Chapter 15

15.1 With full screening, the mean number of mosquitoes caught was 41% of the number caught compared to the control houses (no screens). With screened ceilings, the mean number of mosquitoes caught was 53% compared to those caught in the control houses.

15.2 With moderate depression, the crude and adjusted relative risks for angina pectoris were not significant in the population because the confidence interval contained 1. With severe depression, both the crude and adjusted relative risks were significant in the population – the confidence interval did not contain 1. The adjusted RR implies that the risk of angina pectoris was 2.3 times than that of patients who were not depressed.

15.3 *Relative risk.* With L-arginine + vitamins, RR = 0.42 and the confidence interval does not include 1; therefore, it is significant. We can be 95% confident that women in this group have 42% of the risk of eclampsia compared to women in the placebo group. With vitamins alone, the confidence interval includes zero so it is not significant (but note that the best guess, point estimate, of 0.74). With L-arginine + vitamins compared to vitamins alone, the RR = 0.56 and is significant because the confidence interval does not include 1. We can be 95% confident that the women in this group have 56% the risk of eclampsia compared to women in vitamin-only group.

Absolute risk reduction. All three absolute risk reductions are significant in the population – none of the confidence intervals include 1. Notice how much smaller the absolute risk reductions are compared to the relative risks: 0.17 compared to 0.42, 0.07 compared to 0.74 and 0.09 compared to 0.56.

15.4 (a) They are very often confounding variables. (b) Exercise has greater benefits (reduction in odds for stroke) the earlier in life it is taken. Between 15 and 25, it reduces odds to 33% compared to the non-exercisers and is significant in the population (confidence interval does not contain 1). Also significant when taken between 25 and 40; reduces the odds for stroke to 43%. Exercise is not significant in reducing odds for stroke when taken between 40 and 55. Confidence interval includes 1 (but once again note best guess value of 0.63).

15.5 All outcomes, except last two, have confidence intervals that don't include 1, so we can be 95% confident that they are significant in the population. Odds for each outcome vary from 0.18

to 0.23, so about 20% of the odds for these four outcomes in cervical pessary group compared to expectant management (control) group. The odds for the last two outcomes, chorioamnionitis and pregnancy bleeding, are not significant as the confidence intervals include 1 but note the best guess point estimates of 0.82 and 0.77, each showing a reduction in odds for these two outcomes.

15.6 Being older than 54. Having had a previous joint replacement. Having a walking disability.

Chapter 16

16.1 (a) Is the proportion of males and females who use my genito-urinary clinic the same?; (b) $H_0: \pi_{male} = \pi_{female}$?; (c) reject, p-value <0.05. (d) Do not reject, p-value ≥ 0.05.

16.2 Suctioned blood, and total intraoperative blood, both p-values <0.05.

16.3 Significantly different: Age; Age at menopause; BMI. Not significantly different: age at birth of 1st child; age at menarche; months breastfeeding; mean years of HRT.

16.4 All differences significant except HDL cholesterol (p-value >0.05)

16.5 None of the differences in the medians appear to be significant (all of the p-values are >0.05) except the Maximum pressure procedure where the p-value is considerably <0.05.

16.6 A confidence interval tells you not only about significance but also gives you some idea as to the value of any difference, and is in units which can be easily interpreted, whereas a p-value tells you only about significance.

16.7 (c) False positive with α. False negative with β.

16.8 (b) Because if you decrease α, you inevitably increase β.

Chapter 17

17.1 Observed values (*expected values*)

		Outcome		
		Sub-optimum IQ?		
		No	Yes	Totals
Urinary iodine-to-creatinine ratio	$<150\,\mu/mg$	469 (*482.8*)	177 (*163.2*)	646
	$\geq150\,\mu/mg$	247 (*233.2*)	65 (*78.8*)	312
	Totals	716	242	958

17.2 (a) Because sample size was small. Same reason and can use with 2×2 tables. (b) Cannot reject the hypothesis of no difference among White British between early and late deaths as p-value in not <0.05.

17.3

Step 1. The $(O - E)$ terms from Figures 17.1 and 17.2, are as follows:
$(469 - 482.8)$, $(177 - 163.2)$, $(247 - 233.2)$ and $(65 - 78.8)$, that is, -13.8, 13.8, 13.8 and -13.8

Step 2. Squaring each of these values gives: 190.44, 190.44, 190.44 and 190.44

Step 3. Dividing each of these values by its E value, gives:
$190.44/482.8 = 0.394$, $190.44/163.2 = 1.167$, $190.44/233.3 = 0.816$ and $190.44/78.8 = 2.417$

Step 4. Sum all of the values in the previous step $= 4.794$
So the chi-squared statistic $= 4.794$, which exceeds the critical value for a 2×2 table of 3.84 so that we can reject the hypothesis of no relationship between maternal mild iodine deficiency during early pregnancy and a sub-optimum IQ in children aged 8 years.

17.5 (i) No relationship between social class and whether lump is malignant or not, p-value is >0.05. (ii) There is a relationship between lifetime use of contraceptives, p-value <0.05. (iii) No relationship with amount of alcohol consumed, p-value >0.05. (iv) No relationship with cigarettes smoked, p-value >0.05.

Chapter 18

18.1 Reduced by 58% – 42%.

18.2 See table footnote for reference categories. Parity $= 0$; born anywhere but UK; BMI >35; pre-existing diabetes; antepartum haemorrhage; active smoker, no foetal growth restriction; active and passive smoker, foetal growth restriction; non-smoker, foetal growth restriction.

18.3 For the first three outcomes, we can be 95% confident in rejecting the hypothesis that there is a no significant difference between the tranexamic acid group and the placebo group; p-values are all <0.05. None of the remaining outcomes are significantly different.

18.4 We can be 95% confident in rejecting the hypothesis of no increase (or decrease) in risk from smoking or passive smoking compared to no exposure to smoke, for all factors (p-values <0.05), except for passive smoking from husband, passive smoking at work, both p-values >0.05.

Chapter 19

19.1 The scatter indicates a positive linear association between CD and UCD.

19.2 Top scatter shows negative linear association between the two variables, although there is an outlier on the horizontal axis, which spoils the party a little. The bottom scatter is negative but definitely not linear.

19.3 A scatterplot can help to reveal the shape of an association.

19.4 Both variables must be metric continuous and at least one Normally distributed.

19.5 Starting with stomach cancer, we see a strong and significant correlation in 2001 between stomach cancer and deprivation ($r = 0.379$, p-value <0.01 – see table footnote) and not surprisingly between deaths from stomach cancer and the SMR. Deaths from stomach cancer in 2001 are also significantly associated with mortality and deprivation in the 1900s ($r = 0.299$ and $r = 0.231$, respectively). So there appears to be some carry-over effect (epigenetics?). The causes of deaths that do not show an association between 2001 and the 1900s are (i) breast cancer (not associated with either mortality or deprivation; $r = -0.068$ and $r = -0.019$; p-values of both are >0.05.) and (ii) prostate cancer, similar r and p-values).

19.6 If either variable was ordinal or both metric but I was not sure about linearity.

19.7 The correlation between antibacterial resistance and antibacterial prescribing (i) is significant for all β lactans, both p-values <0.05, at both primary care group and practice levels ($r_s = 0.57$ and $r_s = 0.18$, respectively). (ii) For ampicillin and amoxicillin, it is not significant at primary care group level (p-value *not* <0.05), but it is significant at practice level (p-value <0.05). (iii) For trimethrim, it is not significant at primary care group level (p-value is not <0.05), but it is significant at practice level (p-value <0.05).

19.8 Only significant correlation is among men in countries with low unemployment levels before the crisis (p-value <0.05).

Chapter 20

20.1 Association is about the values of two variables tending to move together; agreement is about the values of two variables being the same. Not necessarily, although variables that agree will be associated.

20.2 Yes. No.

20.3 Contingency table:

		Observer 1		
		<16	≥16	
Observer 2	<16	5	2	7
	≥16	0	9	9
totals		5	11	16

(a) Observed proportional agreement $= (6 + 9)/16 = 0.938$.

(b) Expected values are as follows:

		Observer 1	
		<16	≥16
Observer 2	<16	2.19	4.81
	≥16	2.81	6.19

Expected agreement $= (2.19 + 6.19)/16 = 0.523$.

So kappa $= (0.938 - 0.523)/(1 - 0.523) = 0.870$. From Figure 20.3, chance adjusted agreement is very good.

20.4 There may be no two values which are the same.

20.5 There appears to be a very small amount of negative bias (not easy to see). The spread of values increases as the mean birthweight increases. Incidentally, the authors reported a Spearman's rank correlation coefficient for the two assessments of 0.87.

Chapter 21

21.1 Extending the line back to the vertical axis gives $b_0 = 43$ approx. For slope: vertical distance is from 22 to $43 = 21$. Horizontal distance $= 78$. So slope $b_1 = -21/78 = -0.269$. Slope is negative because line slopes down from left to right. So equation is:

Male smoking prevalence $= 43 - 0.269 \times$ Score on tobacco control scale.

21.2 Bthwt $= 2460 + 11.0 \times$ Mothers' wt

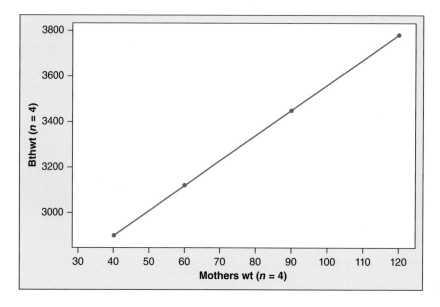

21.3 (a) Best straight line by eye:

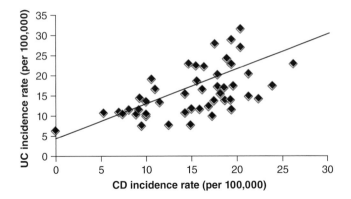

Equation is approx: UCD $= 4 + 25/30 \times$ CD or UCD $= 4 + 0.833 \times$ CD. So if CD increases by 1 unit (1 per 100 000), UCD will increase by 0.833 units (0.833 per 100 000).

(b)

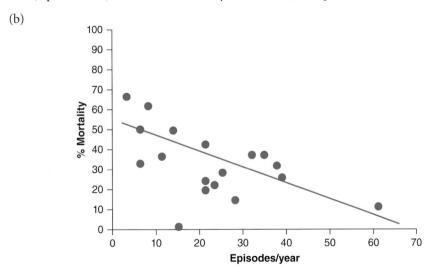

Equation is approx %M $= 55 - 55/65 \times E$ or %M $= 55 - 0.85 \times E$.

A decrease in % mortality of 0.85%.

21.4 b_0 is the sample estimate of the parameter β_0 and b_1 of β_1.

21.5 It has to be metric continuous.

21.6 birthweight $= 2460 + 11.01 \times 80 = 3340.8$ kg

21.7 Paternal BMI (its coefficient is bigger).

21.8 (a) Mothers' weight and height are significant – confidence intervals do not include 0 (and p-values are both <0.05). Age is not significant – confidence interval includes 1 (and p-value >0.05). (b) It does not because it is not significant. (c) R^2 is now 0.129. With only height and weight, adjusted R^2 was 0.126 (Figure 21.10), fit has improved very little. But see section on adjusted R^2 further in this book. (d) Mean birthweight is:

$$\text{mean birthweight} = -77.346 + 8.311 \times 60 + 15.887 \times 150 + 5.487 \times 30 = 2968.974\,\text{g}$$

21.9 (a) R^2 for men $= 0.27$, for women $R^2 = 0.28$ so men – marginally. (b) Men. 2.2 compared to 1.7 for women. Increases because sign on coefficient is positive.

21.10 Without sex, adjusted $R^2 = 0.123$ (Figure 21.10). With sex, adjusted $R^2 = 0.121$. So fit is slightly worse.

21.11 For each variable added to the simple model, adjusted R^2 increases so goodness-of-fit improves each time.

21.12

Subject	Age	D_1	D_2
1	50	1	0
2	55	0	0
3	35	0	1

21.13 Manual and automatic. Manual is preferred if you have an idea as to your main explanatory variable.

21.14 (a) Age; Age^2; Family history of hypertension; Calcium intake. (b) We can be 95% confident that the population parameter on age is between 0.28 and 0.64 (so does not include 0). (c) The blood lead model (largest age coefficient).

Chapter 22

22.1 Because the relationship with a binary model is not linear. And the dependent variable is a probability so has to be between 0 and 1. Logistic regression.

22.2 Using the formula (given in Chapter 12): odds $=$ prob/(1-prob), when Prob($Y = 1$) $=$ 0.4286 when OCP $= 0$, then odds $= 0.7501$. When Prob($Y = 1$) $= 0.227$ when OCP $= 1$, then odds $= 0.2898$. So odds ratio $= 0.2898/0.7501 = 0.386$.

22.3 (a) Yes. Confidence interval does not include 1 (and p-value <0.05).

(b) $P(Y = 1) = -6.467 + 0.102 \times \text{Age}$

(c) When age $= 45$: $P(Y = 1) = e^{-6.647+0.102\times45} = e^{-2.057} = 0.1278.$

Similarly, when Age $= 50, P(Y = 1) = 0.2548.$

(d) Age $= 45$: $[1 - P(Y = 1)] = 1-0.1278 = 0.8722.$ So odds (using formula in Chapter 12) $= 0.8722/(1 - 0.8722) = 6.825.$

Age $= 50$: $[1 - P(Y = 1)] = 1-0.2548 = 0.7452.$ Similarly odds $= 2.925.$

Odds ratio $= 2.925/6.825 = 0.429.$ So a woman aged 45 has just under half the odds of a malignant diagnosis as does a woman aged 50.

(e) Antilog$_e$ $0.1023 = 0.431$ (same as OR, allowing for rounding of values)

(f) change in the odds ratio $= e^{10 \times b1} = e^{10 \times 0.102} = 2.77$.

22.4 Significant (CI does not include 1), with OR $= 1.089$. So each unit increase in BMI increases odds for a malignant diagnosis by 0.089.

22.5 'Ever used OCP' is not significant (CI includes 1). Age and BMI are both significant (confidence intervals do not include 1). With only OCP used in the model, the LL $= -200.009$. With Age and BMI added to the model, LL $= -165.645$, so closer to 0, so better model.

22.6 0.74 the odds.

22.7 As for linear regression, choice is between automatic selection and manual selection.

Chapter 23

23.1

1	2	3	4	5	6	7	8
Day	Number still in study at start of day t	Withdrawn prematurely up to day t	Deaths in day t	Number at risk in day t	Probability of death in day t	Probability of surviving day t	Cumulative probability of surviving to day t
t	n	w	d	r	d/r	p = 1-d/r	S
3	8	0	1	8	1/8 = 0.125	0.875	0.875
8	7	0	1	6	1/6 = 0.167	0.833	0.758
13	6	1	1	4	1/4 = 0.25	0.75	0.569

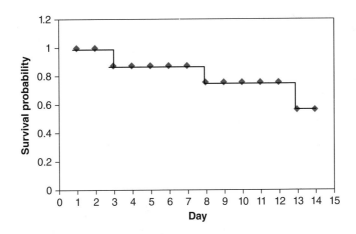

23.2 About 7 months.

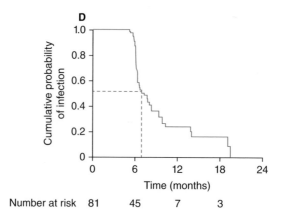

Number at risk   81   45   7   3

23.3 252 days and 266 days.

23.4 The log-rank test tests the hypothesis that there is no difference in the survival experience of the two groups over the whole period of the study. The p-value in this case is 0.0139, which is <0.05, so we can reject the hypothesis. There is a difference in total survival experiences.

23.5 Significant difference between OC and LAC surgery in probability of being free of recurrence. Not a significant difference for overall survival (but p-value only just exceeds 0.05). Significant difference in probability of cancer-related survival.

Chapter 24

24.1 To find all relevant studies. Some may not be in English. Some may be published in obscure journals. Some may not be published (PhDs, conference reports, pharmaceutical company reports, etc.).

24.2 Risk ratio (relative risk) shown by ↑. Size of sample not indicated in this figure.

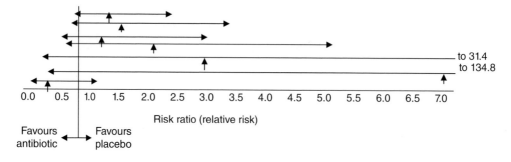

24.3 (a) See text. (b) The authors comment that the plot 'suggests a small degree of publication bias, with a slight under-representation of small studies showing neutral or unexpected protective effects.

24.4 (a) We cannot combine the studies if they are not sufficiently similar. (b) No, $I^2 = 27.7\%$ which is indicative of only moderate heterogeneicty.

Chapter 25

25.1

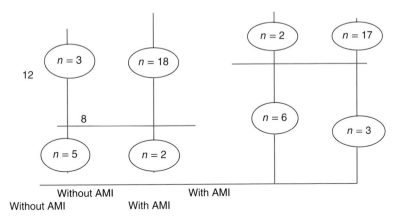

With cut-off = 8, sensitivity = 18/20 = 0.90 or 90%. Specifitity = 5/8 = 0.625 or 62.5%

When cut-off = 12, sensitivity = 17/20 = 0.85 or 85%. Specificity = 6/8 = 0.750 or 75.0%

25.2

PSA cut-off (ng/ml)	Sensitivity	Specificity	(1 − spec)
0.5	0.99	0.13	0.87
1.0	0.96	0.44	0.56
2.0	0.78	0.75	0.25
3.0	0.59	0.87	0.13
4.0	0.44	0.92	0.08
5.0	0.33	0.95	0.05
10.0	0.13	0.99	0.01
20.0	0.05	1.00	0.0

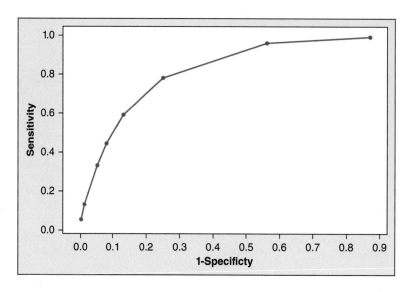

Optimum cut-off is 4 ng/ml

Index

NOTE: Page numbers in *italics* refer to Figures

Medical Statistics from Scratch: An Introduction for Health Professionals, Third Edition. David Bowers.
© 2014 John Wiley & Sons, Ltd. Published 2014 by John Wiley & Sons, Ltd.